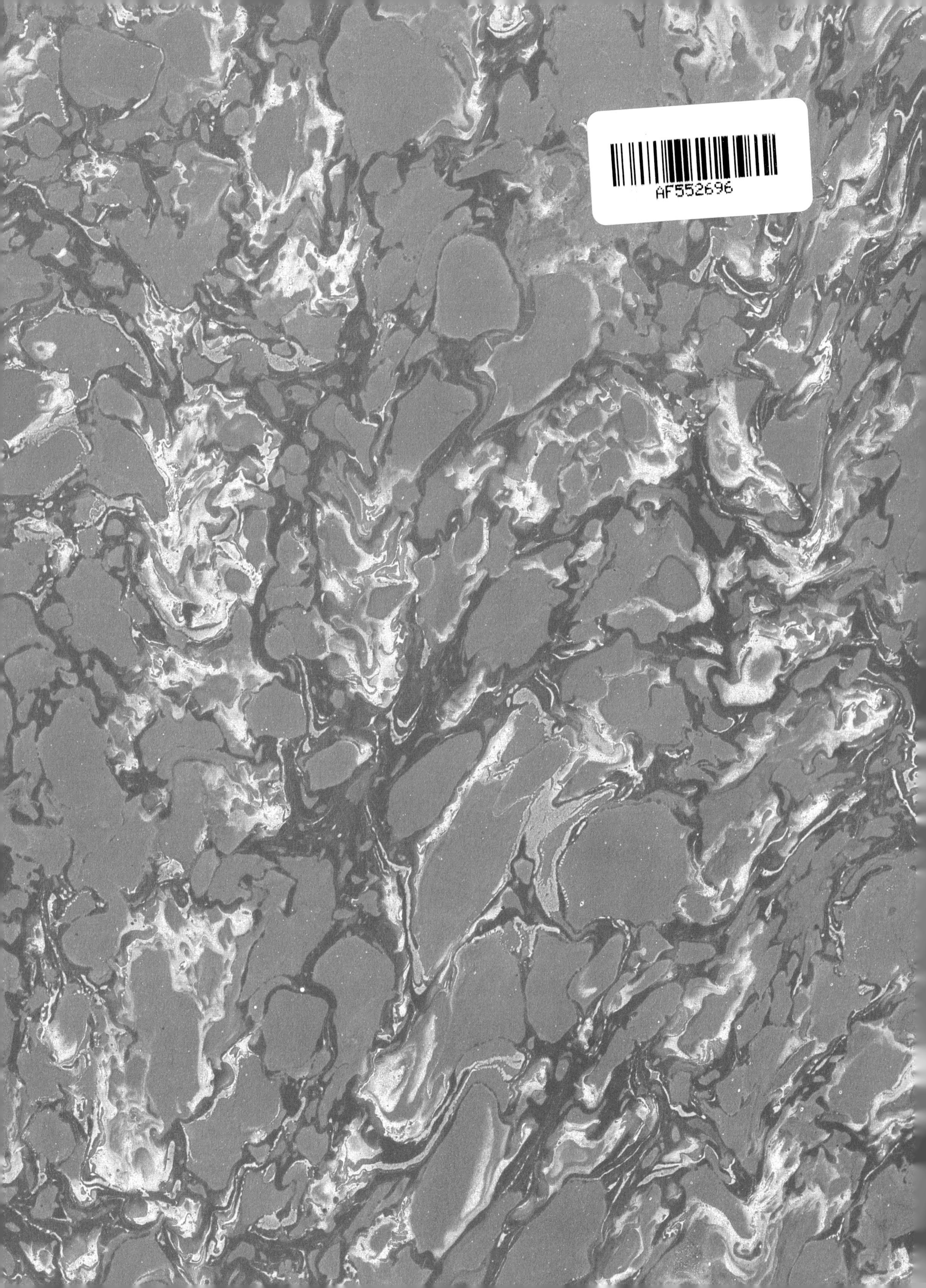
AF552696

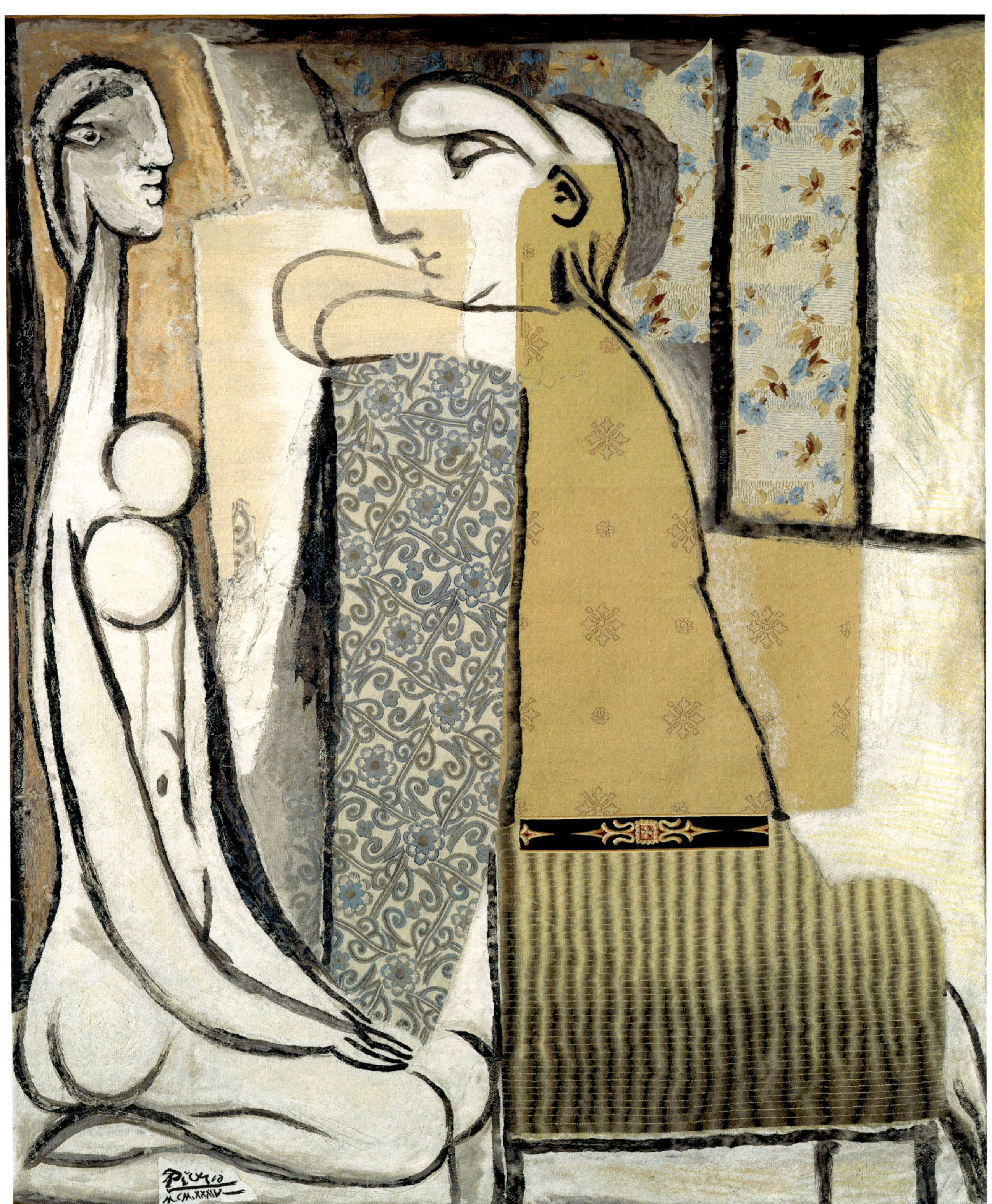
M.CM.XXXIV

helena rubinstein
beauty is power

mason klein

The Jewish Museum, New York
Under the auspices of the Jewish Theological Seminary of America

Distributed by
Yale University Press
New Haven and London

This book has been published in conjunction with the exhibition *Helena Rubinstein: Beauty Is Power*, organized by the Jewish Museum, New York, October 31, 2014–March 22, 2015, traveling to the Boca Museum of Art, April 21–July 12, 2015.

The catalogue is funded through the Dorot Publication Fund and a gift from Helena Rubinstein, L'Oréal Luxe.

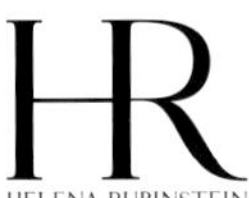

Director of Publications: Eve Sinaiko
Designed by A Practice for Everyday Life, London

Produced and typeset by Marquand Books, Inc., Seattle
marquand.com
Typeset in Accent Graphic and Romain by Maggie Lee
Production assistance by Ryan Polich
Proofread by Diana George and Sylvia Karchmar

The Jewish Museum
1109 Fifth Avenue
New York, NY 10128
thejewishmuseum.org

Distributed by
Yale University Press
302 Temple Street
P.O. Box 209040
New Haven, CT 06520-9040
yalebooks.com/art

Library of Congress Control Number: 2014944850
ISBN 978-0-300-19556-9

The paper for this book meets the guidelines for permanence and durability of the Committee on Production Guidelines for Book Longevity of the Council on Library Resources.

10 9 8 7 6 5 4 3 2 1

Color management by iocolor
Printed and bound in China by Artron Color Printing Co., Ltd.

On the cover: Helena Rubinstein with an African mask, 1934 (see page 116).

Frontispiece:
Pablo Picasso
Confidence, 1934
Tapestry, 76¾ × 67 in. (195 × 170.2 cm)
Private collection

Page 15: detail of a 1957 advertisement for Helena Rubinstein's Circulotion Mask skin treatment; see page 85.

Artwork copyright notices and photograph credits appear on page 167.

contents

6 The Jewish Museum Board of Trustees
7 Donors and Lenders to the Exhibition
8 Foreword
10 Preface and Acknowledgments
16 Beauty Is Power
162 Selected Bibliography
165 Index
167 Image Credits, Copyrights, and Museum Accession Numbers

the jewish museum board of trustees

donors and lenders to the exhibition

***Helena Rubinstein: Beauty Is Power* is made possible by The Jerome L. Greene Foundation.**

Major support is also provided by the Eugene M. and Emily Grant Family Foundation and The David Berg Foundation. Additional generous support is provided by the Leon Levy Foundation, The Horace W. Goldsmith Foundation, The Helena Rubinstein Fund / The Roy and Niuta Foundation, the Helena Rubinstein Philanthropic Fund at The Miami Foundation, and Ealan and Melinda Wingate.

Private Lenders and Galleries
Anonymous
The Africarium Collection
The Arman Marital Trust, Corice Arman, Trustee
Gilbert and Doreen Bassin
Berry-Hill Galleries, New York
Mr. Celestin Clamra, New York
Amy Fine Collins
Nicole and John Dintenfass
Valerie Franklin, California
Daniel Katz Gallery, London
The Myron Kunin Collection, courtesy of Sotheby's
Fred Leighton, New York
Galerie Louise Leiris, Paris
Hersch and Avril Klaff, Chicago
Yvonne Prigent Lacks
Frances and Bernard Laterman
Drs. Daniel and Marian Malcolm, New Jersey
Cameron McMunn-Coffran
Mr. and Mrs. Robert and Diane Moss
Colección Pérez Simón, Mexico
Primavera Gallery
The Ulla and Heiner Pietzsch Collection, Berlin
Michael and Rosemary Roth, St. Louis
Louis Slesin
Suzanne Slesin and Michael Steinberg
Sheldon H. Solow
Staley-Wise Gallery, New York
Gordon Sze
Daniel Wolf and Mathew D. Wolf in memory of Diane R. Wolf
Joe and Cathy Zicherman
Ann Ziff

Institutional Lenders
Allen Memorial Art Museum, Oberlin College, Oberlin, Ohio
Les Arts Décoratifs, Musée de la Mode et du Textile, Paris
Banco Nacional de México
Brooklyn Museum
Carnegie Museum of Art, Pittsburgh
Condé Nast
Detroit Institute of Arts
Fashion Institute of Technology, SUNY, Gladys Marcus Library, Special Collections
Helena Rubinstein, L'Oréal Luxe, Paris
High Museum of Art, Atlanta
Himeji City Museum of Art, Japan
Hirshhorn Museum and Sculpture Garden, Smithsonian Institution, Washington, DC
Indiana University Art Museum, Bloomington
The Kreeger Museum, Washington, DC
Los Angeles County Museum of Art
The Menil Collection, Houston
The Metropolitan Museum of Art, New York
The Museum of Fine Arts, Houston
Milwaukee Art Museum
The Museum of Modern Art, New York
Mount Holyoke College Art Museum, South Hadley, Massachusetts
National Gallery of Art, Washington, DC
National Gallery of Victoria, Melbourne
National Portrait Gallery, Smithsonian Institution, Washington, DC
New Orleans Museum of Art
New-York Historical Society
Philadelphia Museum of Art
Tel Aviv Museum of Art
Williams College Museum of Art, Williamstown, Massachusetts

foreword

When the cosmetics entrepreneur Helena Rubinstein died in 1965 at age 92, she left behind an immense fortune, a vast business empire, and a distinguished collection of art. Her fame survived for many years—not least in the philanthropic Helena Rubinstein Foundation. Her brand exists to this day. Although her artworks were dispersed, many are now in museums. But what was lost over time was a sense of the woman herself.

Helena Rubinstein was an extraordinary person: a self-made woman whose career spanned nearly a century. Her business innovations created the modern beauty industry, defined women as an autonomous market, and forged a link between the commercial world and the realm of women's empowerment. Forward-thinking and entrepreneurial, she changed our concepts of commerce and culture, and explored the ways in which the two interact.

But why should an art museum devote an exhibition to Rubinstein? True, her art collection was significant and unusual, and deserves to be rediscovered; but more important is the way her love of art intersected with a celebration of diversity. A visionary of the twentieth century, Rubinstein built her cosmetics empire on the idea that women must be free to invent their own identity, rather than trying to meet an arbitrary, fixed standard of beauty.

Art was, for her, a model of that expressive freedom. She collected enthusiastically and bought in quantity. Above all, she shared the works she owned with the public, displaying them in her salons and offering lessons in art appreciation along with classes on how to apply makeup. In her eclectic congeries of works were Mexican folk portraits, exotic jewelry, signature sculptures and paintings by the leading modernists, furniture in materials from Lucite to mother-of-pearl, and a breathtaking selection of figures and masks from Africa and Oceania. The thread connecting these varied works is her abiding interest in the face as a work of art.

At the Jewish Museum we have often investigated the permeable boundaries between popular culture and art, so it is natural for us to celebrate Helena Rubinstein's extraordinary accomplishments. A Jewish girl from the Polish shtetl who became one of the most powerful business leaders in the world, she represents a kind of individual achiever peculiar to the twentieth century, one who ignores all obstacles on the path to self-invention, and yet combines vaulting ambition with a deep commitment to public service, education, and the arts. Her lesson was that in the modern world there is no longer just one convention or definition of beauty; rather, beauty is something each of us defines for ourselves.

When Mason Klein proposed an exhibition on the life of Rubinstein and her art collections, he did so with this idea in mind. *Beauty Is Power* is a complex exhibition, neither purely biographical nor only focused on artworks. Such hybrid projects are a forte of the Jewish Museum, and we are fortunate to see this one realized so splendidly.

Claudia Gould
Helen Goldsmith Menschel Director
The Jewish Museum

preface and acknowledgments

The idea of organizing an exhibition on Helena Rubinstein was sparked by several wishes. Not least was the desire to tell the story of a remarkably ambitious woman who built the first global beauty empire, while employing herself and her salons to promote her modern image and style. Despite Rubinstein's fabled biography, she had become vintage. It was time to revisit someone about whom at least a full generation had little knowledge, especially after the French company L'Oréal bought her brand in the 1980s and ceased selling her products in the United States. With the absence of the brand, there also has been little occasion to appreciate her eccentric style, her longstanding patronage of art, and the endlessly eclectic trove of paintings and objects that she accumulated. Daunting, however, was the fact that her multitude of possessions had been dispersed at auction soon after she died in 1965. It was a challenge to sleuth out and reassemble so much that had been scattered or whose whereabouts were unknown.

Yet the point of this project was never to assess Rubinstein's status as a connoisseur, which she never professed to be, but rather to clarify her progressive role as a collector and purveyor of taste, and to explore her dual effort to promote modernism and democratize beauty. She first introduced her salons and their up-to-the-minute modernist decor to New York in 1915, a time of enormous cultural change, when the fight for women's suffrage was coinciding with the breakthrough of aesthetic modernism. Her respect for each consumer's distinctive character and the value she placed on subjectivity reflected both these revolutionary forces. Today, we continue to define Western standards and ideals, which have begun to dominate, if not homogenize, the global beauty industry. Rubinstein's encouragement of ethnicity and internationalism anticipated the imperative need to acknowledge the full variety of paradigms of beauty available throughout the world.

Rubinstein's skill in entrepreneurship and her prowess as a dealmaker remain legendary. Working at the beginning of the twentieth century with her first husband, the literary figure Edward Titus, she became acutely aware of the role of advertising in awakening the fantasies of ordinary people. If today her press advertising appears quaint and outdated, it was extraordinarily effective in its time, and remains a fascinating window into the culture of beauty in the last century. Nevertheless, Rubinstein could not compete with the media blitz of full-color, sexually charged images launched by the Revlon company after World War II, in print and on television.

Rubinstein's work was marked by an attempt to reach and empower women—a striking contrast with the postwar approach of the cosmetics business, characterized by media exploitation. The stigma that today attaches to the industry does not stain her reputation. As an unprecedented female CEO of an international company and an industry innovator, she had long been concerned with workers' rights and with educating her public. Among other things, she was one of the first advocates for a nutritional diet and for the use of sunscreen. Above all she was an ardent promoter of a woman's autonomy and quest for self-awareness and expression.

Beauty Is Power (an advertising slogan that she first employed in 1904) is both an exhibition about the woman—a complex, multifaceted person who controlled her image rigorously—and an exploration of her ironic fascination with how beauty was defined. She famously claimed that there were no ugly women, just lazy ones. However rooted in commerce, the opinion speaks as much to her own work ethic as to her publicity genius. From the procession of varied portraits she commissioned of herself over the decades to her heterogeneous collections, Rubinstein professed inclusiveness rather than exclusiveness. She wore costume jewelry with as much flair as emeralds. It was perhaps when she stopped caring about taste that she became her most creative. The potpourri of fashions and styles she mixed together reflected the constant shifts within modernism as well as her own restless embrace of whatever caught her eye and fancy. In reimagining the beauty industry, she emphasized a belief in change and, above all, expressive individualism. *Beauty Is Power* is a testament to that spirit.

I wish to thank Claudia Gould, Helen Goldsmith Menschel Director, who supported this idea from its inception, and I join her in thanking the lenders and sponsors who made the exhibition possible. I also extend my appreciation to my many colleagues at the Jewish Museum, without whom a project of this magnitude could not have materialized, especially Ruth Beesch, Deputy Director for Program Administration; Jens Hoffmann, Deputy Director for Exhibitions and Public Programs; Ellen Salpeter, Deputy Director for External Affairs; Norman Kleeblatt, Susan and Elihu Rose Chief Curator; Nelly Silagy Benedek, Director of Education; Elyse Buxbaum, Director of Institutional Giving; Al Lazarte, Director of Operations; Susan Wyatt, Senior Grants Writer; Niger Miles, Audiovisual Coordinator; Julie Maguire, Senior Registrar; and Jessica Nilsen, Assistant Registrar.

Rebecca Shaykin, Leon Levy Assistant Curator, deserves enormous credit for managing numerous aspects of the exhibition, while also serving as the chief coordinator of loans. Her crucial contributions cannot be overstated, and she accomplished them with unfailing grace and levelheadedness under pressure. I thank as well our intern Danielle Satran, Blanksteen Curatorial Interns Justine Bunis, Rebecca Levinsky, and Lily Shoretz, and Alex Kelly, Shoshanna and David Wingate Curatorial Intern, as well as Bradford Robotham for his photography, Robin Sand for photo research, and Lucie Steinberg for assistance with the archive.

For her intelligence, energy, and sheer brio, I am indebted to Eve Sinaiko, Director of Publications. I had the privilege of working with the design team A Practice for Everyday Life, whose exhibition and book design were conceptually in tune with the project's ideas and content: I thank the designers, and the architects, Feilden Fowles.

I would also like to thank the following individuals and institutions for their support: Suzanne McCullagh, Anne Vogt Fuller and Marion Titus Searle Chair and Curator of Prints and Drawings, Art Institute of Chicago; Alberto Barral; James Berry Hill at Berry-Hill Galleries, New York; David A. Cassera at Cassera Arts Premiers; Amy Schichtel, Executive Director, Willem de Kooning Foundation; Clare Gidwitz, Gagosian Gallery; Makiko Yamada, Curator, Himeji City Museum of Art; Andrea Caratsch, Galerie Andrea Caratsch, Zurich; Franck Prazan, Galerie Applicat-Prazan, Paris; Valerie J. Fletcher, Senior Curator, Hirshhorn Museum and Sculpture Garden; Christian Schmidt, Galerie Jablonka, Zurich; Jennifer McCarthy Elliott, Independent Curator; Diana Howard, Independent Curator; Judy A. Greenberg, Director, The Kreeger Museum; Florence Puech, Helena Rubinstein L'Oréal Luxe, Paris; Josef Helfenstein, Director, The Menil Collection; at The Metropolitan Museum of Art: Thomas P. Campbell, Director; Sabine Rewald, Jacques and Natasha Gelman Curator in the Department of Modern and Contemporary Art; Rebecca Rabinow, Curator, Department of Modern and Contemporary Art; Alisa LaGamma, Curator in Charge of the Department of the Arts of Africa, Oceania, and the Americas; Yaëlle Biro, Assistant Curator for the

Arts of Africa; Harold Koda, Curator in Charge, and Elizabeth Q. Bryan, Associate Research Curator, The Costume Institute; and Jan Glier Reeder, Consulting Curator for the Brooklyn Museum Costume Collection at The Metropolitan Museum of Art; Olivier Gabet, Director, Musées des Arts Décoratifs; Pamela Golbin, Chief Curator, Fashion and Textile, Twentieth Century Collections, and Evelyne Possémé, Chief Curator, Art Nouveau / Art Déco, Musée de la Mode et du Textile, Les Arts Décoratifs; Phyllis Magidson, Curator of Costumes and Textiles, Museum of the City of New York; Gary Tinterow, Director, and Toby Kamps, Curator of Modern and Contemporary Art, Museum of Fine Arts, Houston; Etheleen Staley, Staley-Wise Gallery, New York; Mme Christiane Falgayrettes-Leveau, Director, and Bonny Gabin, Curator, Musée Dapper; Cécile Debray-Amar, Curator, Modern Art, Musée National d'Art Moderne, Centre Pompidou; Harry Cooper, Curator of Modern and Contemporary Art, and D. Dodge Thompson, Chief of Exhibitions, National Gallery of Art; Dilys Blum, Senior Curator of Costume and Textiles, Philadelphia Museum of Art; Francisca Cruz, Curator, The Ulla und Heiner Pietzsch Collection, Berlin; Doron Lurie, Curator, Tel Aviv Museum of Art; Elisha Booker at Stair Galleries; Barbara Haskell, Curator, Whitney Museum of American Art; Joseph Baillio, Senior Vice President, Wildenstein & Co.; and Laurence Kanter, Chief Curator, Yale University Art Gallery.

The bounteous cooperation and generosity of Robert and Diane Moss, Madame Rubinstein's great-niece and former president of the Helena Rubinstein Foundation, have been unwavering. Much appreciation also goes to Michael Steinberg and to Suzanne Slesin, Rubinstein's step-granddaughter, for her varied efforts on our behalf, as well as for her book *Over the Top: Helena Rubinstein: Extraordinary Style, Beauty, Art, Fashion, and Design*, an inspiring reminder of Madame's extravagance; and similarly to Louis Slesin, Madame's step-grandson.

I have benefited enormously from the extensive research compiled by Lindy Woodhead in her book *War Paint: Madame Helena Rubinstein and Miss Elizabeth Arden: Their Lives, Their Times, Their Rivalry*, upon which the documentary *The Powder and the Glory* (2009) by Ann Carol Grossman and Arnie Reisman was based. Among the coterie of experts who have explored Madame's cultural significance, I owe special thanks to Marie J. Clifford, whose work has focused on how Rubinstein's gendered mercantile practice interwove profoundly with her marketing of modernism; Kathy Peiss, whose sage historical analysis of cosmetics and the development of female identity was enlightening; and the dialogue and encouragement I received from Michèle Fitoussi, the author of the most recent biography, *Helena Rubinstein: The Woman Who Invented Beauty*.

My endeavor also required the network of information provided by many auction houses, whose enormous assistance I gratefully acknowledge, especially Sotheby's and Christie's. I am truly indebted to Heinrich Schweizer, head of Sotheby's Department of African and Oceanic Art, who was invaluable in helping us secure many loans; Elizabeth Gorayeb, Vice President, Specialist, Impressionist and Modern Art, Sotheby's; Beth Wassarman, Senior Business Director, Jewelry, Sotheby's; Jennifer Roth, Senior Vice President, Fine Art, Sotheby's; Rachel Schaefer, Assistant, Impressionist and Modern Art, Sotheby's; Caitlyn Frank, Assistant, Impressionist and Modern Art, Sotheby's; Molly Eckel, Sales Administrator and Assistant, Fine Art, Sotheby's; Fergus Duff, Private Client Group, Sotheby's London; Andrew Strauss, Senior Director, Department of Impressionist and Modern Art, Sotheby's Paris; Cyanne Chutkow, Deputy Chairman, Impressionist and Modern Department, Christie's; Samantha

Shaffer, Bid Coordinator, Christie's; and Rahul Kadakia, Senior Vice President, Jewelry, Christie's.

Many of the works reproduced in this book are in private collections. I would like to convey my deep appreciation to all those collectors, galleries, and individuals who graciously provided us the opportunity to reproduce works in their possession. I am grateful too to the archivists and image specialists who gave of their time: Juliet Jacobson and April Calahan of Special Collections, Gladys Marcus Library, Fashion Institute of Technology, SUNY, which today houses the Helena Rubinstein Foundation archive; Lisa Luna, Associate Editor, Hearst Corporation; Leigh Montville, Associate Director, Condé Nast Licensing; and Andrew Gutterson, Sales Executive, Corbis.

To all who have helped in immeasurable ways I wish to express my appreciation. I am particularly grateful to friends and family: Alice Attie and Royce Howes, Deborah Bell, Lowery Stokes Sims, Maurice Berger and Marvin Heiferman, Ronit and Bill Berkman, Anouk Cézilly and Marc Sillam, Wendy Grossman, John and Helga Klein, Eunice Lipton and Ken Aptekar, Amy Schewel, Jill Silverman, and Sandford Starkman. In particular, I thank my wife, Elizabeth Sacre, for her unstinting counsel, editorial input, and unwavering confidence.

Perhaps I was fated to curate a show on Madame Rubinstein, given the mother I had, a woman who cultivated her own beauty and, like Rubinstein, fostered an individualist sense of style. I therefore dedicate *Beauty Is Power* to Irene Klein, who admired Rubinstein and many other strong-minded women.

Mason Klein
Curator
The Jewish Museum

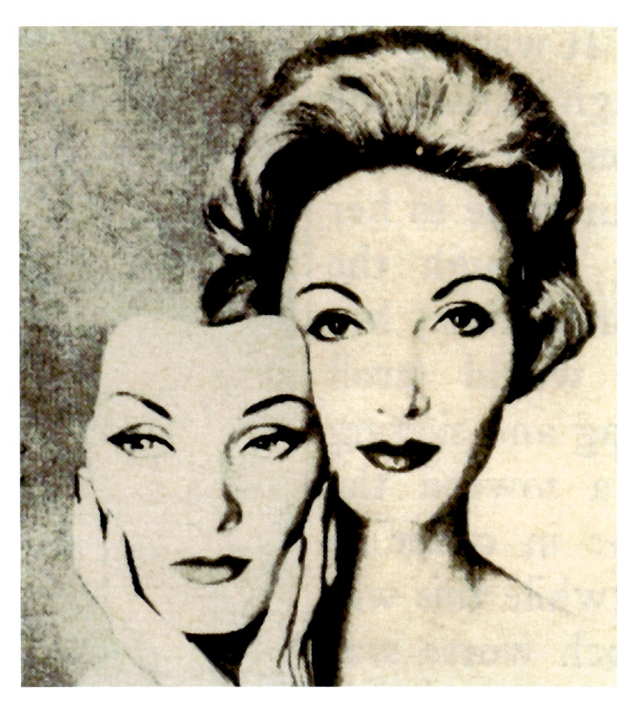

beauty is power

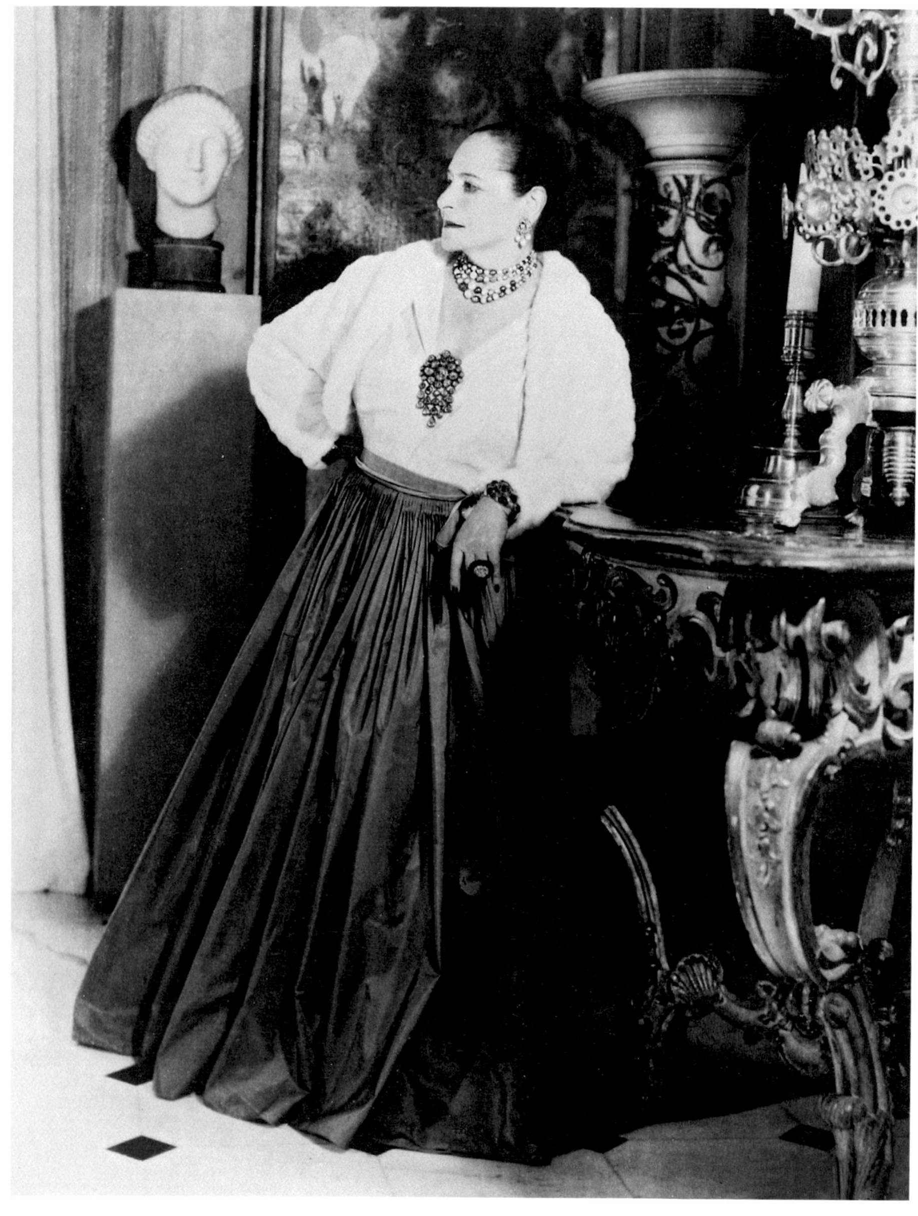

A classic portrait of Madame Rubinstein, 1958, elegantly dressed for the evening in a satin skirt and white mink bolero jacket, her hair in a soignée chignon. She is bedecked with multiple strands of black and white pearls and her signature pendant earrings, an antique brooch, cuffs, and a regal ring containing a 9.5-carat diamond surrounded by diamonds and ruby beads.

By her death in 1965 Helena Rubinstein was well into her seventh decade of business. Her cosmetics empire extended to four continents, and she had become a global icon of female entrepreneurship, as well as of art, fashion, and philanthropy.[1] Her business had challenged the myth of beauty and taste as inborn, or something to which only the wealthy were privy. As an innovator in the field of cosmetics, she had insisted that the entitlement of the few become the enrichment of the many, and she had boldly confronted the parochial constraints faced by women at the turn of the century.

A model of independence, and arguably the first modern self-made woman magnate, Rubinstein produced and marketed the means for ordinary women to transform themselves, to become acquainted with their own subjectivity, and to enhance the quality of their everyday lives through the appreciation of art and design. By enabling women to improve their appearance and define themselves as self-expressive individuals, she contributed to their empowerment. In short, Helena Rubinstein helped make women modern.

The Democratization of Beauty

Rubinstein rose from extremely modest beginnings in small-town Jewish Poland. Born Chaja Rubinstein in 1872, she came of age as the twentieth century was beginning, during a period of social reforms that challenged cults of control—whether domestic, economic, or sartorial.[2] By 1896, having fled the prospect of an arranged marriage, she found her way from Krakow to Vienna to Melbourne. She returned to Europe in 1906 and then went to the United States, where she reached the peak of her success. She witnessed the halcyon days of Edwardian London, the extravagance and optimism of the Belle Epoque before World War I, the literary and artistic avant-garde of interwar Paris, and the shifts of aesthetic and political influence after World War II, as Paris and London yielded to New York. This peripatetic life exposed her to the broadest range of cultural change. Her personality was judgmental and her management style autocratic, but these traits never made her conventional. She believed in itinerancy as a means of solving problems. Throughout her life she periodically pulled up roots, and continued to travel well into her nineties.

During the early decades of the twentieth century, in both Europe and the United States, a number of businesses developed, geared to the emerging market of products and services for women. Some of these were established by women who were themselves first-generation feminists, although they did not always see themselves in those terms. These included Rubinstein, Elizabeth Arden, and Coco Chanel, not to mention entrepreneurs such as Annie Turnbo Malone and Madam C. J. Walker, who pioneered the African American market, selling their products door to door. These strong, independent women largely developed the beauty industry. Ironically, today the industry is dominated by men, who are often cited for failing to grasp essential gender-related issues implicit to their trade, such as aging and self-esteem.[3] While one can fault some of the advertising claims made by early women entrepreneurs, their mercantilism was indisputably designed to empower women, well before the rise of contemporary debates on the industry's role in liberating or objectifying women.

Rubinstein was distinctive in some key respects. More than the others, she made herself an icon of the products she sold, and her own self-created taste a model for the idea that the modern woman could and

1 The exact number of salons Rubinstein opened in the course of her career is unknown, but based on advertisements in magazine and newspaper archives, at one time or another they were in more than thirty cities, including Atlantic City, Auckland, Boston, Cannes, Chicago, Detroit, Hollywood, London, Los Angeles, Melbourne, Mexico City, Miami, Milan, Montreal, New Orleans, New York, Newark, Newport, Palm Beach, Paris, Philadelphia, Rio de Janeiro, Rome, San Francisco, Seattle, Southampton, Sydney, Toronto, and Vienna. She also sold her products throughout the United States, Canada, and Europe in department stores.

2 Rubinstein's date of birth is contested and she seems to have given different dates at various times. This is typical of her tendency to invent fabrications about herself. In addition, the archives and records of her life and her business are incomplete, riddled with discrepancies. It is therefore difficult to establish chronology with any certainty. Much research remains to be done, but Lindy Woodhead provides the most thorough documentation available; see Lindy Woodhead, *War Paint: Madame Helena Rubinstein and Miss Elizabeth Arden—Their Lives, Their Times, Their Rivalry* (Hoboken, NJ: John Wiley & Sons, 2003).

3 See, for example, Anita Roddick, *Body and Soul: Profits with Principles, The Amazing Success Story of Anita Roddick and The Body Shop* (New York: Crown Publishers, 1991).

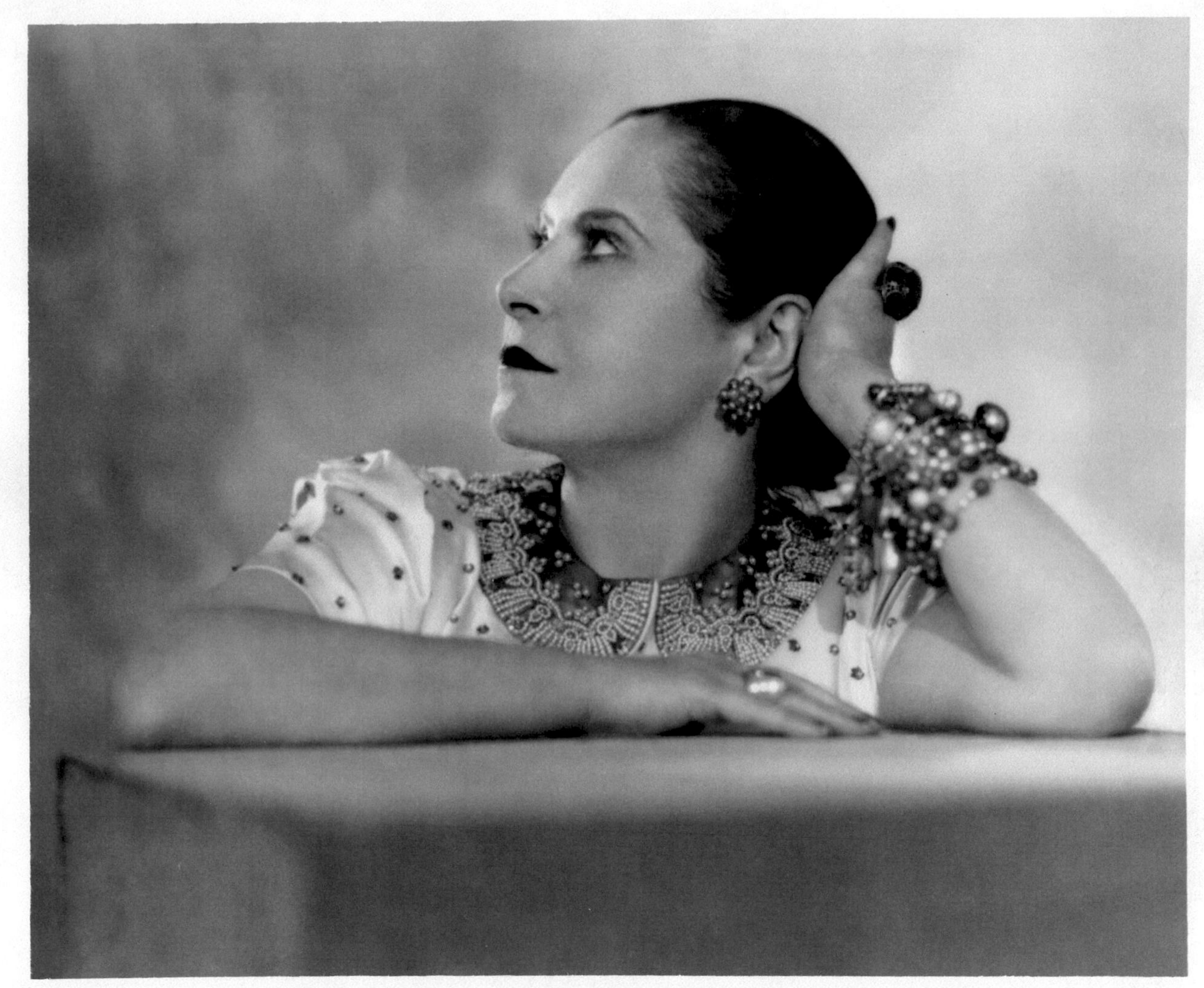

Rubinstein in the 1930s.

should curate herself. She attached her name and personal identity to a range of businesses and products associated with women's beauty and health.

Beginning with her first corporation, Helena Rubinstein & Company, founded in Melbourne, Australia, in 1903, her salons provided virtually every conceivable beauty treatment. Services included skin analysis, full body and facial massage, makeup, deportment and exercise classes, hairdressing, and lectures on the latest advances in the field.[4] She published instructional books and innumerable brochures that offered advice on the dangers of suntanning, the necessity of nutrition and exercise, and other topics. She continually rolled out new products: by the 1930s these included 629 creams, lotions, powders, rouges, lipsticks, nail and eye treatments, perfumes, colognes, soaps, and masks that served specialized needs. Rubinstein even attempted to market products for men; well ahead of other companies she launched the House of Gourielli (named for her second husband, Artchil Gourielli) in 1941.

Over time she grew more audaciously independent and creative, sanctioning ideas of diversity in terms of beauty and art that challenged traditional notions of taste. Lacking a formal education, she acquainted herself with the history of art and style, and even assembled a celebrated collection of miniature period rooms that she displayed in her home and at one point in her beauty salon.

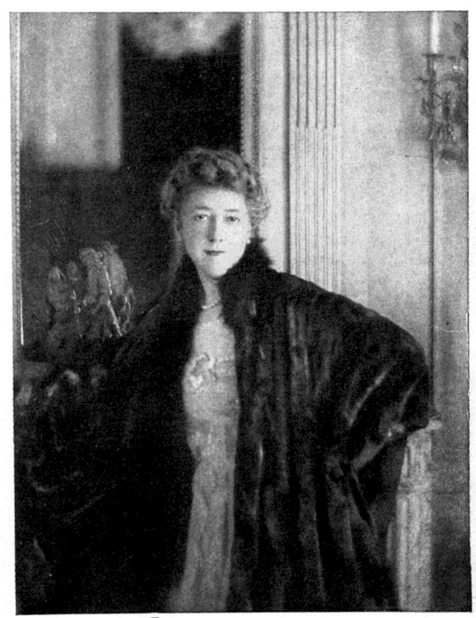

Elsie de Wolfe, c. 1913, frontispiece to *The House in Good Taste*. De Wolfe added her signature below the photograph of herself that appears at the beginning of the book, conjuring, perhaps, what has since become known as a "signature designer." The portrait was taken by Baron de Meyer, an established fashion photographer who worked for *Vogue*.

In conjuring her commercial beauty parlors in the tradition of the domestic European literary salon, Madame, as she was universally called (even by her family), was invoking a social institution—centuries old in Italy and France—in which advanced ideas were exchanged under the guidance of an elegant, educated patroness.[5] This heritage allowed Rubinstein to merge beauty, art, and modernism under a mercantile umbrella, one that was also feminine. The resulting synthesis allowed her to cultivate her various identities as a fashionable *salonnière* and an expert in beauty, business, and style. Toward that end, Rubinstein created her beauty salons and her home as social, aesthetic, and performative spaces where feminine expression could assert itself in counterpoint to the ongoing social and aesthetic eruptions that characterized modernism.

Today's fashion and beauty industries are marked by a conscious embrace of narcissism and decadence, but that is a more recent trend. These businesses, formed in the late nineteenth and early twentieth centuries, coincided with the quest for female autonomy and self-expression. As such, they were engines of modernism and liberation; Rubinstein's achievements must be viewed in this light. Her efforts to reach women are far different from today's media exploitation. The self she created served as the beacon of a subtle but emboldened femininity, a combination that appealed to progressive women.

Part of that attraction transcended cosmetics to include what Rubinstein referred to in 1923 as "exterior decoration"—what came to be called interior design. The concept was first popularized at the beginning of the century by such women as Elsie de Wolfe, who established it as a profession, catering at first to the wealthy but also reaching out to a broader clientele. While neither de Wolfe nor Rubinstein was radical, each advocated for individualism, encouraging women to be open to new principles and to trust their own instincts.[6] Rubinstein considered her beauty salon a place where a woman could learn not only how to improve her looks, but also how to reconceive her standards of taste, to understand

4 Woodhead, *War Paint*, 50.

5 The tradition of the progressive literary or political salon is intimately bound up with the history of feminism, beginning in the seventeenth century in France, and even earlier in Italy, within the smaller courts. In Germany, emancipated Jewish women found such gatherings to be unique opportunities to counter gender and anti-Semitic restrictions.

6 Born in New York in 1865, de Wolfe was a socialite, actress, and doyenne of home decorating. She referred to herself as "an ugly child born in an ugly age" and set out to remedy the problem. In 1913 she published the first book for consumers on interior decor, the immensely successful and influential *The House in Good Taste* (New York: Century, 1913, repr. New York: Rizzoli, 2004), see xvi, 4.

design, color, and art.[7] Though both women encouraged consumer fantasy, they also inspired their female clients to make choices that expressed their own personalities.[8]

When Rubinstein first established her salons at the turn of the century, she served as an exemplar of discernment. As she began to collaborate with artists and designers, her role evolved. She probably never really conceived of herself as an authority, but gradually became an impresario of style and a creative challenger of traditional "good taste." "My seemingly unconventional taste has been frequently commented upon," she acknowledged in 1964. "The explanation is simple, really: I like different kinds of beautiful things and I'm not afraid to use them in unconventional ways."[9]

Through her openness to the new and willingness to experiment she underscored her own eccentric individuality, using her body, her art, her homes, and her salons to promote her personality, and vice versa. She and her brand became associated with her heterogeneous collection of African, Oceanic, modern European, folk, and Latin American art.

She was an early proponent of this last, collecting the Brazilian artist Cândido Portinari and numerous Mexican artists, most prominent of whom was Frida Kahlo.[10] Toward the end of 1940, with the war on her mind, Rubinstein decided to get away, and booked a cruise to Mexico, Panama, and South America. It was a chance to explore the Latin American market for her beauty products and salons, and of course to buy art and jewelry. In Mexico, Madame paid a visit to Kahlo and Diego Rivera and became intrigued by their art, which she acquired in addition to work by many of the country's unknown naive portraitists and local artists such as Jesús Ray. Apart from the obvious appeal that Kahlo's exoticism and personality held for her, Rubinstein responded to local art, and soon began collecting works by little-known artists (see page 131). Rubinstein subsequently opened several establishments in South America, which fared surprisingly better than those of Arden, who had followed suit.

Madame's genuine fascination with an immense range of cultures and artistic approaches was reflected in her clothes, art, furniture, and jewelry. Through carefully considered publicity, she made her personal aesthetic taste an integral feature of her business. Conversely, she used the private domestic space of her several homes to dramatically define and champion a multicultural identity and a nonhierarchical assessment of beauty. At the same time, her line of beauty products offered a wide array of choices to young and older women, and those with dark as well as fair complexions. Together with a kaleidoscopic variety of styles in the decor of her salons and homes, this served to level snobbish taste and democratize who and what could be considered beautiful.

In addition to these innovations, Rubinstein added a patina of science to her presentation of beauty products and the self-improvement programs offered at her salons. Perhaps, as an immigrant with little formal education, she felt the need to evidence a rigorous approach to her work. She emphasized her scientific credentials, however aggrandized, and offered credible proof that her products had been tested and proven effective.[11] Such characteristics differentiate her from her lifelong rival, the doyenne of WASP taste and old-world culture, Elizabeth Arden, whose predilections in art and decor tended toward the parochial and elitist. (Her beloved racehorses were her passion.) In contrast, Rubinstein took pleasure in new styles and the provocative, even cheeky ways in which they could be mixed. She was not only an early patron of modern art, fashion, and decor, and a leading collector of African and Oceanic art of the early twentieth century, but was ahead of her time in decoratively

7 Helena Rubinstein, "Exterior Decoration," *Arts and Decoration* 18, no. 3 (January 1923): 52, 56.

8 See Penny Sparke, "The 'Ideal' and the 'Real' Interior in Elsie de Wolfe's 'The House in Good Taste of 1913,'" in *Journal of Design History* 16, no. 1 (2003), 65.

9 Helena Rubinstein, *My Life for Beauty*, rev. ed. (New York: Simon and Schuster, 1966), 91.

10 See Hayden Herrera, *Frida: A Biography of Frida Kahlo* (New York: Harper & Row, 1983), 219.

11 Rubinstein anticipated the industry's later emphasis on scientific research and development, concentrating particularly on hormone rejuvenation. In the mid-1930s her company launched Hormone Twin Youthifiers, a cream "to stimulate and rebuild new, younger skin cells." As she grew older, hormone treatments interested her more. She researched female hormone extracts, producing numerous products, including Estrogenic Hormone Cream with Progesterone and Ultrafeminine, which became one of the first beauty products to be approved by the Food and Drug Administration. See Maxene Fabe, *Beauty Millionaire: The Life of Helena Rubinstein* (New York: T. Y. Crowell, 1972), 121; Woodhead, *War Paint*, 230.

Rubinstein and Arden both introduced many beauty products before the 1938 Food, Drug and Cosmetic Act (FDCA) was enacted in the United States. The beauty industry's advertising claims subsequently began to be scrutinized more carefully, and product labels had to comply with such distinctions. Rubinstein was forced to change the name of her Valaze Skin Food to Wake Up Cream; see Woodhead, *War Paint*, 205; Florence E. Wall, *The Principles and Practice of Beauty Culture*, 4th ed. (New York: Keystone Publications, 1991). Restrictions placed by the Food and Drug Administration on estrogen levels in American over-the-counter hormone creams may have been the reason Rubinstein altered her original Hormone Twins cream, introducing a hormone cream called Tree of Life in 1956.

Rubinstein herself often claimed to have entered medical school, but to have left when she found the medicinal smells and the sight of blood unbearable. When she settled in Paris in 1912 she did enroll in clinical studies in dermatology at the St. Louis Hospital for a time; see Woodhead, *War Paint*, 88.

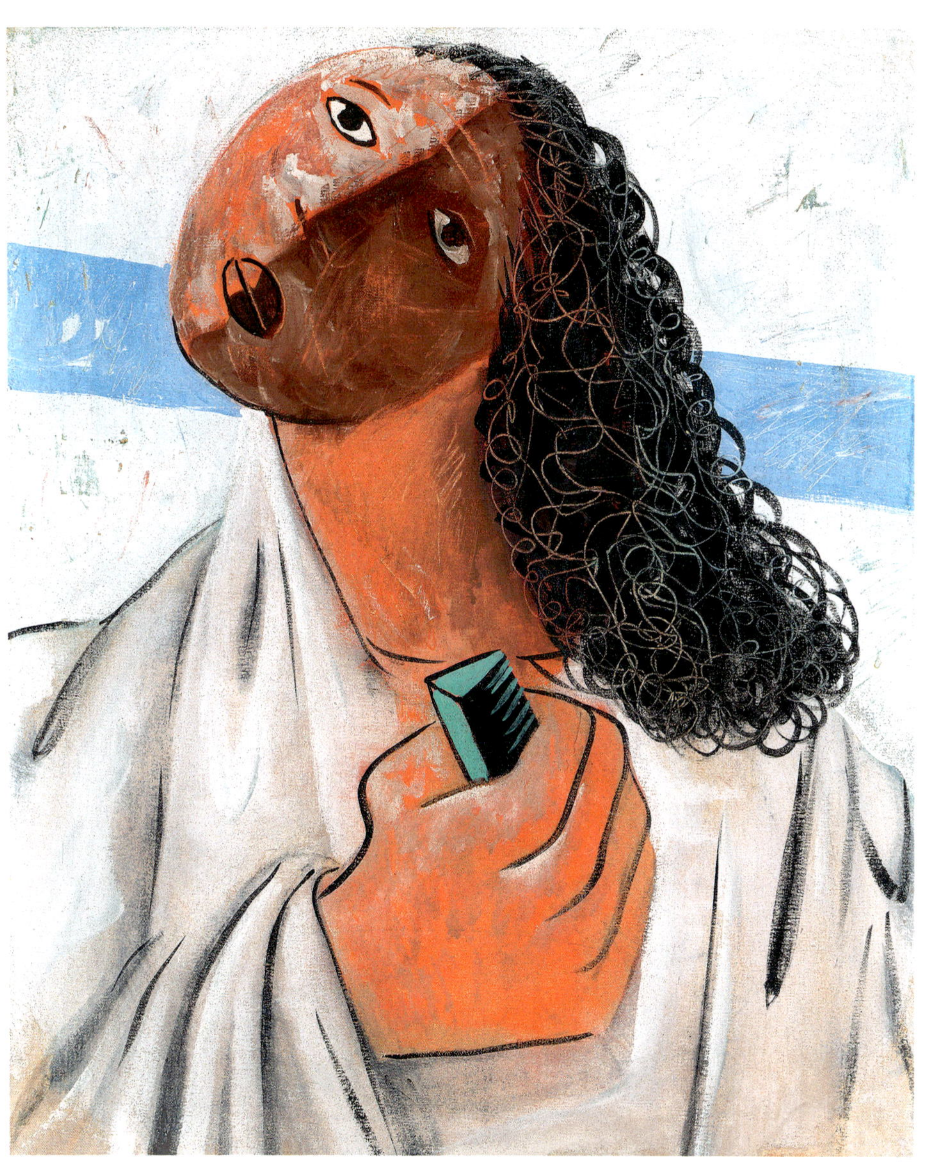

Cândido Portinari
Young Woman Combing Her Hair, 1941
Tempera on canvas, 28½ × 23½ in. (72.4 × 59.7 cm)
Collection of Hersch and Avril Klaff, Chicago

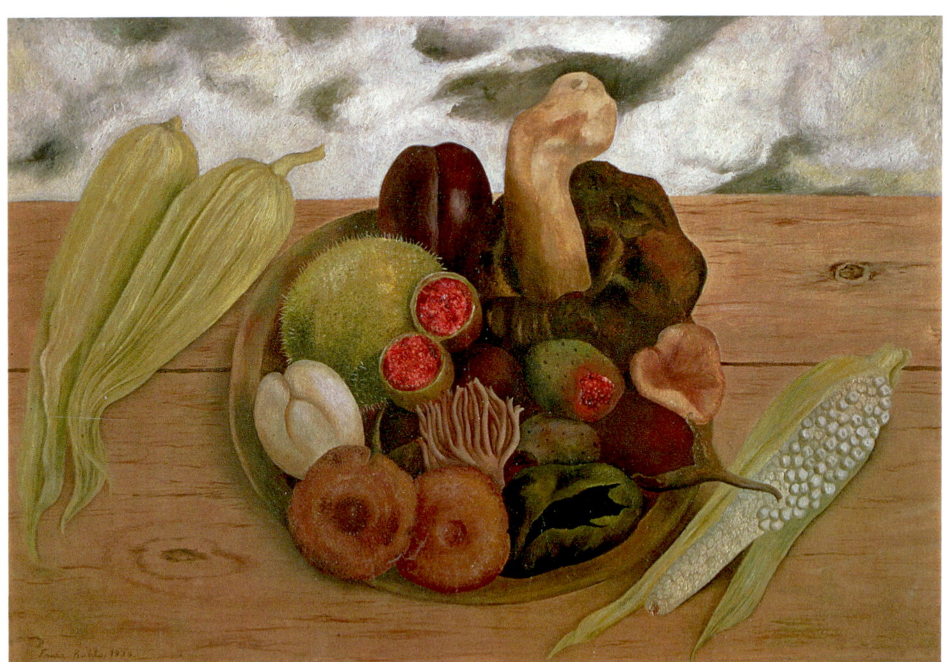

Frida Kahlo
The Fruits of the Earth, 1938
Oil on Masonite, 16 × 24 in. (40.6 × 61 cm)
Collection of the Banco Nacional de México, México DF

Rubinstein discovered Kahlo's work during a visit to Mexico in 1940. She felt an immediate personal connection to Kahlo, drawn to her eccentric style and sympathetic to her tumultuous life. "It seemed to me," she wrote to the artist in 1941, "that even in the short time we had together, a bond of simpatico was established—your life, your situation impressed me profoundly, and I think of you often."

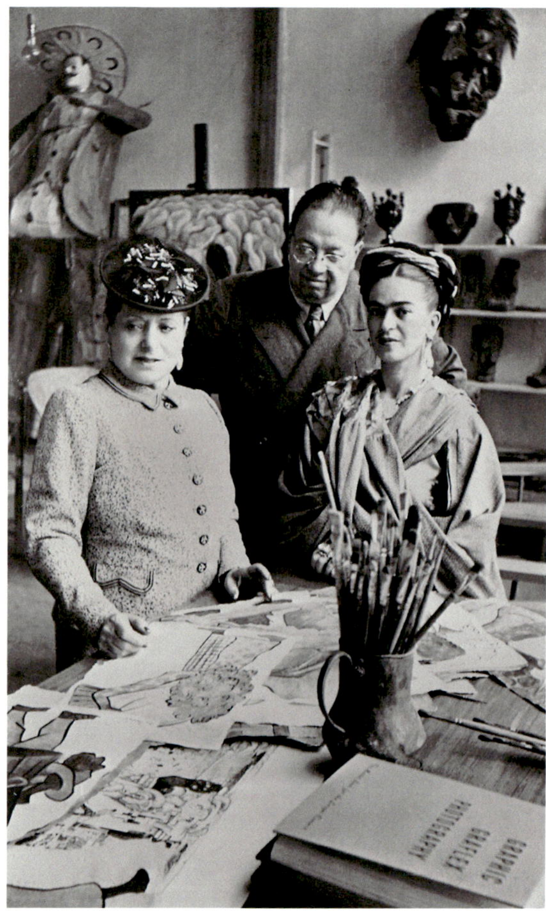

Rubinstein visiting Diego Rivera and Frida Kahlo, probably 1940.

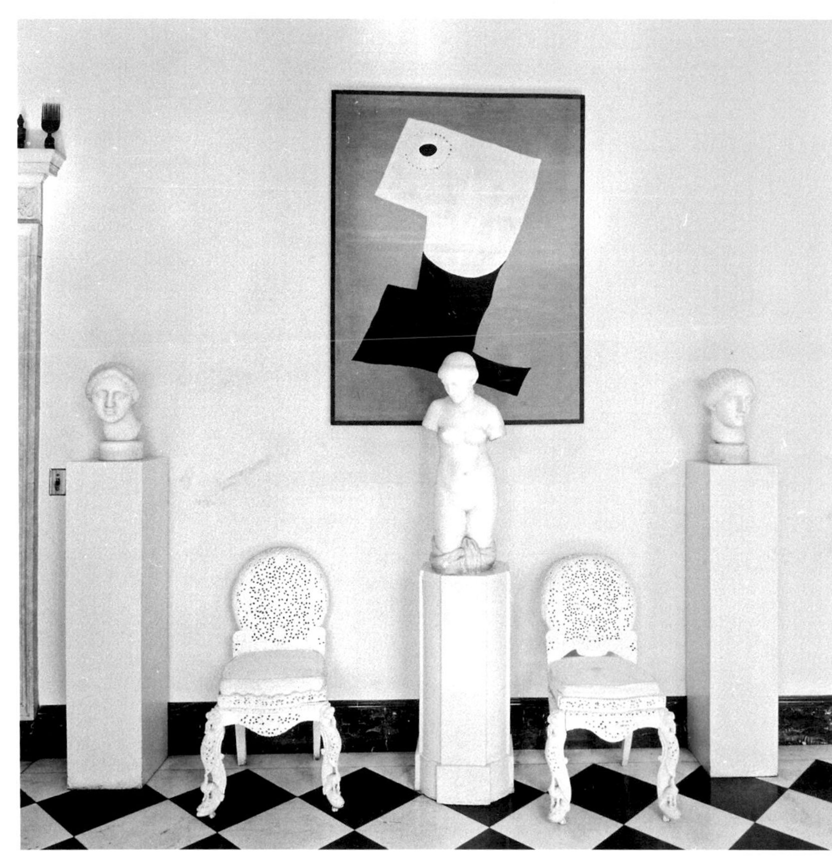

The foyer of the 625 Park Avenue apartment, with Joan Miró's *Portrait*, Elie Nadelman sculptures, and an African comb.

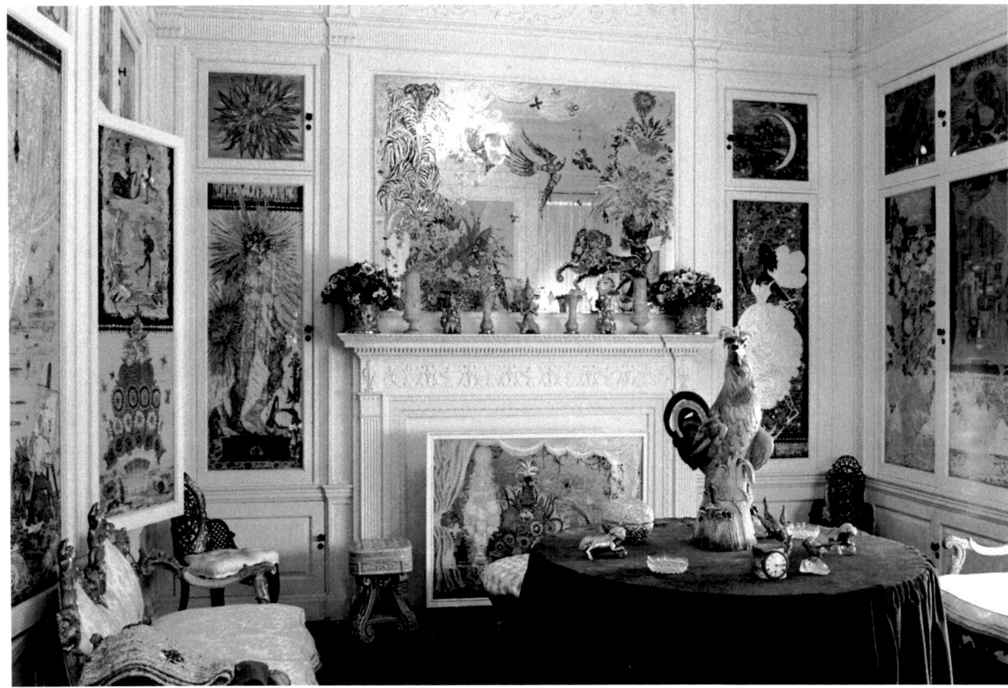

The library in Helena Rubinstein's apartment at 625 Park Avenue in the 1940s, with painted-glass panels by Federico Pallavicini, each of which symbolizes an event in Madame Rubinstein's life.

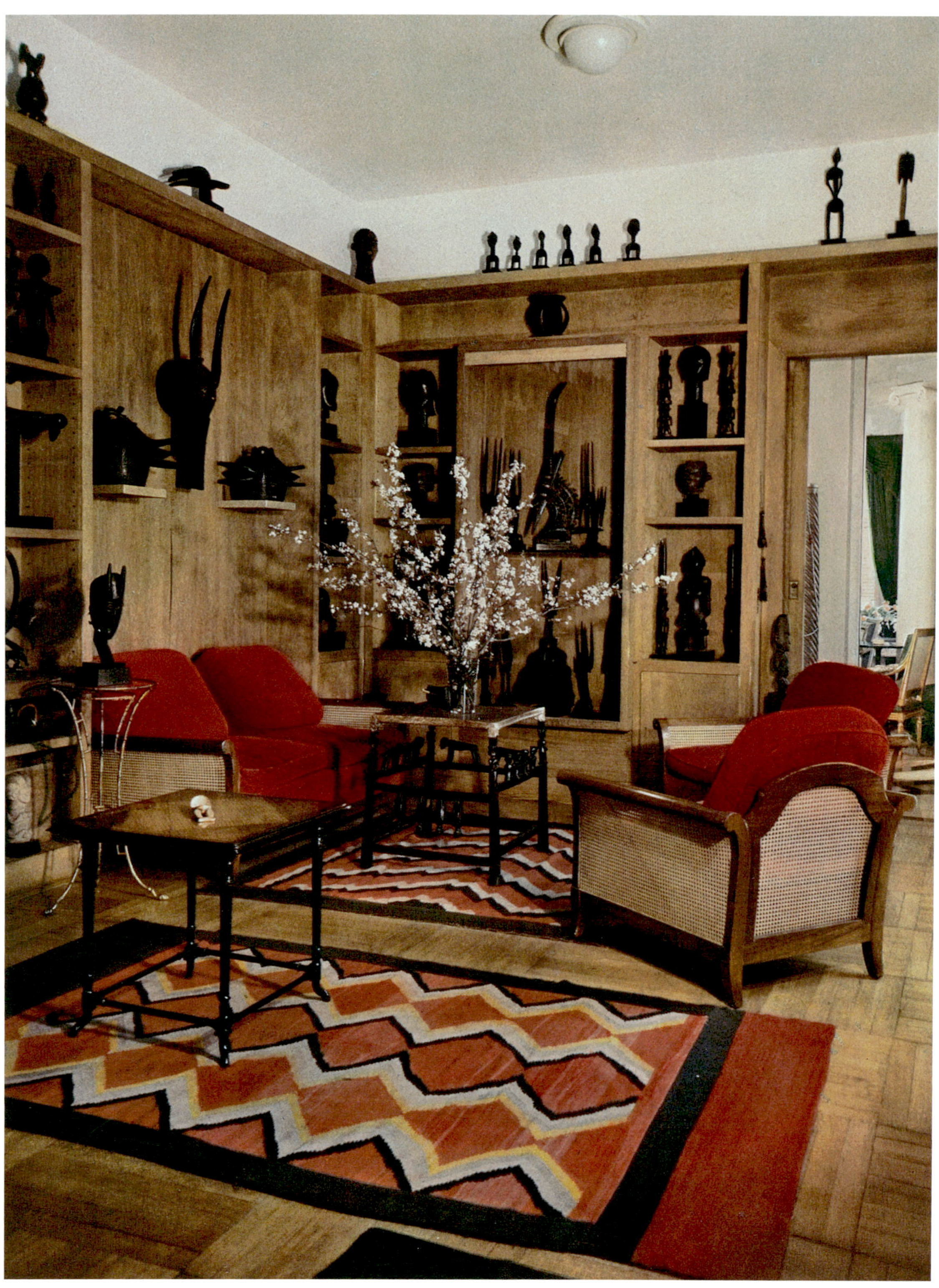

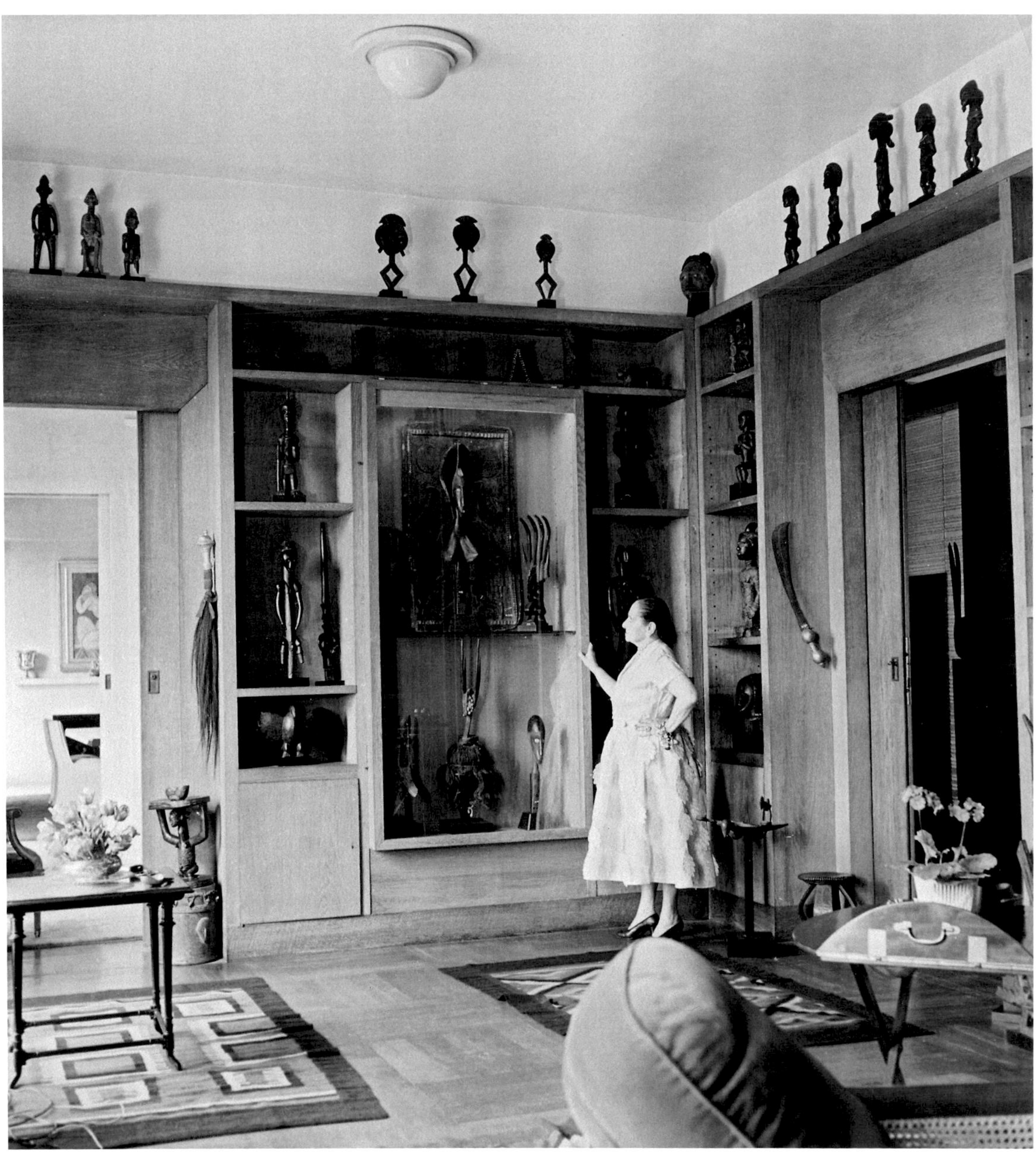

Helena Rubinstein in the library of her Paris apartment on the Ile St.-Louis, 1951. On display is a fragment of her extraordinary collection of African and Oceanic art. Madame arranged and rearranged her collections incessantly. At left is the same room in about 1955.

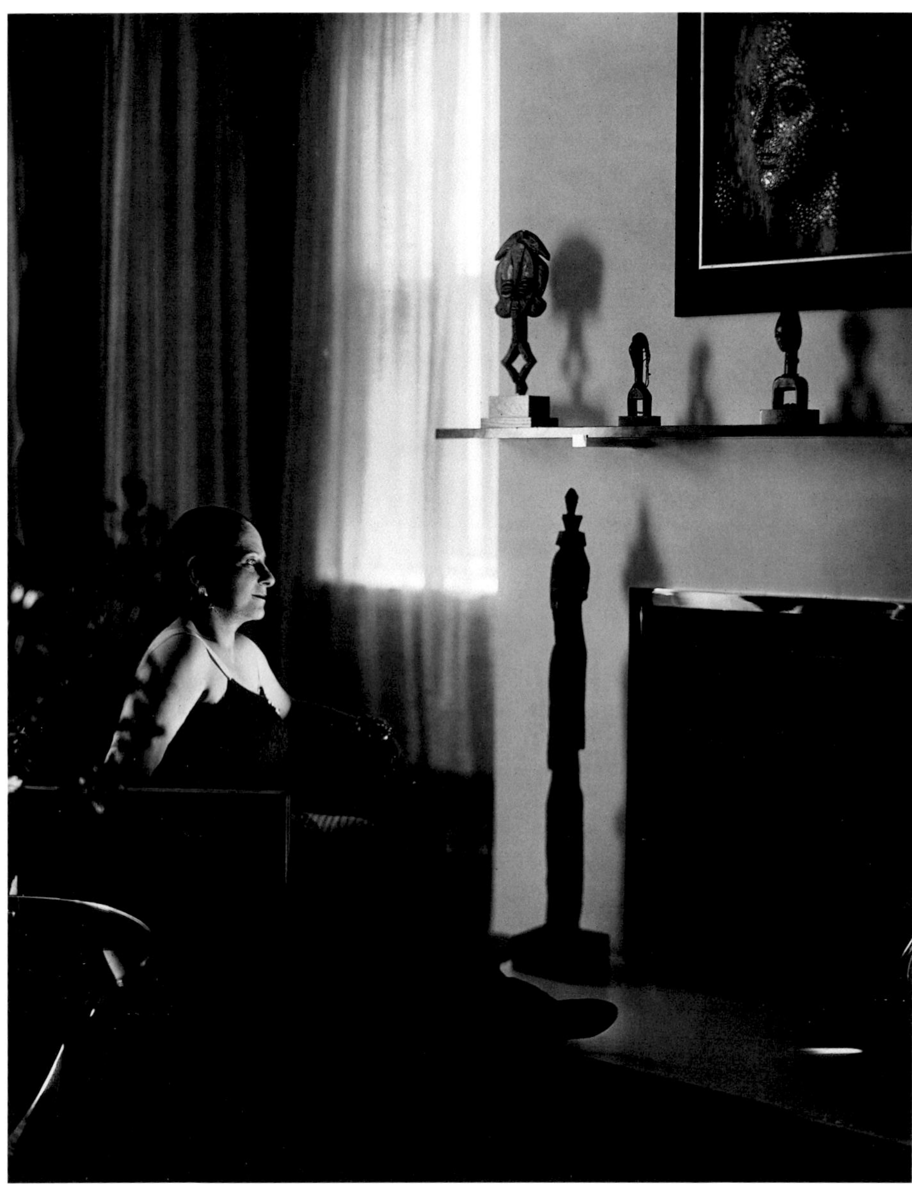

Rubinstein in her New York apartment at 895 Park Avenue, designed by Donald Deskey, c. 1935.

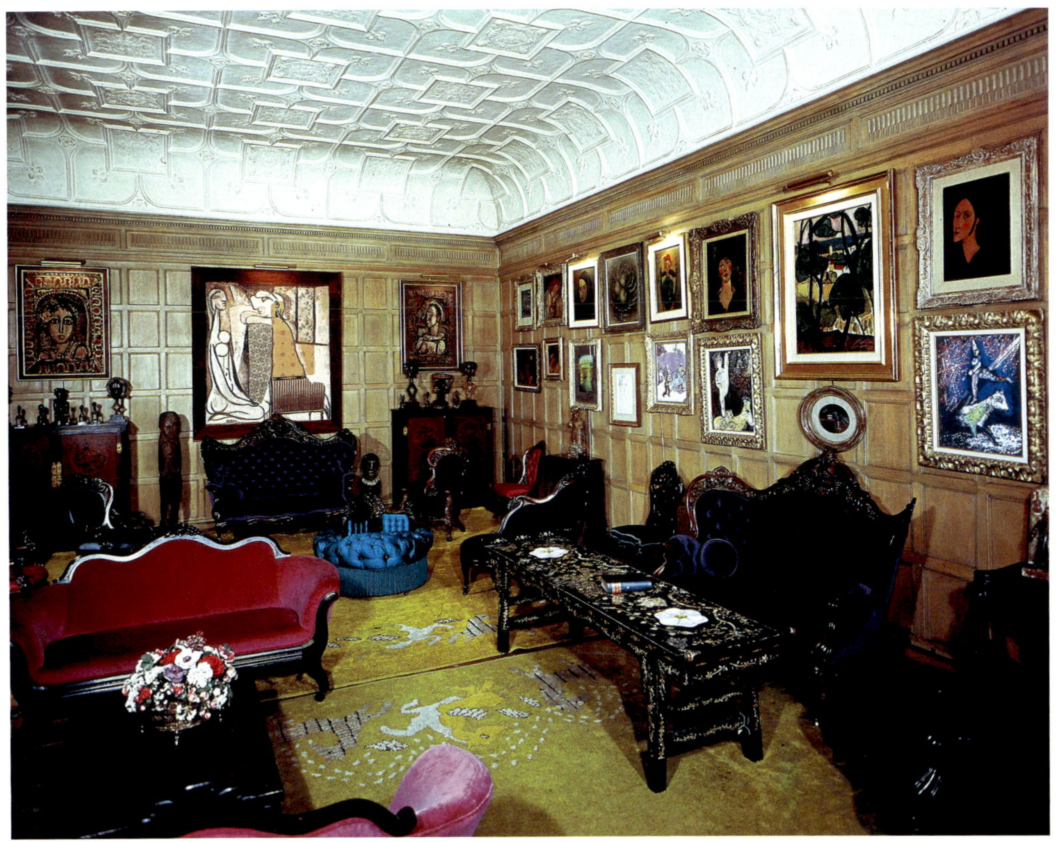

Each of Rubinstein's many homes was more lavish and extravagant than the last. Her apartment at 625 Park Avenue was on three floors and was packed with art. *Above*: Her living room with paintings and tapestries by Picasso, Rouault, Matisse, Chagall, Modigliani, and others, sculptures from Africa and Oceania, and a Lurçat carpet. *Below*: The private art gallery on the top floor in 1950.

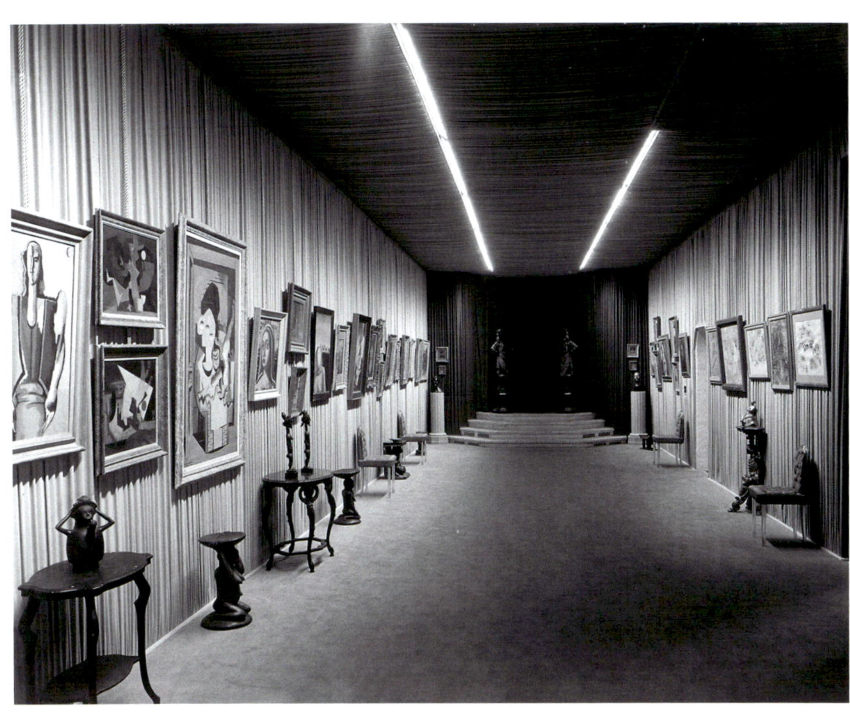

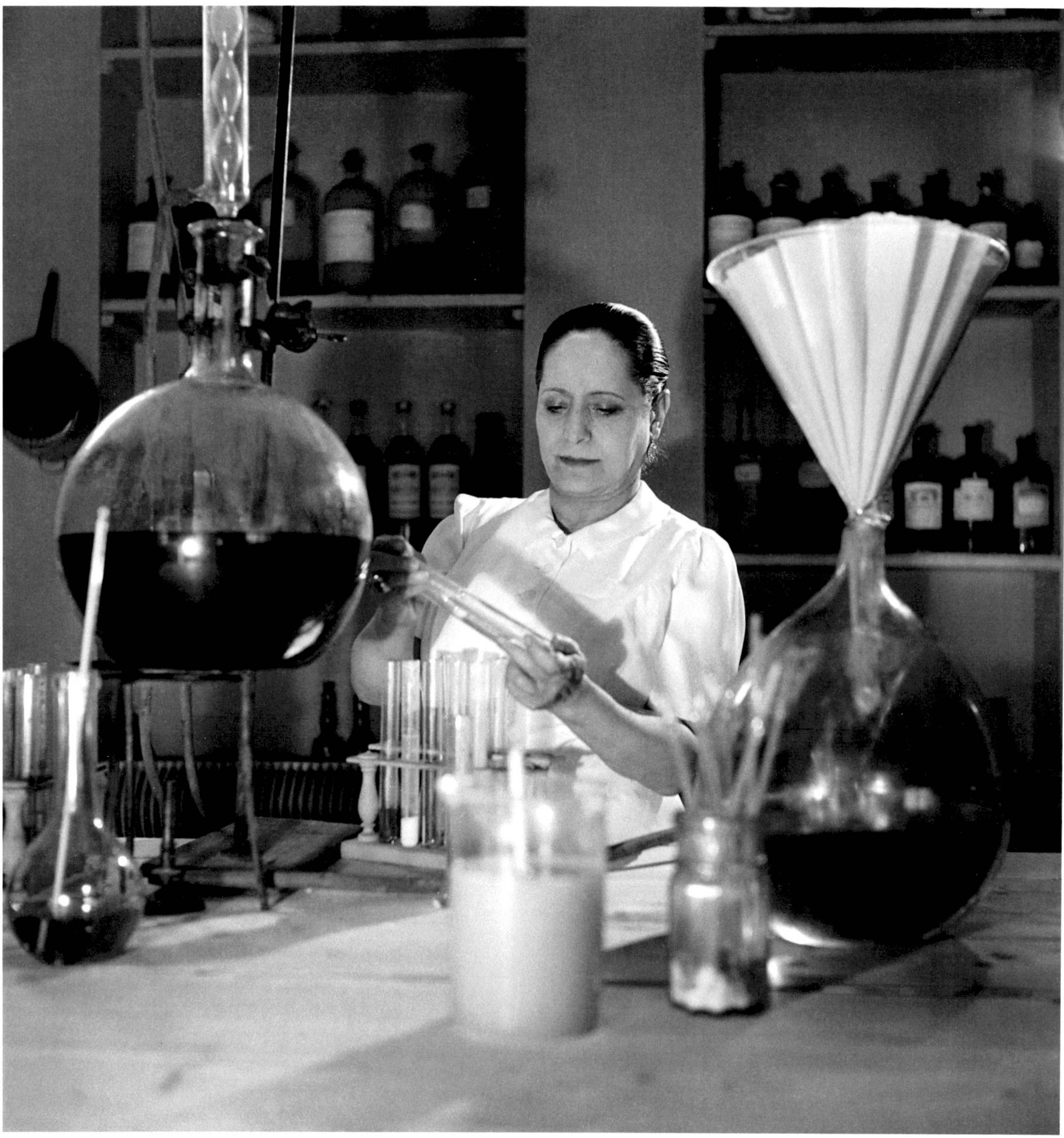

Rubinstein in her laboratory in Saint-Cloud, France, 1939. As a cosmetics entrepreneur—or beauty scientist, as she preferred to think of herself—Rubinstein carefully marketed her professional image, advertising herself as both a researcher and a beauty queen, living proof of the efficacy of her wondrous potions. Here, she poses in a deliberately unglamorous white lab coat, looking serious and professional.

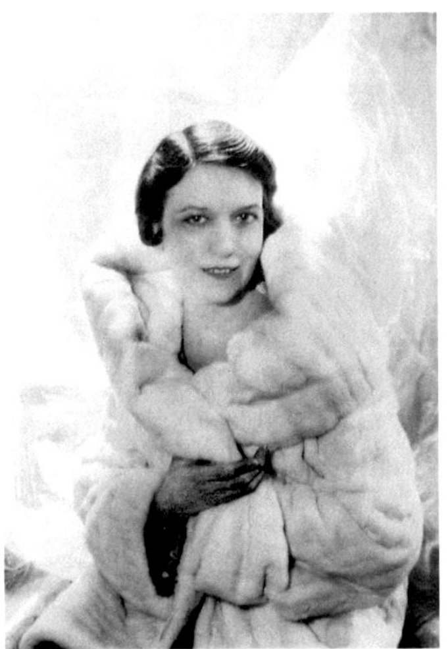

Elizabeth Arden photographed by Cecil Beaton, 1930.

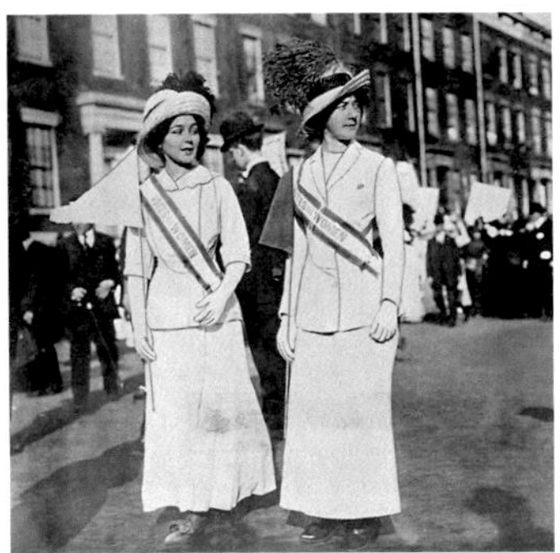

American suffragists march to demand the vote, 1912.

mingling Western and non-Western art.[12] While Arden was forced to compete with Rubinstein's fashionably chic persona, she always exuded a reserved elitism.

Although both beauty queens appealed to a wealthy clientele, Rubinstein differed profoundly from Arden, whose snobbishness, referred to by one biographer as "tendencies . . . typical of the era in which she grew up," seemed to gravitate to similarly minded friends, such as the Duke and Duchess of Windsor.[13] Arden's public image of exclusivity was expressed metaphorically by the inimitable red door of her salons. Also typical of the era were a casual, confident anti-Semitism and racism. Arbiters of taste like Arden and Chanel were not just conscious of their social set, but maintained a similar dislike of Jews—allegedly, in Chanel's case, instilled in her convent years and hardened by her association with society elites.[14] In retaining her Jewish surname, Rubinstein was making an unusual and aggressive statement in opposition to this. She calculated, correctly, that she could appeal to a wider market either despite or because of her Jewishness. During an age of unprecedented mobility, in which untold numbers of women were entering the work force, beauty salons were an affordable luxury. Rubinstein seems to have intuited the presence of this potential niche market.

After her initial successes in Melbourne and Sydney, and then in London and Paris, she was forced at the outbreak of World War I to move to New York, where she opened her first salon in 1915. Her timing was fortuitous; two revolutionary events had just occurred there: the Armory Show of avant-garde European art in 1913, and a major rally of women suffragists in New York in 1911. Tens of thousands of women had marched, with some wearing lip rouge as a badge of emancipation. Indeed, the 1910s could not have been a more promising period to enter the beauty industry. This was especially true in the United States, where entrenched puritanical attitudes toward makeup were suddenly being challenged, and where an unprecedented influx of young immigrant women into the work force created a market that was demanding autonomy—not only the independence that went with a paycheck but also the fundamental right to define their appearance.

It has been estimated that in 1916 only twenty percent of Americans used toiletries or cosmetics.[15] Rubinstein, who had already established a successful global business, saw a further opportunity in the United States, with its exploding population and the rising consumerism of its new middle class. Modest soap manufacturers were about to grow into huge beauty companies, as people became convinced of the importance of appearance and hygiene; no less transformative was the proliferation of images made possible by the modern technologies of electricity, photography, and mechanized printing. And of course there was the cinema: close-ups required cosmetics, particularly eye shadow and mascara, previously unused in America. In preparation for her film *A Fool There Was*, Theda Bara came to Rubinstein for advice in creating what came to be known as the vamp look. It was mascara, as much as pose or hairstyle, that made Bara the "siren of the Silent Screen."[16] Glamour was being introduced into people's lives in unprecedented ways, and it led to a hunger for a new kind of education of the senses. As a consequence, the American beauty industry was booming by the 1920s.

Rubinstein and Arden were in the same business for more than a half-century. Both established thriving international companies, which they ran themselves, and both were culturally transformative. Their mutual avoidance was legendary: neither woman once directly engaged

12 In 1938 *Vogue* referred to Rubinstein's home as a "Collector's Fantasy," identifying her as "an adventurous soul who deviates from established routes," noting how she paired modern and antique furniture, European paintings with African sculptures, to create an "assemblage." "Collector's Fantasy," *Vogue* 92, no. 4 (August 15, 1938), 120.

13 Lindy Woodhead, *War Paint*, 146, 280.

14 Hal Vaughan, *Sleeping with the Enemy: Coco Chanel's Secret War* (New York: Knopf, 2011), 101.

15 Kathy Peiss, *Hope in a Jar* (New York: Henry Holt, 1998), 50.

16 Rubinstein, *My Life for Beauty*, 63.

the other. As rivals they possessed little in common other than overbearing temperaments and certain phobias and eccentricities, which they could afford to indulge.[17] Both were from modest, if not poor backgrounds, though Arden's route from her Canadian origins scarcely compares to the dramatic odyssey that Rubinstein embarked upon, leaving her home in Krakow while still a teenager. Whereas Rubinstein retained her name, Florence Nightingale Graham became Elizabeth Arden. The latter's tastes and interests were clearly more conservative, as she avidly sought acceptance among the social elite. Such preoccupations mattered less to Rubinstein, who, besides being more hands-on in her business, did not like parties and small talk. Both, however, sold their products at premium prices. Although the two entrepreneurs emerged during the infancy of what later came to be called feminism—the assault on patriarchy and the demands of the women's suffrage movement—neither one had a sustained involvement with such social issues.

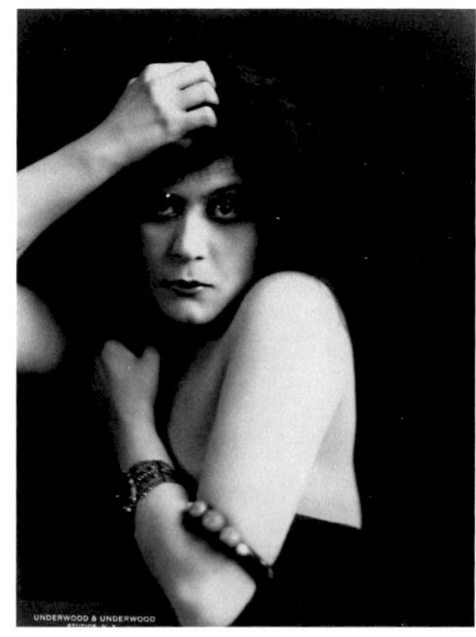

Theda Bara, the original vamp, c. 1915.

Social pedigree, though, maintained its importance for Arden, and was a requirement for those who wished to rise within her company.[18] Rubinstein, in contrast, mainly employed her family, whom she could trust. Arden, whose relatives were never much help in her business, snippily referred to the Rubinstein clan as the "Polish Mafia."[19]

Rubinstein could hardly have claimed WASP credentials, but her choice to create a brand with an overtly Jewish name is notable. Outside of the financial field, few eponymous brand names were Jewish in origin. Interestingly, she chose to change her given name, Chaja, to Helena, making herself the namesake of the great mythic beauty.[20]

She used her international celebrity and wealth as a foil against the ingrained anti-Semitism of her time. In 1941, for example, when she sought to rent a triplex apartment at 625 Park Avenue, one of Manhattan's most prestigious addresses, she was told that the building did not accept Jewish tenants; she responded by buying the building. Scarcely unaware of her ethnicity, Rubinstein nevertheless allegedly also made disparaging comments about Jewish taste or certain neighborhoods, such as her first family apartment on Manhattan's West End Avenue, an area she characterized as "too Jewish." She was not herself a practicing Jew.[21]

When it came to assembling her art collections, Rubinstein acquired what she liked and learned as she went. She knew many artists and drew upon their guidance. To buy African and Oceanic art, she turned to noted collectors with whom she would negotiate, often rather persuasively. In the early 1930s, for example, she obtained the *Bangwa Queen*, a celebrated Cameroon Grasslands statue, from the Paris dealer Charles Ratton by swapping a group of earlier acquisitions.

By the 1930s Madame had become a fixture in the art world, known for an independent, deliberate unconventionality. She mixed disparate tastes and cultivated an eclectic style, becoming increasingly intrigued by Surrealism, with its endlessly mutable fantasies (see page 47). She would design and redesign the rooms of her salons and homes, mixing, regrouping, or rotating her various collections from one to another. While some of her private homes, in Paris and New York, became ever more public platforms for the display of her collections, her public salons never ceased exuding a sense of domesticity, appointed with recent acquisitions and the latest in decorative arts.

She had little interest in the conventional standards of connoisseurship. Though her art collection had some important pieces, it is best judged as a whole, particularly in terms of its cultural diversity; it was an eccentric assortment of Latin American, African, and Oceanic artists,

17 For the definitive biography of both figures, see Woodhead, *War Paint*.

18 Woodhead, *War Paint*, 372. Arden fundraised for elite cultural causes such as the Opera Guild and the Friends of the Philharmonic and participated in charity events, but never had a foundation. Rubinstein, in contrast, established the Helena Rubinstein Foundation in 1953; among many other contributions to the arts and sciences, it endowed a fellowship program at the progressive Whitney Museum of American Art's Independent Study Program. The Helena Rubinstein Pavilion for Contemporary Art opened in Tel Aviv in 1959, and is now part of the Tel Aviv Museum of Art. She also supported programs in education, community services, and health, with a special interest in those that benefited women and children and assisted disadvantaged communities.

19 Woodhead, *War Paint*, 153. Among Madame's numerous sisters, Ceska was set up in Australia, Pauline in Paris, Manka in America; her cousin Lola worked at the Chicago salon. Another sister, Stella, later replaced Pauline as head of the Paris salon. Various cousins and second cousins also were employed, most prominently a niece, Mala, whom Madame mentored to become her key surrogate, and who changed her surname to Rubinstein. A nephew, Oscar, assumed a substantial executive position. One sister, Regina, stayed in Poland and perished in the Holocaust, along with most of the 60,000 Jews of Krakow. *War Paint*, 255.

20 Woodhead suggests that Helena is an anglicized version of the Hebrew Chaja; see *War Paint*, 33.

21 See Woodhead, *War Paint*, 108, 247.

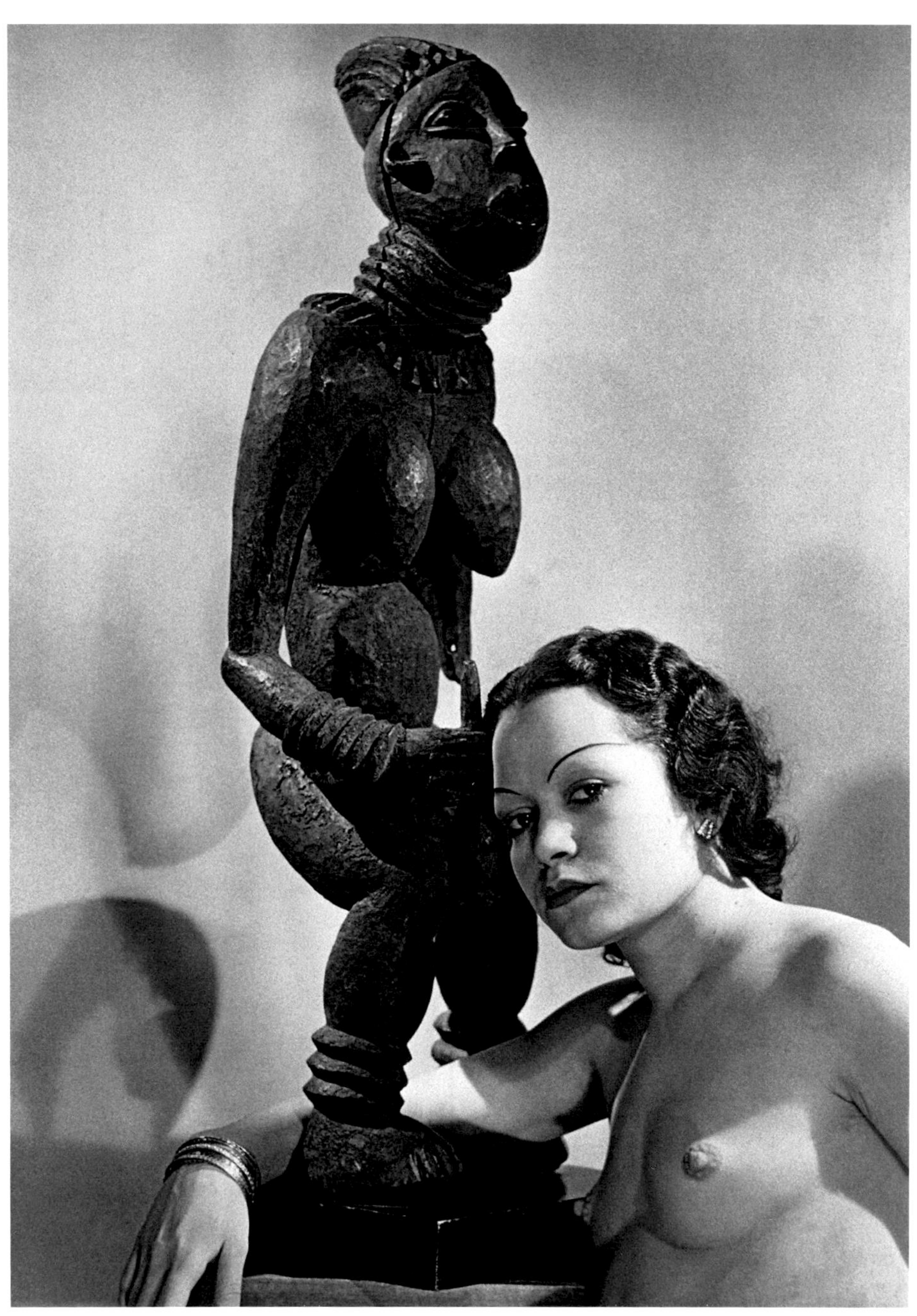

Man Ray
Untitled (*Bangwa Queen* and model), c. 1934
Gelatin silver print, 11¾ × 9 in. (29.9 × 22.9 cm)

Rubinstein lent the *Bangwa Queen*, a jewel of her collection, to her friend Man Ray for this photograph. It is one of several by the Surrealist artist that juxtapose fair-skinned models with non-Western sculptures, provoking questions about race and aesthetics. The twentieth century saw a radical redefinition of female beauty in both art and fashion. Rubinstein's love for African and Oceanic art was unusual in her milieu; for her, ideals of beauty were less fixed than was the norm.

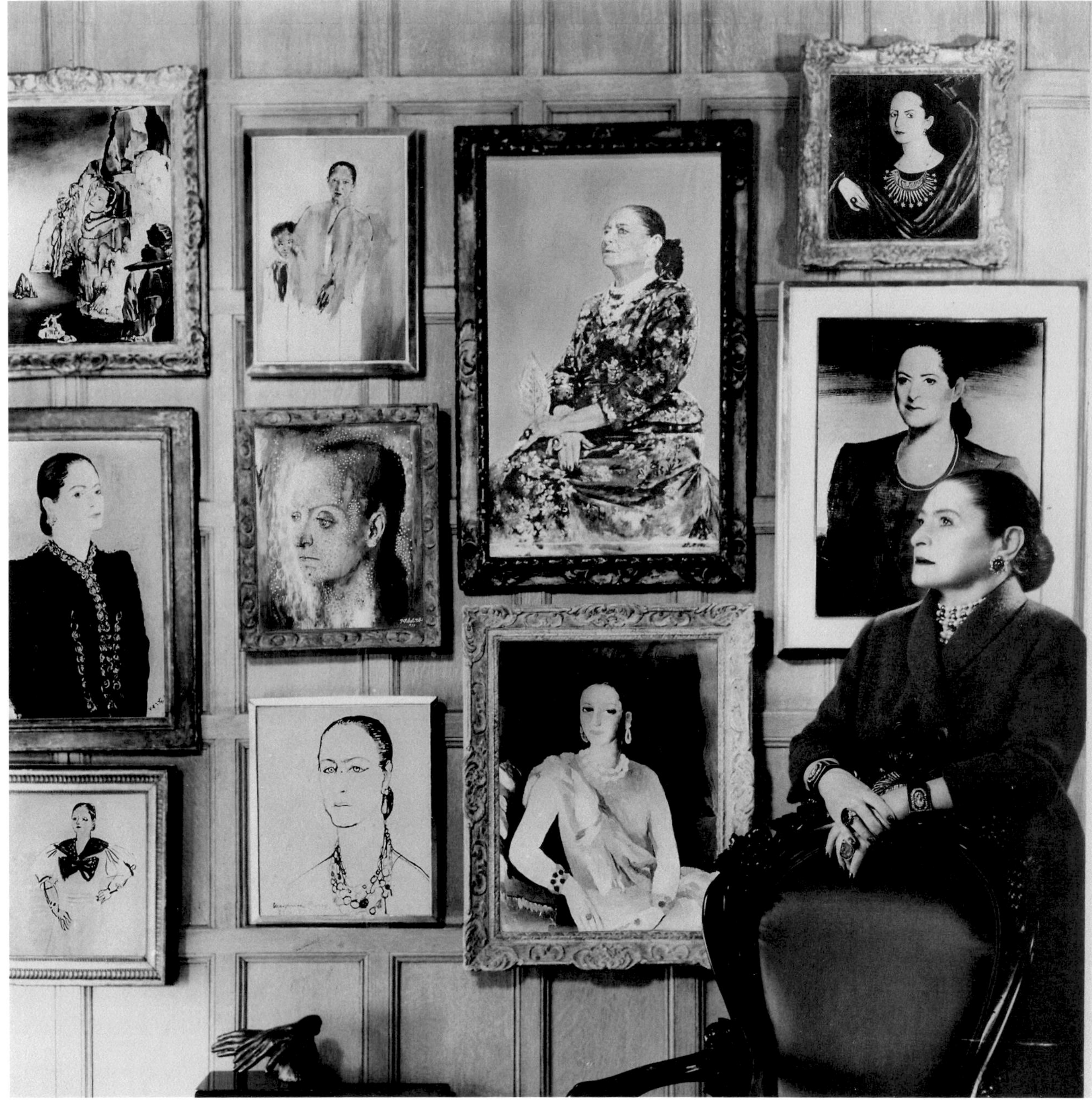

Rubinstein in front of a montage of some of the many portraits she commissioned throughout her life; left to right, from top: Salvador Dalí, 1943; Christian Bérard, 1938; Graham Sutherland, 1957; Roberto Montenegro, 1941; Marcel Vertès, c. 1940; Pavel Tchelitchew, 1934; Cândido Portinari, 1939; Raoul Dufy, c. 1935; Margherita Russo, 1953; and Marie Laurencin, 1934.

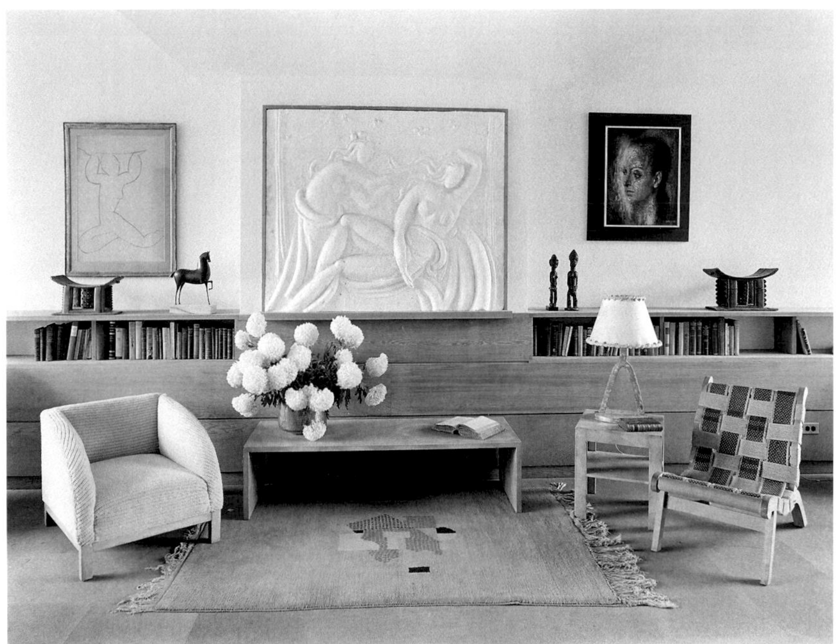

The beauty salon at 715 Fifth Avenue had a library, designed to look like the living room of a home. In 1936 it was filled with art: Elie Nadelman's plaster bas-relief, *Two Nudes*, c. 1911, is at center, flanked by Pavel Tchelitchew's *Head of Helena Rubinstein Encrusted with Sequins*, 1934, Nadelman's bronze horse, c. 1914, African figures and headrests on the shelf, a Jean-Michel Frank lamp, and a carpet designed by Fernand Léger and produced by Maison Myrbor. The drawing of a caryatid at left, thought at the time to be by Amedeo Modigliani, is a fake.

modernist masterworks by Constantin Brancusi, Pablo Picasso, Joan Miró, Fernand Léger, Henri Matisse, Elie Nadelman, and an uneven array of other works.[22] Yet her enthusiasm for the new scarcely biased her against historical precedents. She was enthralled by the permutations of design, material, palette.

Naturally, she was particularly attracted to portraiture. The theater of the face was her daily occupation, and the evocation of personality her business. The countless variables of the genre never ceased to fascinate her, encouraged by a strong dose of self-promotion—she had her own portrait photographed and painted countless times. But crucially, her promotion of individualism was founded on the notion of difference, rather than on a single standard of beauty. In her business she claimed to read the face of each individual client in personal terms, and to teach the art of transforming one's appearance—painting one's own face as if creating a "cosmetic self-portrait" (see page 43). Her encouragement of difference was matched by a parallel compulsion to collect multiples. "Quality is nice," she liked to say, "but quantity makes a show."

She had an irrepressible impulse to assemble a potpourri of objects—mounds of pearls and emeralds, costume jewelry, luxurious fabrics, Venetian Rococo mirrors, or her celebrated collection of opaline glass (see pages 44 and 69). She had first discovered the thrilling diversity of the world during her youthful voyage by ship from Europe to Australia. From Genoa to Naples, Alexandria, Bombay, Calcutta, and Ceylon, the ship had called at colorful port markets teeming with treasures, wending its way to Perth, then Adelaide, and finally Melbourne. The exotic inclinations stimulated by this voyage paved the way for her attraction to non-Western art and her taste for abundance.

Still, the urge to accumulate was perhaps as much a consequence of her rootless and multicultural identity as it was an expression of her boundlessness, her urge toward inclusion, and the democratization of beauty. As the social historian Kathy Peiss has observed, "As a Jewish woman, she was especially perceptive about the varying beauty needs and skin types of women of different ethnic origins. Every woman, Madame observed, could 'make herself attractive along the lines of whatever is most characteristically herself.'"[23]

Persona

The beauty industry is based on the principle of self-invention. Madame, in consciously personifying this idea, made self-promotion a seamless part of her business. She never passed up an opportunity to have her face associated with her brand; any publicity was good. She was constantly interviewed and rarely ended a session without giving the reporter a packet of products or a ring from her jewelry-laden fingers (chosen in advance for

22 David Nash, who worked at the Parke-Bernet auction house in 1966, when Rubinstein's estate was sold, characterized her as more "acquisitive" than a connoisseur—an assessment that Madame would probably have considered fair; Nash, quoted in the 2007 documentary *The Powder and the Glory*, directed by Ann Carol Grossman and Arnie Reisman.

23 Peiss and Rubinstein, quoted in Suzanne Slesin, *Over the Top: Helena Rubinstein, Extraordinary Style, Beauty, Art, Fashion and Design* (New York: Pointed Leaf Press, 2006). Peiss is one of the few scholars to discuss Rubinstein's sensitivity toward difference.

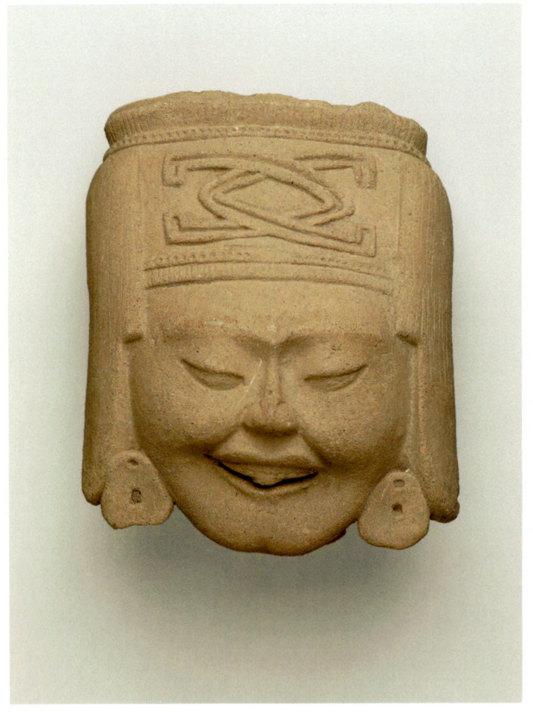

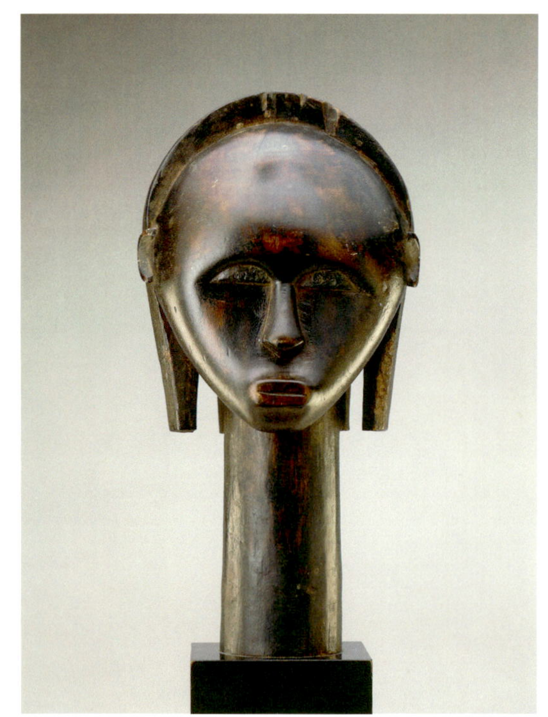

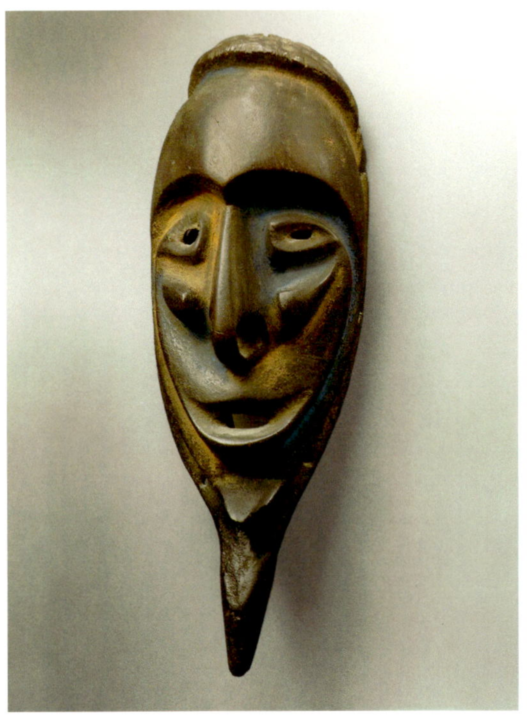

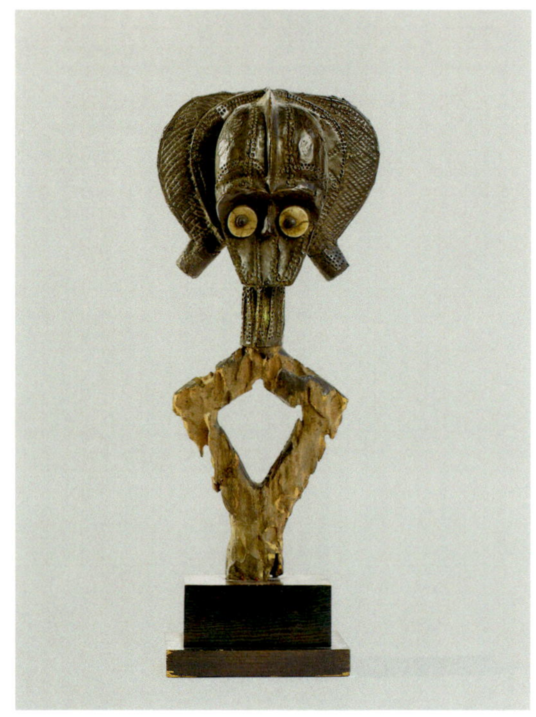

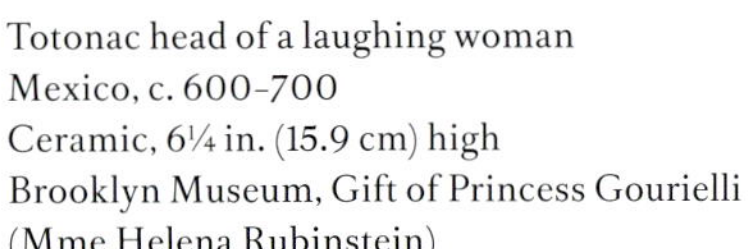

Totonac head of a laughing woman
Mexico, c. 600–700
Ceramic, 6¼ in. (15.9 cm) high
Brooklyn Museum, Gift of Princess Gourielli (Mme Helena Rubinstein)

Dance mask
Vanuatu, Vao or Rano Island, Malekula, Melanesia, nineteenth century
Wood with traces of pigment, 14½ in. (36.8 cm) high
Collection of Valerie Franklin, California

Fang head
Gabon, nineteenth or twentieth century
Wood, 12 in. (30.5 cm) high
Detroit Institute of Arts, Founders Society Purchase, Eleanor Clay Ford Fund for African Art and Mr. and Mrs. Walter Buhl Ford II Fund

Bakota reliquary guardian figure
Gabon, Makoku, date unknown
Wood and copper, 20½ in. (52.1 cm) high
The Arman Marital Trust, Corice Arman Trustee

Janus club (*U'u*)
Marquesas Islands, eighteenth or nineteenth century
Hardwood, 56¼ in. (142.9 cm) high
Collection of Valerie Franklin, California

Rubinstein's vast collections included works from West Africa, pre-Columbian Mexico, and the islands of Polynesia and Melanesia. She often chose sculptures and paintings of faces and masks—the subject of her life's work—and rejected any single, standardized notion of beauty.

Maori roof gable ornament (*Tekoteko*)
New Zealand, Polynesia, Arawa Tribe, eighteenth century
Wood, obsidian, pigment, 37 in. (94 cm) high
Collection of Valerie Franklin, California

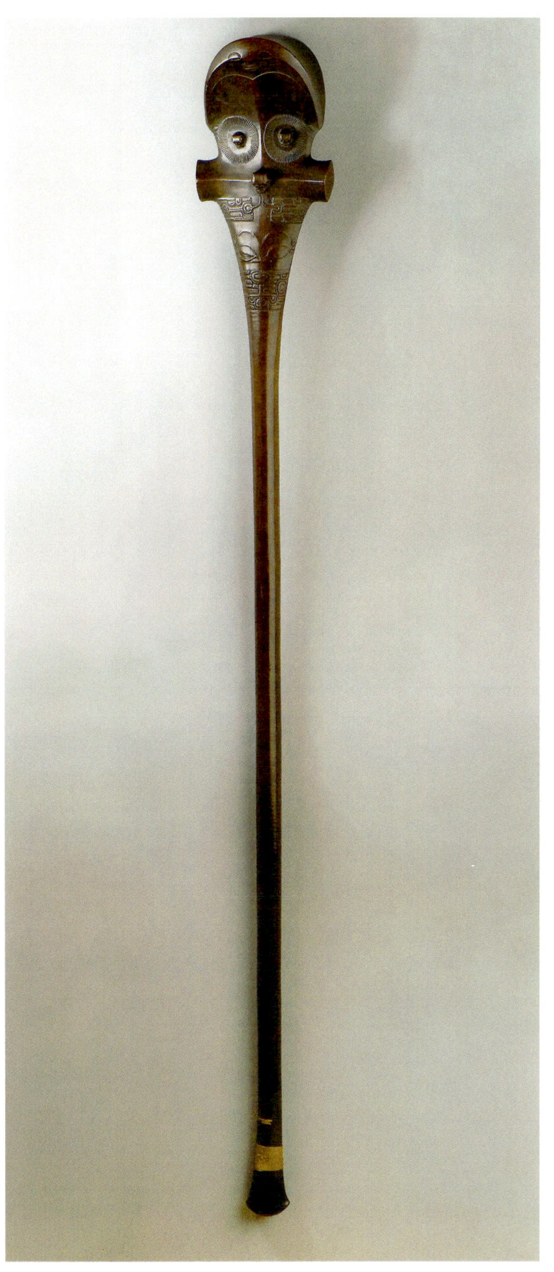

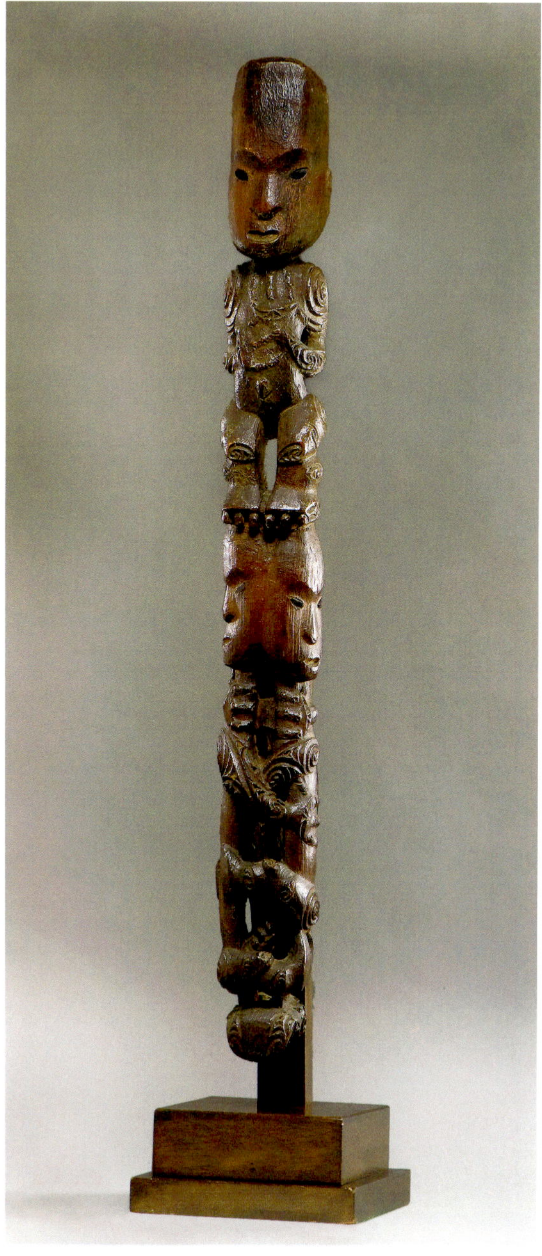

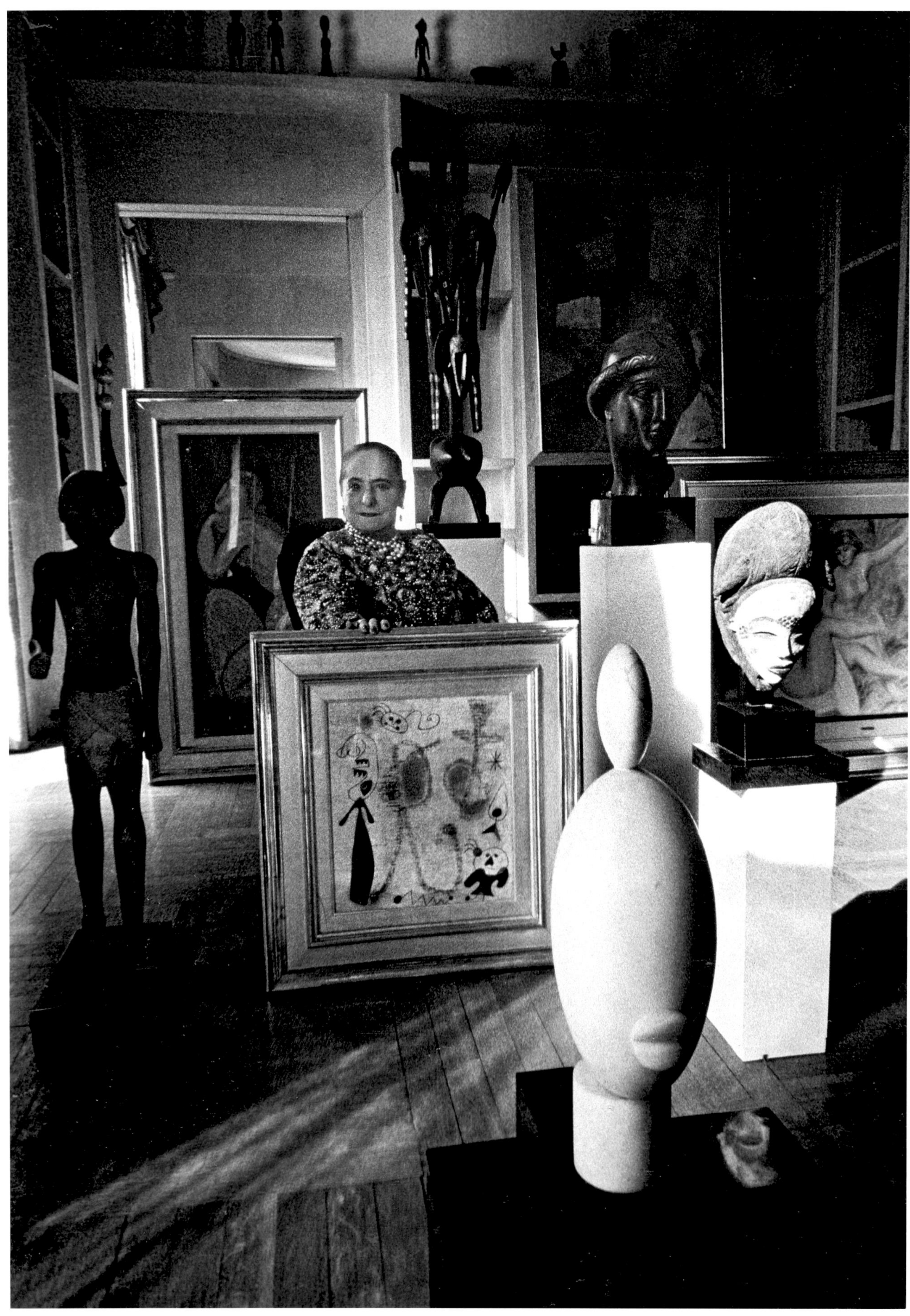

Helena Rubinstein in her Paris apartment, surrounded by works of Western and African art.

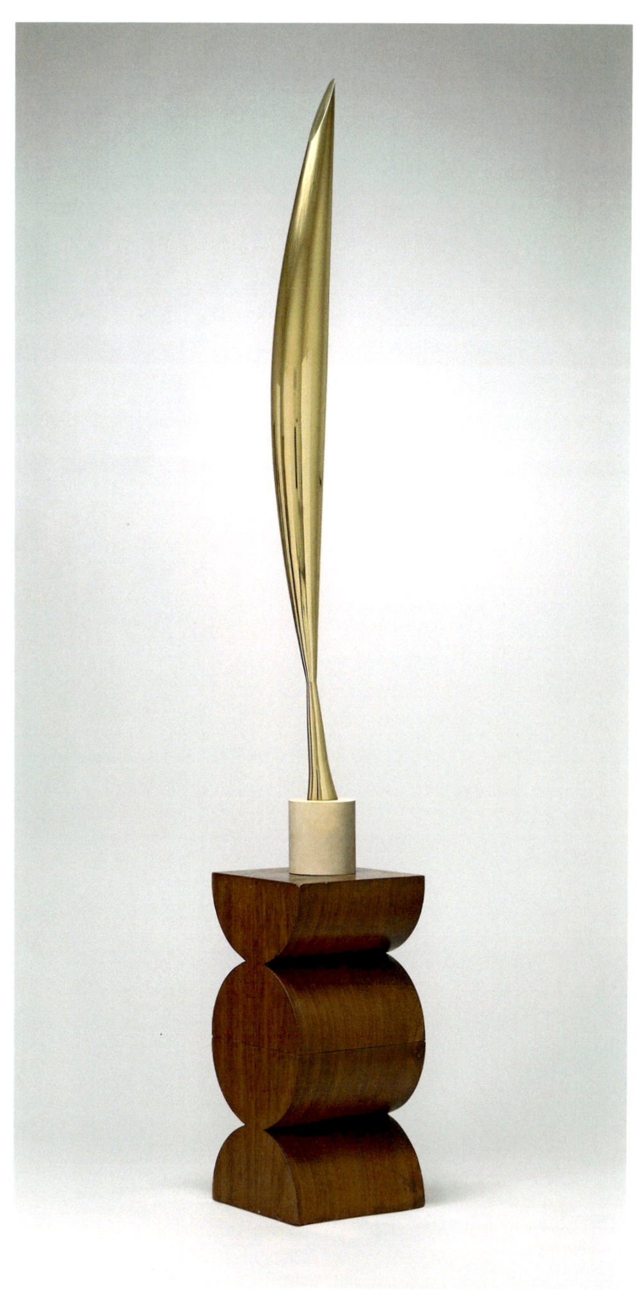

Constantin Brancusi
Bird in Space, 1927
Brass, cast stone, and wood, 113¼ in. (287.7 cm) high
National Gallery of Art, Washington, DC, given in loving memory of her husband, Taft Schreiber, by Rita Schreiber

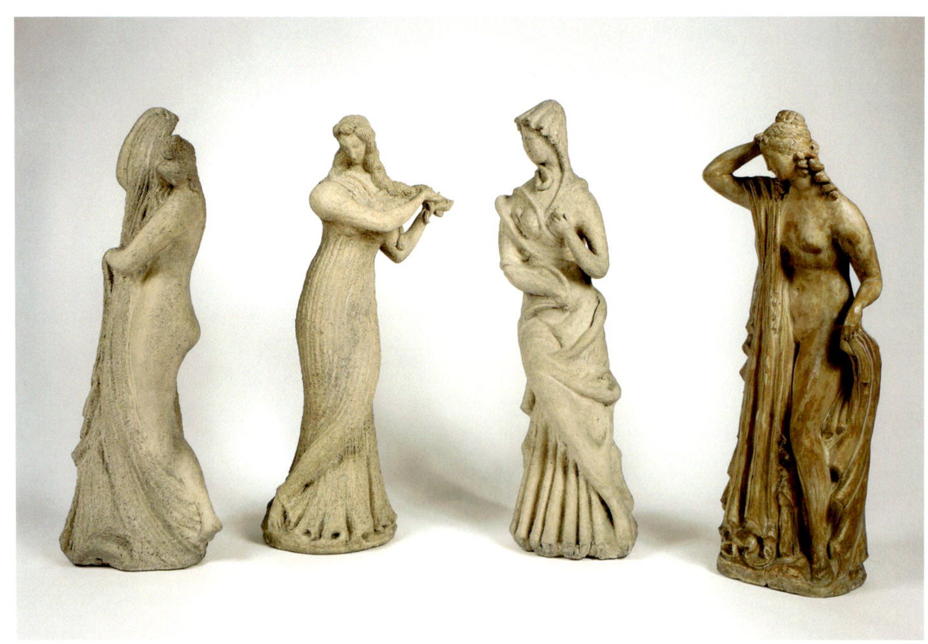

Elie Nadelman
The Four Seasons, c. 1912
Terracotta, each 31 in. (78.7 cm) high
New-York Historical Society

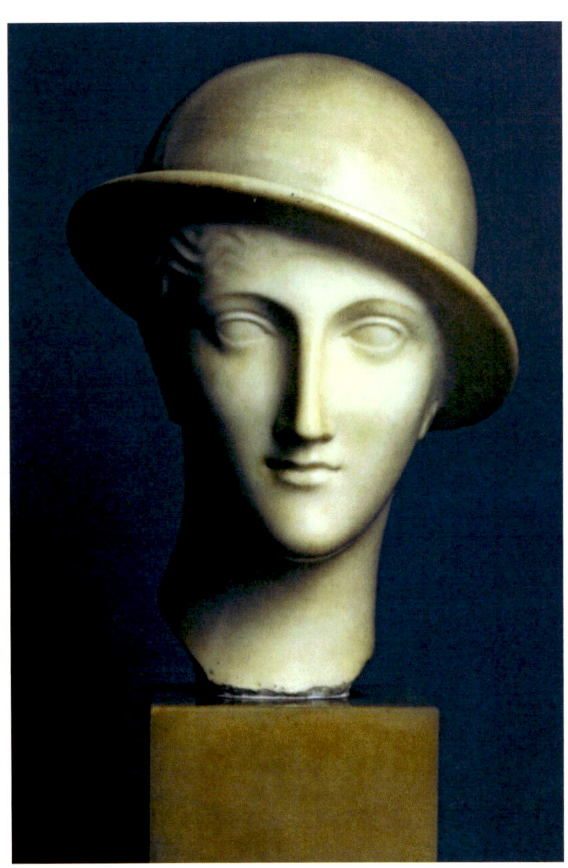

Elie Nadelman
Mercury Petassos I, c. 1914
Marble, 16 in. (40.6 cm) high
Mr. and Mrs. Robert and Diane Moss

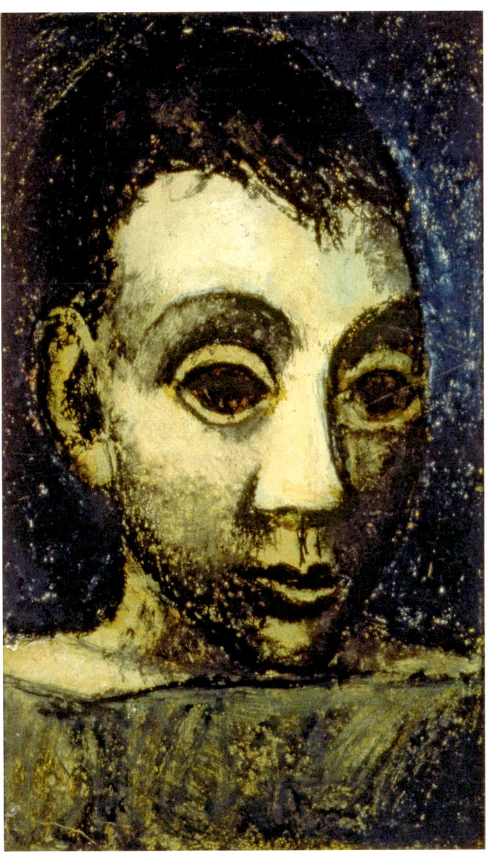

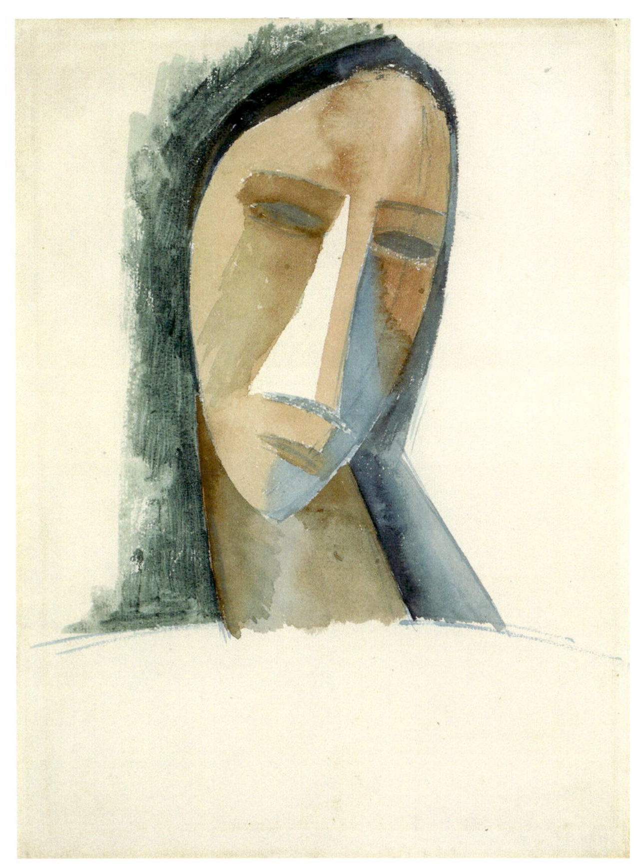

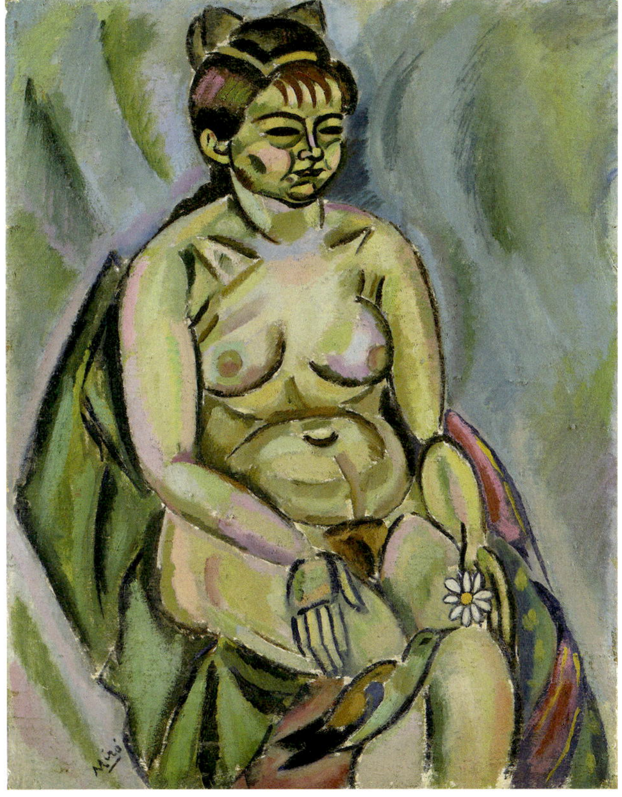

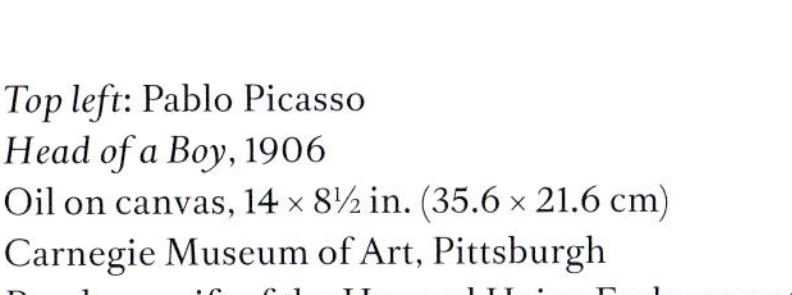

Top left: Pablo Picasso
Head of a Boy, 1906
Oil on canvas, 14 × 8½ in. (35.6 × 21.6 cm)
Carnegie Museum of Art, Pittsburgh
Purchase: gift of the Howard Heinz Endowment

Top right: Pablo Picasso
Head of a Woman, 1908
Watercolor on paper, 12½ × 9½ in. (31.8 × 24 cm)
Metropolitan Museum of Art, New York, Jacques and Natasha Gelman Collection, 1998

Bottom right: Joan Miró
Seated Nude Holding a Flower, 1917
Oil on canvas, 32 × 25¾ in. (81.3 × 65.4 cm)
Metropolitan Museum of Art, New York, Jacques and Natasha Gelman Collection, 1998

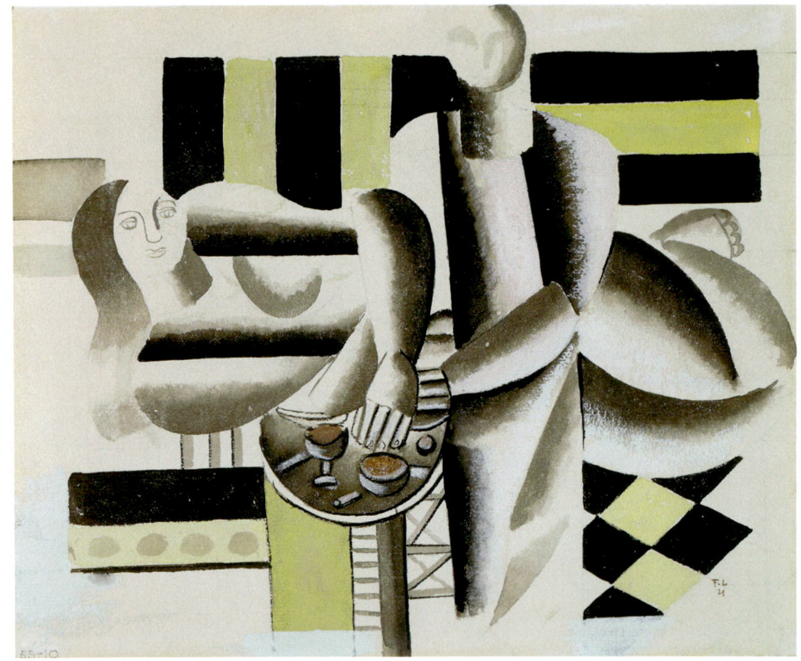

Fernand Léger
Interior, study for *The Three Women*, 1921
Watercolor on paper board
9⅞ × 12¼ in. (25.1 × 31.1 cm)
The Museum of Fine Arts, Houston,
Gift of Madame Helena Rubinstein

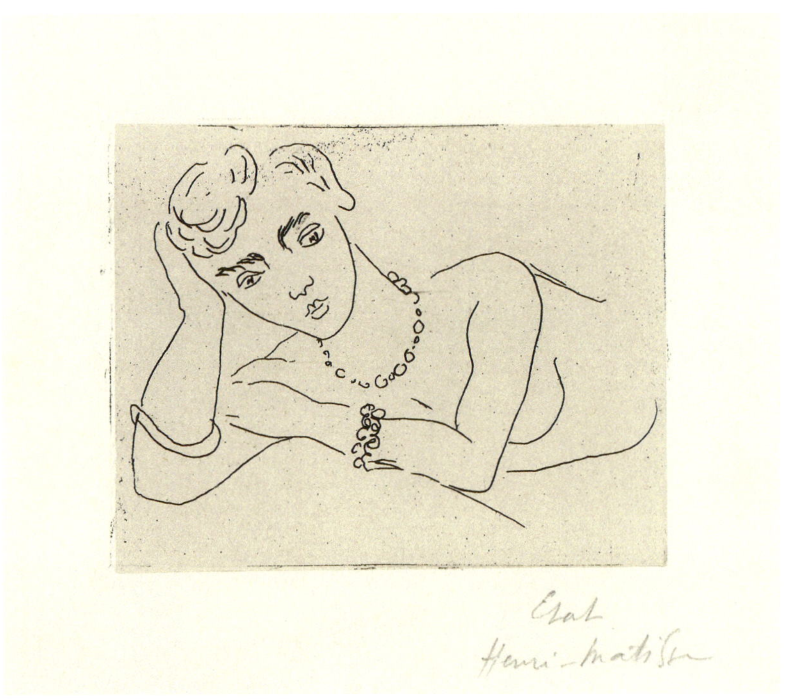

Henri Matisse
Reclining Nude, with Necklace, 1925
Etching on paper, 3⅝ × 4¾ in.
(9.2 × 12.1 cm)
The Museum of Modern Art, New York,
Stephen C. Clark Fund, 1951

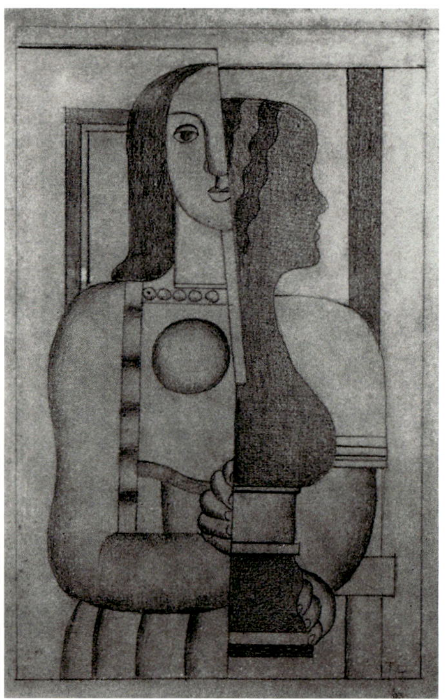

Fernand Léger
Woman, 1927
Pencil on paper, 10½ × 6¾ in. (26.7 × 17.2 cm)
Location unknown

Léger's distinctive adaptation of the visual language of Cubism is eloquently illustrated in this drawing. Here the very notion of style—whether hair, textile, clothing, or architecture—is seen as fluid within a woman's world of possibilities.

Joan Miró
Untitled, 1934
Gouache with chalk on black paper,
25⅝ × 19⅝ in. (65.1 × 49.9 cm)
Collection of Frances and Bernard Laterman

Joan Miró
Women, Birds, Stars, 1943
Gouache, watercolor, pastel,
and pencil on paper, 25½ × 19⅝ in.
(64.8 × 49.9 cm)
Location unknown

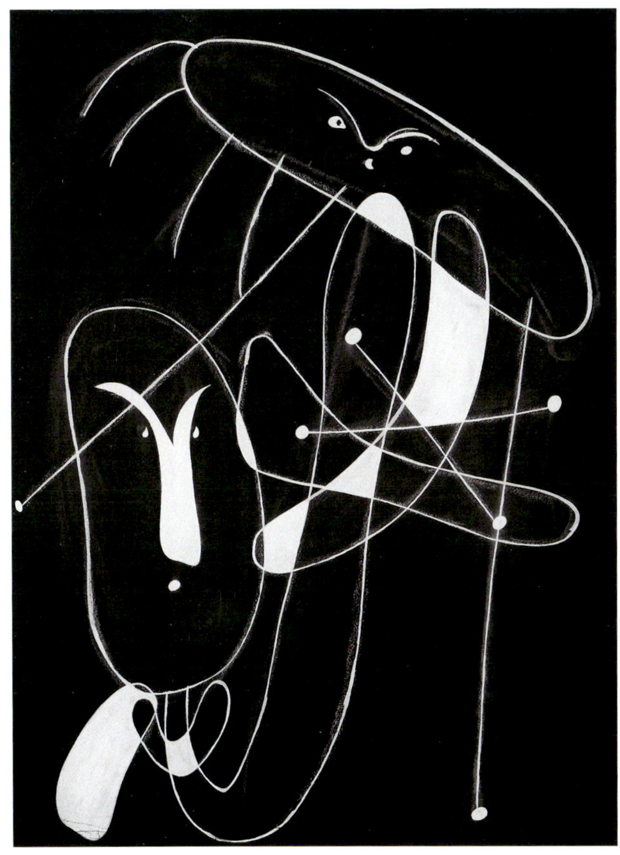

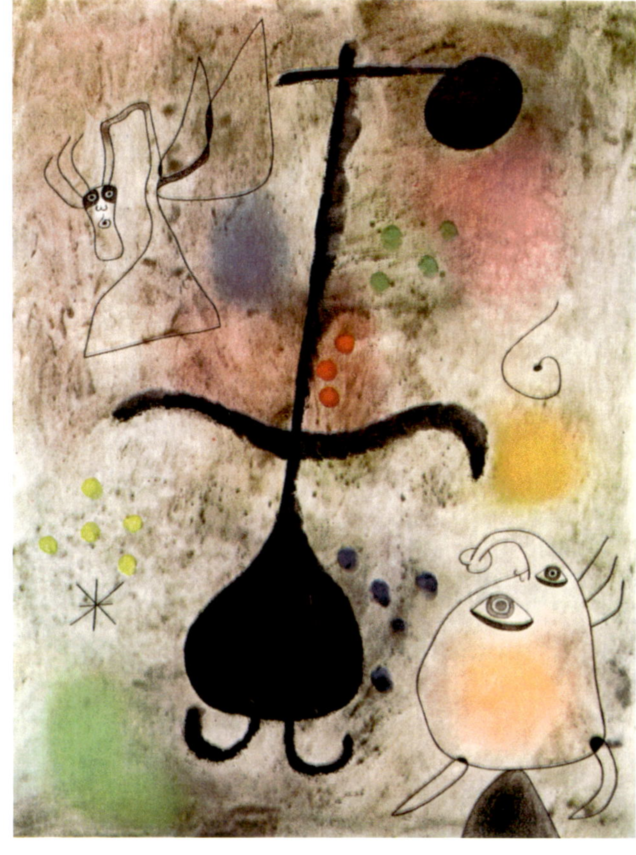

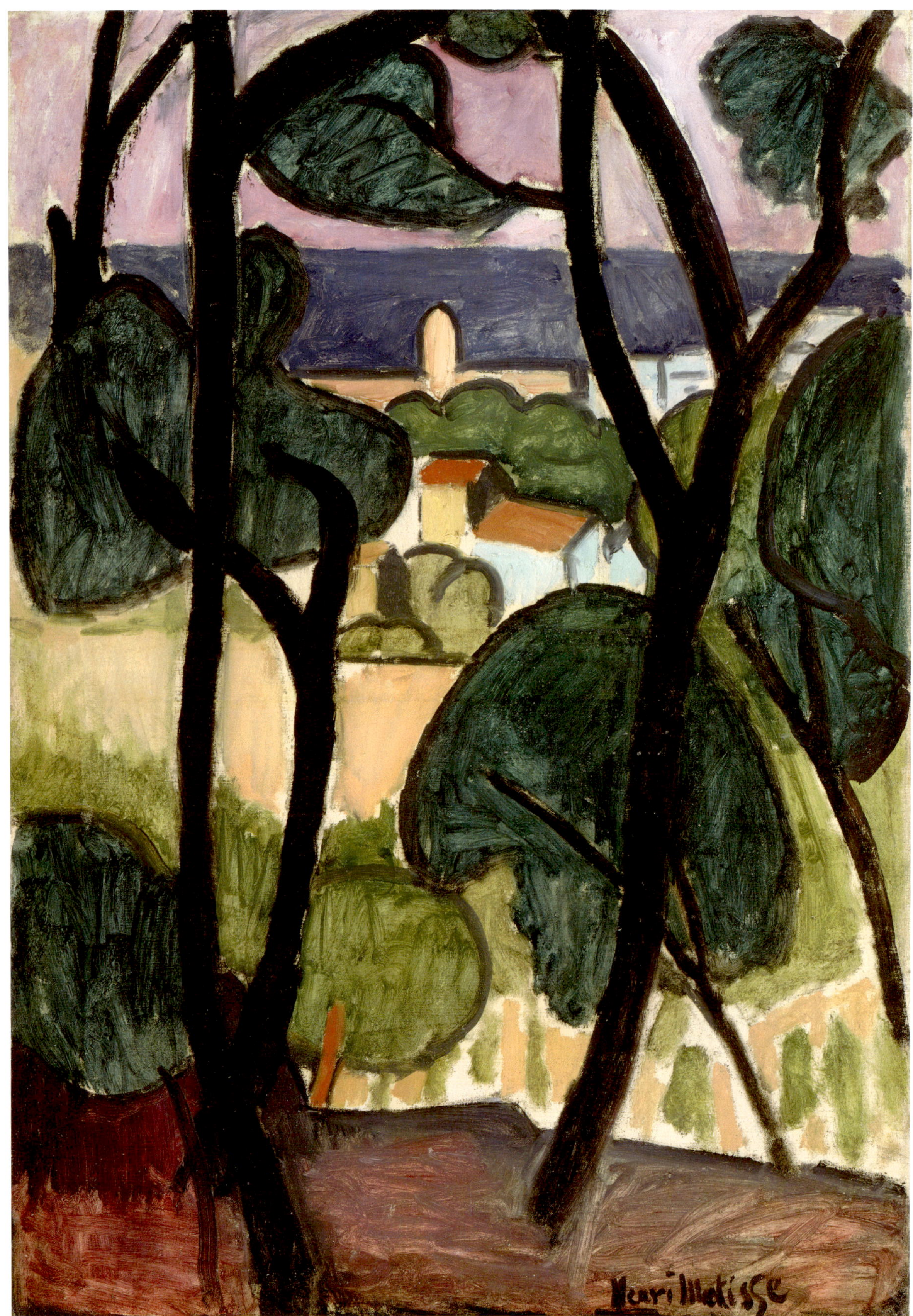

Henri Matisse
View of Collioure, 1907
Oil on canvas, 36¼ × 25⅞ in. (92.1 × 65.7 cm)
Metropolitan Museum of Art, New York,
Jacques and Natasha Gelman Collection, 1998

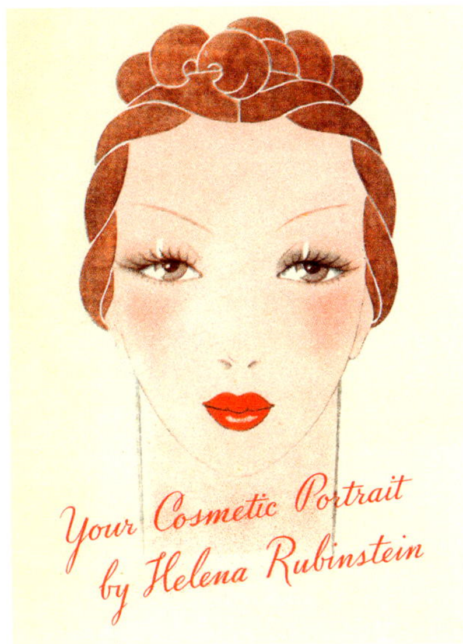

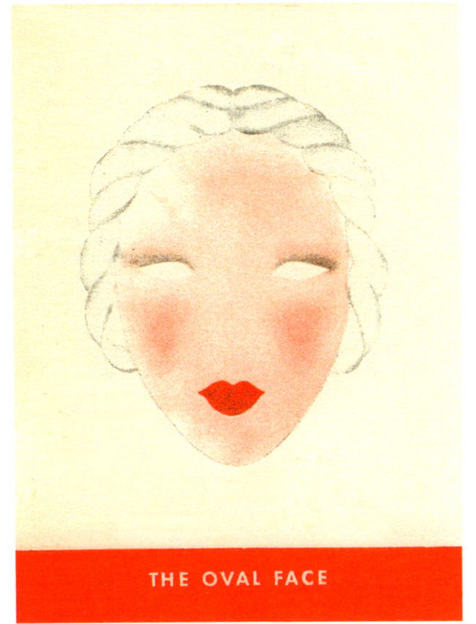

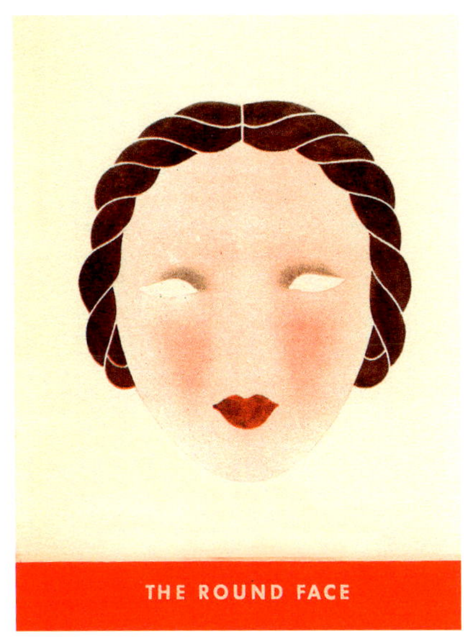

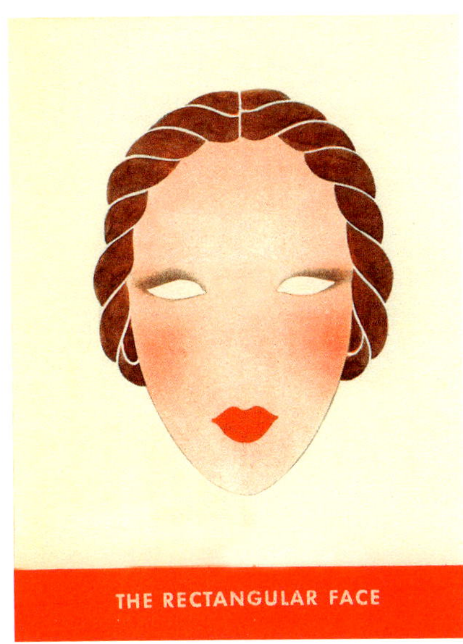

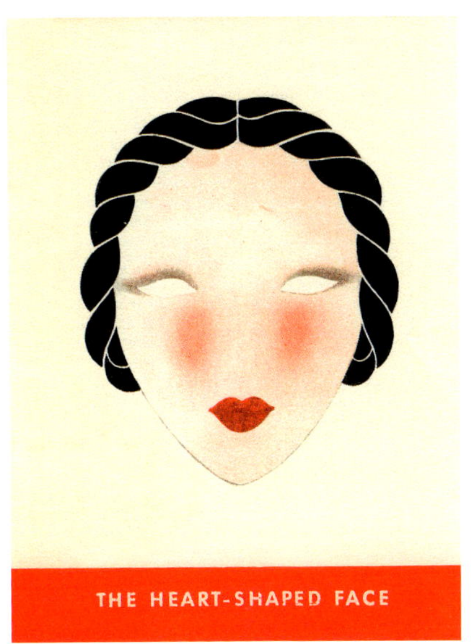

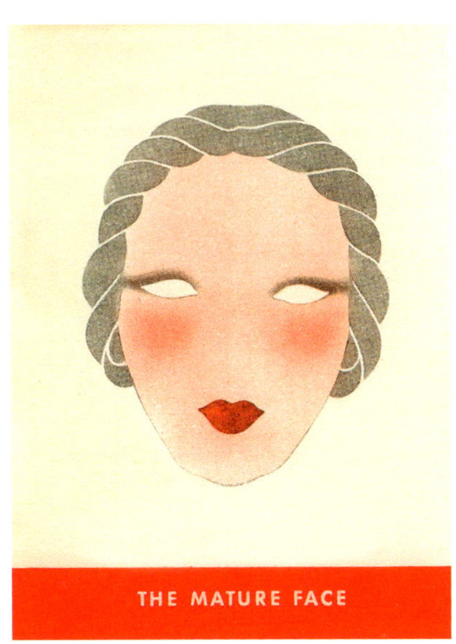

Your Cosmetic Portrait by Helena Rubinstein, booklet, 1935: the oval, round, rectangular, heart-shaped, and mature face.

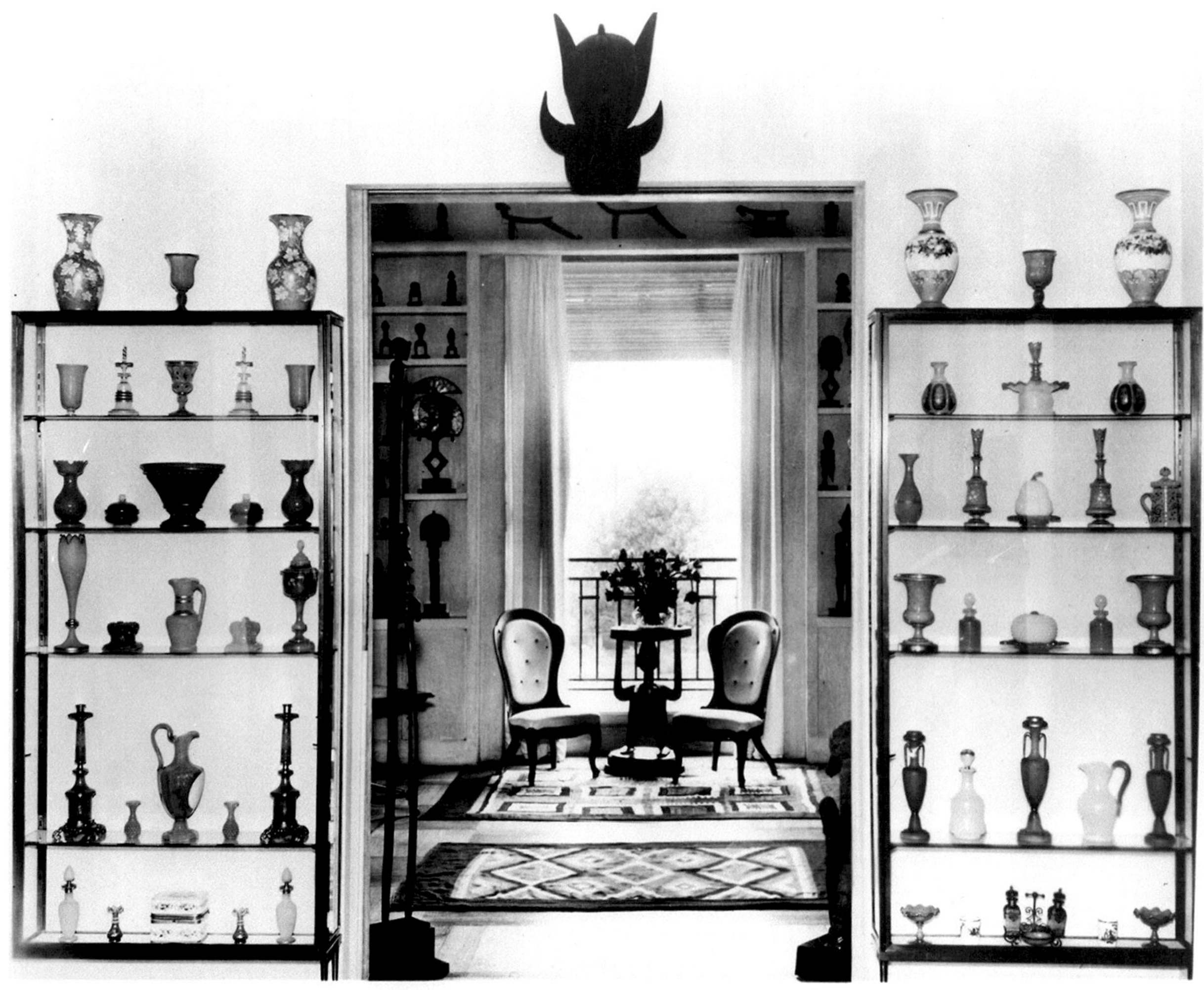

Rubinstein collected opaline glass, a type of nineteenth-century opaque or translucent glass known for its subtle variability. She was fascinated by its luster and by its myriad forms and colors. Her apartment on the Ile St.-Louis in Paris displayed shelves of glass in one room and African art in the next.

A Lesson in Loveliness

By Helena Rubinstein

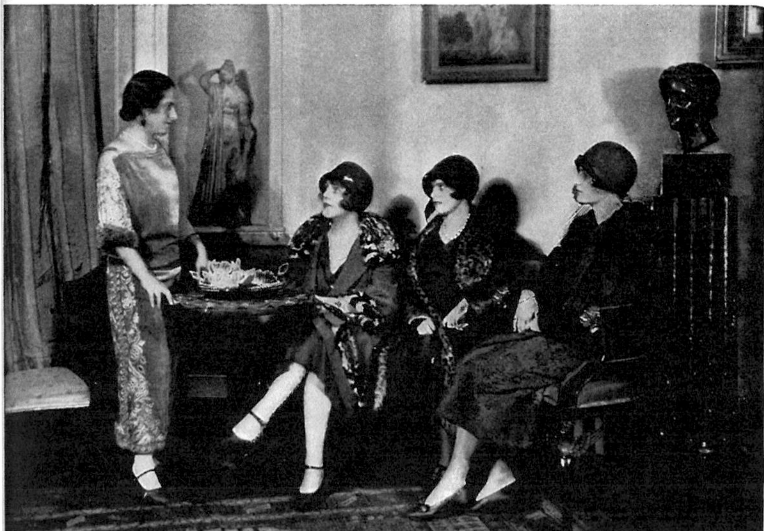

Three socially prominent members of New York's younger set—Mrs. Austin Sherman, Jr., Miss Blanche Strebeigh and Miss Mary Smedberg in consultation with Madame Helena Rubinstein, world renowned Beauty Specialist.

—beauty is such a fragile thing. When I look on a young skin, so exquisitely fresh, so delicately transparent, with the wonderful elasticity that is Youth, I am always impelled to warn its possessor against two great enemies—Neglect and Improper Treatment.

I have travelled all over the world and I consider that among you American women there is a higher percentage of Beauty than anywhere else. But the tragedy of it is you are so negligent of your precious possession. Either you let *unaided* Nature take its course, or you use creams and lotions with little or no thought as to their intrinsic worth or their suitability to your particular quality of skin.

Every day, women young and old, come to me with the heart-breaking evidence of Neglect or Improper Treatment . . . Coarsened Pores, Blackheads . . . Crowsfeet, Lines, Wrinkles . . . Sagging Muscles, Double Chin.

And I have invariably found that the ones with Coarsened Pores and Blackheads have depended upon soap and water alone, or upon heavy, clogging creams, expecting them to do for their skins, what only the most active preparations can do. And in nine cases out of ten, these skins, in a drastic effort to become fine-grained, show ugly little red lines . . . broken veins resulting from the use of ice instead of a gentle astringent.

But why will so many, many women with dry, sensitive skins, deliberately pave the way for lines and wrinkles by adhering to a strict soap-and-water regime, or the use of drying creams and lotions? Perhaps it is because they do not realize the harshening effects of soap and water alone, and it never occurs to them that any cream could possibly be drying in its effect. The crying need of the dry, sensitive skin is for *proper* stimulation, to be followed by rich nourishing creams, bracing balsams and soothing lotions.

Then there are the Flabby Faces, Puffy Eyes and Pendulous Chins, sometimes on quite young people too, and all too often the result of Improper Treatment. A passive preparation *rubbed* upon the surface of Drooping Cheeks or chin, simply stretches the skin and accentuates the droop, but when stimulating, firming, molding preparations are *manipulated* into the underlying tissues and muscles, the unlovely droops and puckers are on the road to complete disappearance.

Let me warn you, my dear young beauty-seekers that it is a wise woman who "knows her own complexion," knows when and how to properly cleanse it, stimulate it, nourish, brace and protect it; *knows that she cannot expect an indiscriminately chosen cream or two to gain or regain for her that most precious of possessions—Beauty.*

For a *certain* knowledge of her skin and its varying needs, for that priceless advice on the attainment or the preservation of Beauty the wise woman comes to her Beauty Specialist, whom she chooses not haphazardly, but because, by her record of past achievements, the Beauty Specialist has proven to the world her right to speak and her right to administer.

An Invitation

Mme. Rubinstein invites you to visit the Salon de Beaute Valaze nearest you, where you will receive, without charge, individual study and expert advice from Mme. Rubinstein herself or from one of her trained assistants.

If however, it is inconvenient for you to visit any of the Salons de Beaute Valaze, write to Mme. Rubinstein at her New York Salon, 46 West 57th Street, and tell her about your problem. She will advise you without charge.

Send for edition H "Secrets of Beauty."

The Valaze

Beauty Preparations

created by

Helena Rubinstein

World-renowned Beauty Specialist

The Valaze Beauty Preparations are highly specialized so as to include the proper treatment for every skin during all the seasons of the year. For over a quarter of a century the Valaze Beauty Preparations have been given the preference by sophisticated and highly discriminating women all over the world.

The Average Skin

Valaze Cleansing and Massage Cream—cleanses the skin quickly, easily, delightfully. **$1.25, $2.50**

Valaze Beauty Grains—the penetrative soap substitute which removes blackheads and other impurities and refines the skin texture. **$1.00, $2.00**

Valaze Beautifying Skinfood (clear-skin cream)—clears, purifies, whitens; removes tan, sallowness and other discolorations. **$1.00, $2.50**

Valaze Refining Lotion—a remarkable preparation for refining the texture of the skin and eliminating broken veins. **$3.00, $5.00, $10.00**

The Oily Skin

Valaze Blackhead and Open Pore Paste—washes the skin free of blackheads and other impurities; refines the skin texture; closes the pores. **$1.00, $2.00**

Valaze Liquidine—beautifying astringent lotion which removes oiliness and "shine." **$1.50, $2.75**

The Dry, Sensitive Skin

Valaze Grecian Anti-wrinkle Cream (Anthosoros)—richly nourishes thin, dry, wrinkled faces and throats. Prevents and removes crowsfeet; pads out hollows. **$1.75, $3.50**

Valaze Herbal Cream—compounded of rare herbs, marvelously soothing to fine, sensitive skins. **$5.00, $10.00**

Valaze Extrait—exquisite anti-wrinkle lotion for thin, dry, sensitive skins. Erases crowsfeet and other lines. **$2.50, $5.00**

Valaze Protective Preparations

Valaze Sun and Windproof Balm—neutralizes the effects of the violet rays of the sun which cause sunburn, tan and freckles. A most becoming powder foundation. **$1.00, $1.75**

Valaze Sun and Windproof Cream—possesses all the efficacious qualities of the Balm, but to a greater degree, and is used for extreme exposure. **$1.00, $2.00**

Famous Valaze Rejuvenators

Valaze Eau Verte—instantaneously rejuvenating stimulant for sluggish, faded dry skin. **$3.00, $6.00**

Valaze Eau Qui Pique—instantaneously rejuvenating stimulant for sluggish oily skin. **$3.00, $6.00**

Valaze Georgine Lactee—the marvelous youthifying muscle and tissue tightener which overcomes double chin, puffy eyes and drooping cheeks without drying the skin. **$3.00, $6.00**

The Valaze Cosmetics

—not only emphasize beauty but safeguard it. They are irreproachable in quality and so marvelously blended as to harmonize perfectly with one's natural coloring.

Valaze Beauty preparations obtainable at all smart shops.

Visit the Salon de Beaute Valaze nearest you. One Valaze Beauty Lesson Treatment will prove a revelation to you!

NEW YORK - - 46 West 57th Street
CHICAGO - 30 North Michigan Avenue
BOSTON - - - 234 Boylston Street
DETROIT - - 1540 Washington Blvd.
NEWARK - - - - 951 Broad Street
LONDON 24 Grafton Street, Piccadilly
PARIS 126 Rue du Faubourg St. Honore

"A Lesson in Loveliness, by Helena Rubinstein," advertisement in the form of an editorial, *Harper's Bazaar*, June 1925.

the purpose). She deployed her persona to maximum effect, especially through photography. The staging and controlling of celebrity photography was a new technique in Rubinstein's lifetime, and she contributed a good deal to its refinement. Thus, as she was well aware, her identity was largely constructed.

After World War II the cultural climate changed. In using her persona as the primary vehicle of her firm's promotions, Rubinstein had always been able to anticipate and adapt, but she had never made full use of broadcasting. She had a strong Eastern European accent, ill-suited to radio, and was even more uncomfortable with television, a medium geared to youth and difficult to control. With the resurgence of the American economy, the beauty industry expanded into mass retail, and Charles Revson, Estée Lauder, and others joined its ranks. The restrained advertising of Arden and Rubinstein's generation was overtaken by a more eroticized style, and their luxurious, time-consuming salon treatments began to appear quaint to a busy postwar clientele. The Revlon brand in particular invested heavily in advertising and made broad use of the explosive popularity of magazines, radio, and television. Its full-color photographs in magazines and stores across the country were noted for their provocative and extravagant tone. Indeed, after the war, the newcomers to the beauty industry began to appeal more convincingly to men and women whose daily reality was sitting at a desk by marketing a consumable style that played on the desire to fulfill fantasies through the construction of a self-image.[24] The fame and glamour of figures such as Rubinstein and Arden began to yield to this revolution in media and an increasing focus on youth. A person as baroque as Madame began to seem a bit passé.

Nevertheless, when Helena Rubinstein died in 1965, age 92, she was still in sole command of her global cosmetics empire and still very much a force in the world of fashion, style, and image. By the time of her death she had salons in cities worldwide and homes in London, Paris, New York, the south of France, and Greenwich, Connecticut, all but the last functioning as showcases for her decorative fantasies, replete with swelling and rotating collections. She had influenced generations of women, not only in terms of self-image, but also as a role model of individuality.

In her memoir, *My Life for Beauty*, written the year before she died, Rubinstein edited her past as creatively as she had lived it. As her son, Roy Titus, wryly noted, "The story of her life was secondary to her. She never talked about herself."[25] Her life had traversed nearly a century, from 1872 to 1965, an age of belief in modernity and in the power of the image.

Throughout her career Rubinstein recorded her image constantly—in photographs and in portraits commissioned from dozens of painters—fulfilling a perennial desire to be seen, to have her presence in the world noted (see page 32). Aging mattered little: she simply used photo retouching to retrace the outlines of her face or silhouette (see page 51). In middle age she brought her own staff photographer when she attended events and approved pictures for circulation.

A Family Photograph

Madame was famously unforthcoming with details of her early life, and few photographs exist from her years in Poland. She was the eldest surviving child of twelve siblings, four of whom died early; the remaining eight were all girls. One may conjecture that in a family that had lost all the male children, it fell upon Helena to take up the mantle and become

24 For the standard analysis of American style and culture, see Stuart Ewen, *All Consuming Images: The Politics of Style in Contemporary Culture*, rev. ed. (New York: Basic Books, 1988). Ewen notes that style "was understood as a tool for constructing personhood. Style was a way of saying who one was or who one wished to be. The emerging market [in the twentieth century] in stylized goods provided consumers with a vast palette of symbolic meanings, to be selected and juxtaposed in the assembling of a public self," 79.

25 Roy Titus, introduction, Rubinstein, *My Life for Beauty*, 7.

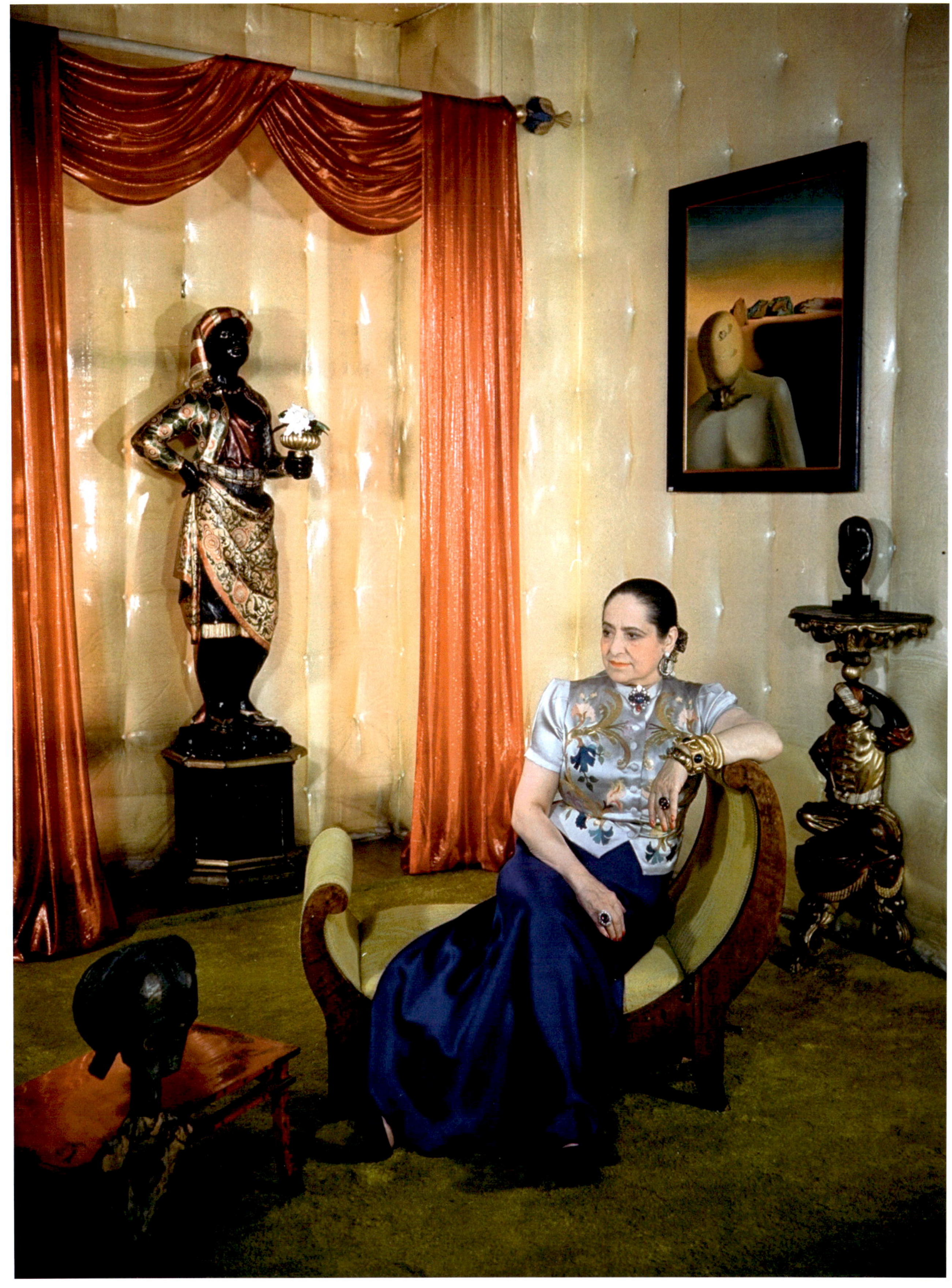

Rubinstein on an Empire loveseat in her apartment at 895 Park Avenue, 1941. Salvador Dalí's *The Average Bureaucrat*, 1930, hangs on the quilted cellophane wall; nearby, a gilt eighteenth-century Venetian console table with the figure of a seated Moor bears a Fang sculpture. In a niche is another Moor. In the foreground stands a Bakota reliquary head. The photograph is from a *Life* magazine feature article on Rubinstein, displaying her eclectic taste.

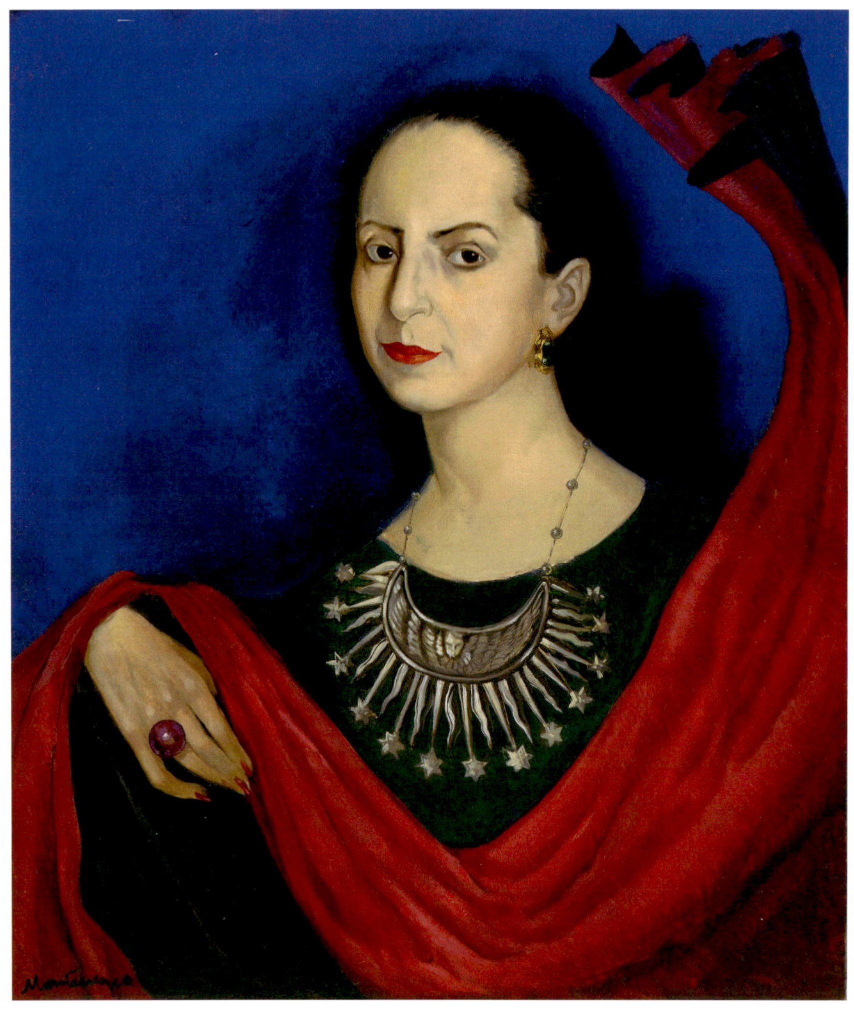

Roberto Montenegro
Helena Rubinstein in a Mexican Silver Necklace, 1941
Oil on canvas, 31½ × 28 in. (80 × 71.1 cm)
National Portrait Gallery, Smithsonian Institution, Washington, DC

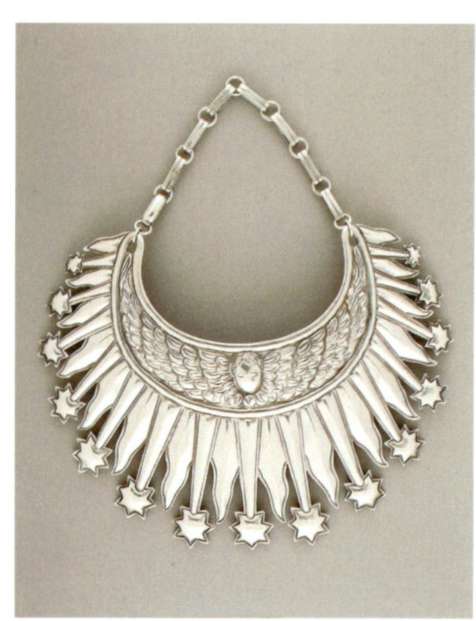

William Spratling
Helena Rubinstein Necklace, c. 1940
Silver, pectoral: 7 × 9 in. (17.8 × 22.9 cm), chain: 8 in. (20.3 cm) long.
Los Angeles County Museum of Art, Gift of the Goddard Family in Memory of Phyllis Goddard

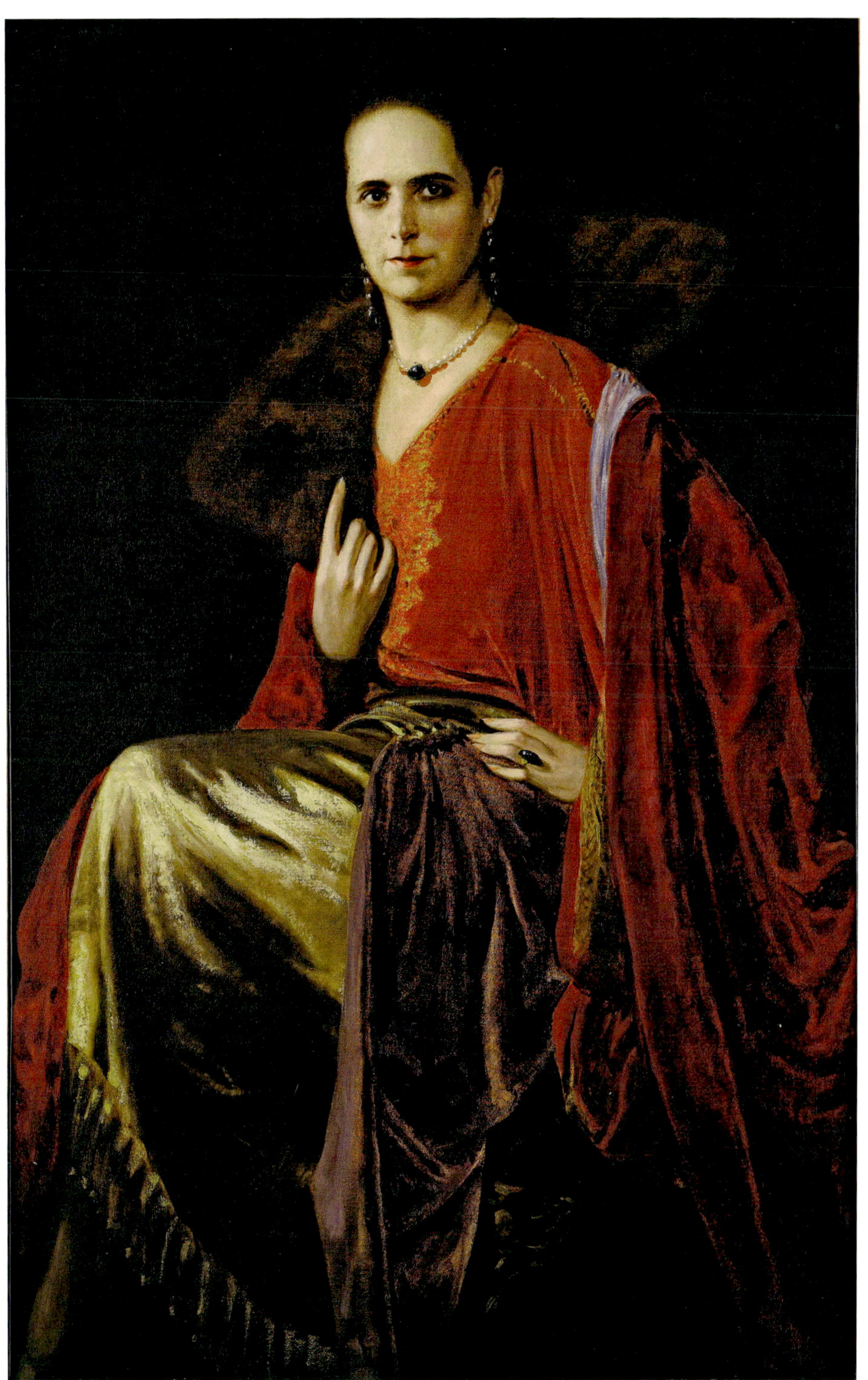

George Maillard Kesslere
Portrait of Helena Rubinstein, 1926
Oil on canvas, 54¼ × 35¼ in. (137.8 × 89.5 cm)
Private collection

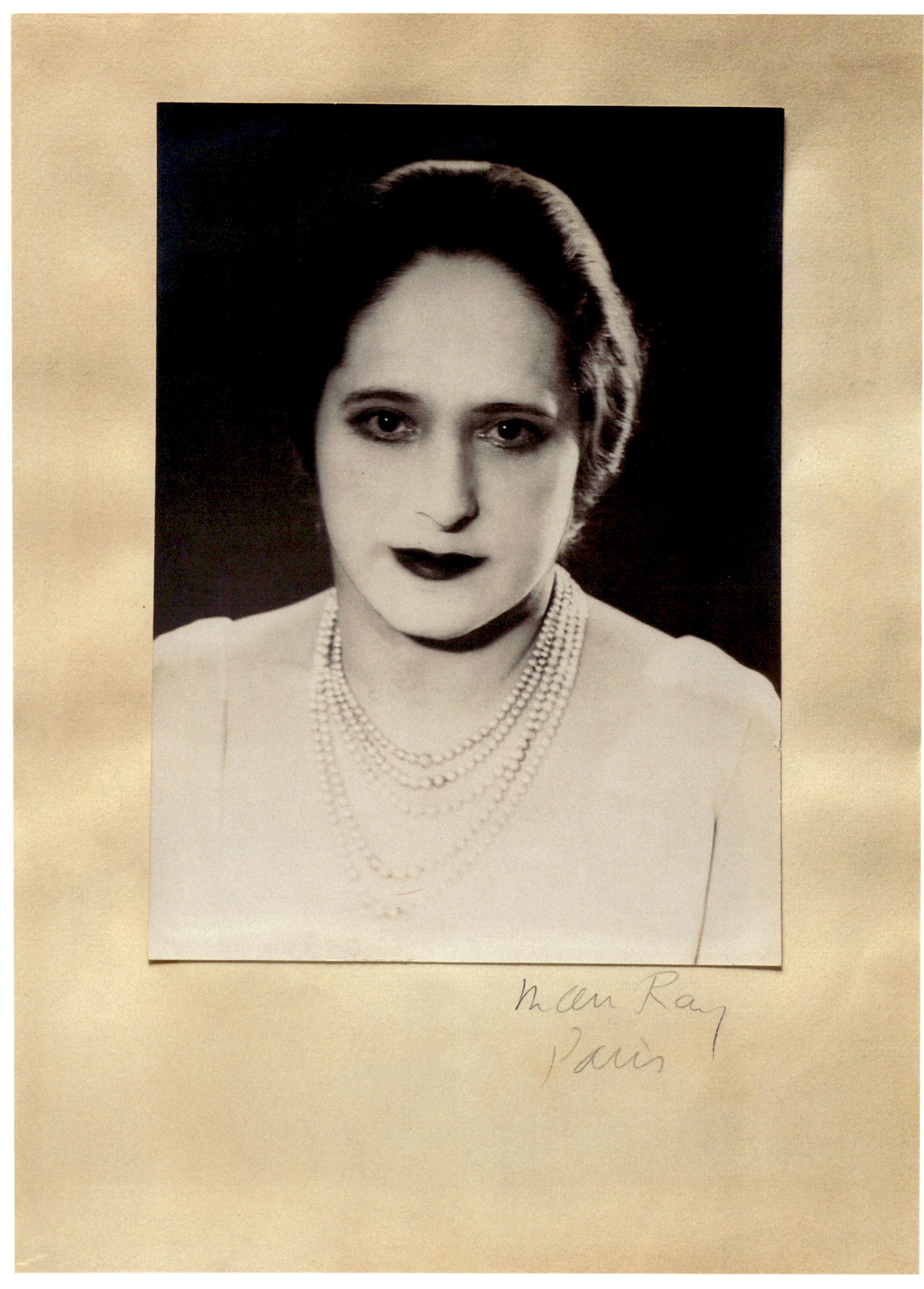

Man Ray
Helena Rubinstein, c. 1924
Gelatin silver print
Private collection, New York

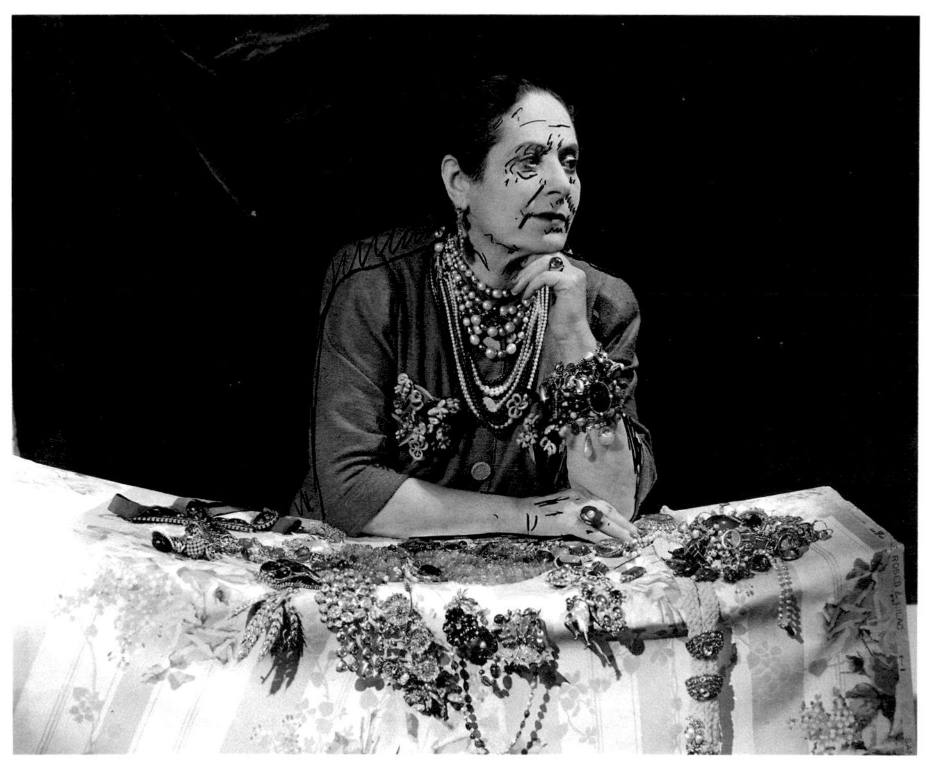

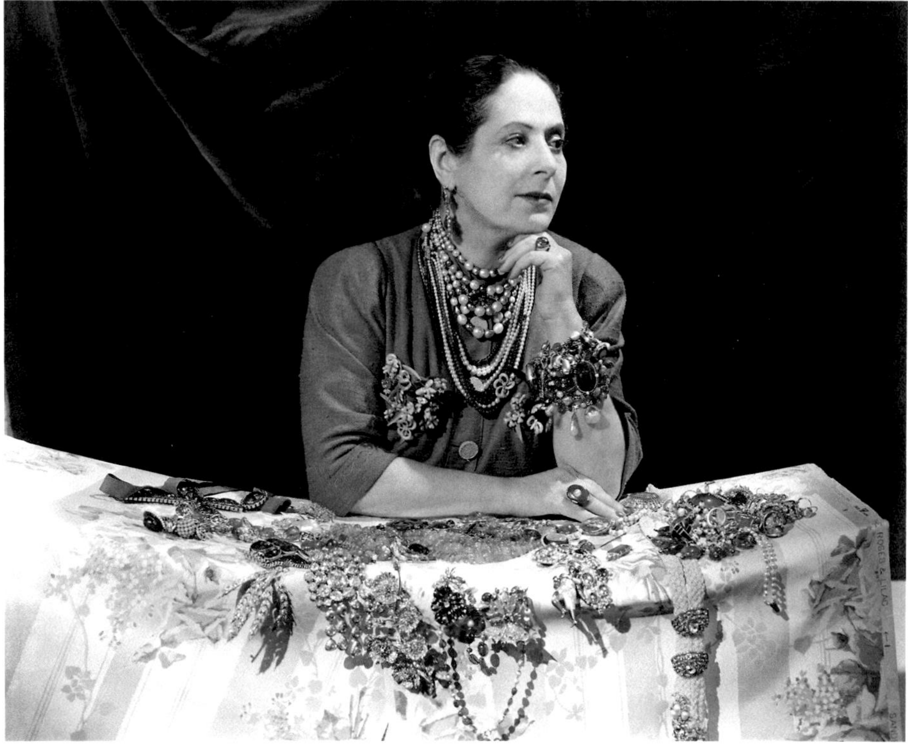

Around 1932 Cecil Beaton photographed Rubinstein for *Vanity Fair*, wearing a Schiaparelli suit with cork buttons and pockets embroidered with glass flowers. Rubinstein controlled her image with care, and such photographs were often retouched. *Above*: Markup for retouching. *Below*: The final photograph.

a de facto son.[26] A rare family picture from about 1888 reveals her natural affinity for the camera. Nineteenth-century photographic portraits are rarely interpreted like paintings: they are not considered subjective depictions so much as a mechanical record, documentation of some truth. But it is difficult not to see in young Helena's pose and mien the spirited rebellion with which, soon after this, she rejected a marriage with an older man, arranged by her father. Such disobedience was intolerable in an Orthodox Jewish family in nineteenth-century Krakow; Helena was banished from home and sent to live with a maternal aunt, Rosalie Silberfeld Beckman.[27]

Whatever motives one might attribute to her subsequent quest for autonomy and her ceaseless drive to succeed, in this photograph Helena exudes a self-assurance that invites scrutiny. Standing at center, she dominates the group, clearly aware of her own beauty and presence—although she was a mere 4 feet, 10 inches tall. While her sisters wear provincial ruffled frocks with high Victorian collars, Helena's dark dress is sophisticated and adult, with a mannish white collar and a fitted bodice that accentuates her figure. Her younger siblings wear their hair down, but hers is up, like her mother's. Already she has flair and a sense of style—promising signs of the independence of a young woman who owns her femininity, her identity.

The photograph speaks to us, yet its message can only be oblique. "Photography's program of realism," Susan Sontag has written, "implies . . . the belief that reality is hidden. And being hidden, is something to be unveiled."[28] As such, the image invites us to conjecture as to its potential multiple meanings, as if they were masked—surely an apt metaphor for cosmetics.

Unorthodox

Little is known of Helena's life in the eight years between her leaving home to live with her aunt and her sailing to Australia in the summer of 1896.[29] In some accounts she considered studying medicine or nursing. However she occupied those years, she eventually found that life in Krakow offered few prospects. By the time of her departure for Australia, she had moved to Vienna to live with another aunt, Helena Silberfeld, whose husband was a furrier. The family fur business introduced her to the world of retail, and she acquired some basic business skills. Vienna was also a center for the study of dermatology at the time; perhaps her interest in skin care was kindled then.[30]

Naive and socially inexperienced as she may have been on her arrival, her time in Vienna—probably two to three years—surely inspired her. At the turn of the twentieth century it was a city where beauty, art, and fashion aggrandized a particular kind of quasi-feminist liberalism, not politically, in terms of women's rights, but in a modernist utopian sense. That is, challenges to gender roles, to class divisions, and to traditional taste were common.[31] While Rubinstein would not have taken part in the cultural vanguard, she was exposed to the city's unusual mixture of provincialism and cosmopolitanism. Within fin-de-siècle Vienna an eruptive modernism and nascent feminism were manifest in the most divergent and contradictory ways, from the discoveries of Sigmund Freud to the paintings of Gustav Klimt. It was the new, modern woman who was poised as a central figure within culture.

Viennese women were known throughout Europe for their stylishness, but were also among the first to embrace clothing reform, rejecting

26 In her memoir, Rubinstein refers to just one brother who died in infancy. According to Woodhead, Gusta gave birth to twelve children, only eight of whom survived; two were boys, Aaron and Abraham, who both died young; see Rubinstein, *My Life for Beauty*, 13; Woodhead, *War Paint*, 30.

27 The arranged marriage may have been an effort to thwart her romance with a non-Jewish medical student. Rubinstein virtually avoids discussion of this in her memoir, simply saying, "Father was furious!" Rubinstein, *My Life for Beauty*, 18. Interestingly, the archive of the Helena Rubinstein Foundation in the Special Collections at the Fashion Institute of Technology Library, State University of New York, includes no photographs of Helena's father, apart from one early photograph of her parents together.

28 Susan Sontag, *On Photography* (New York: Farrar, Straus and Giroux, 1977), 107–8.

29 Rubinstein often altered dates. According to her memoir, *My Life for Beauty*, she arrived in Australia at age 18 in 1888. Woodhead clarifies the various departure dates; see *War Paint*, 33; also see Slesin, *Over the Top*, 212.

30 Woodhead, *War Paint*, 35.

31 On Vienna, see Carl E. Schorske, *Fin-de-Siècle Vienna: Politics and Culture* (New York: Vintage, 1980).

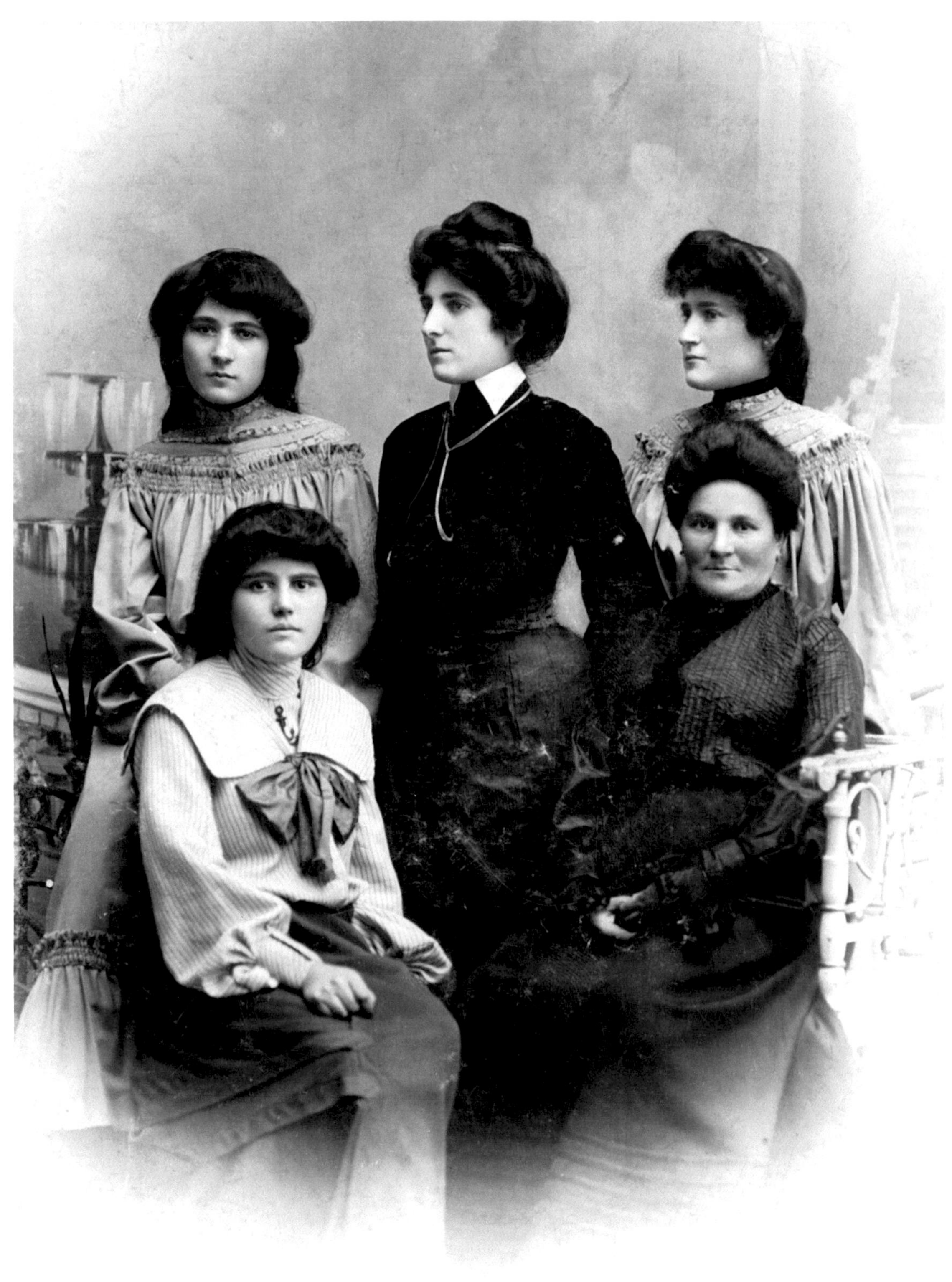

Helena, at center, with her mother, Augusta, seated at right, and three of her seven sisters. She is probably about seventeen or eighteen here.

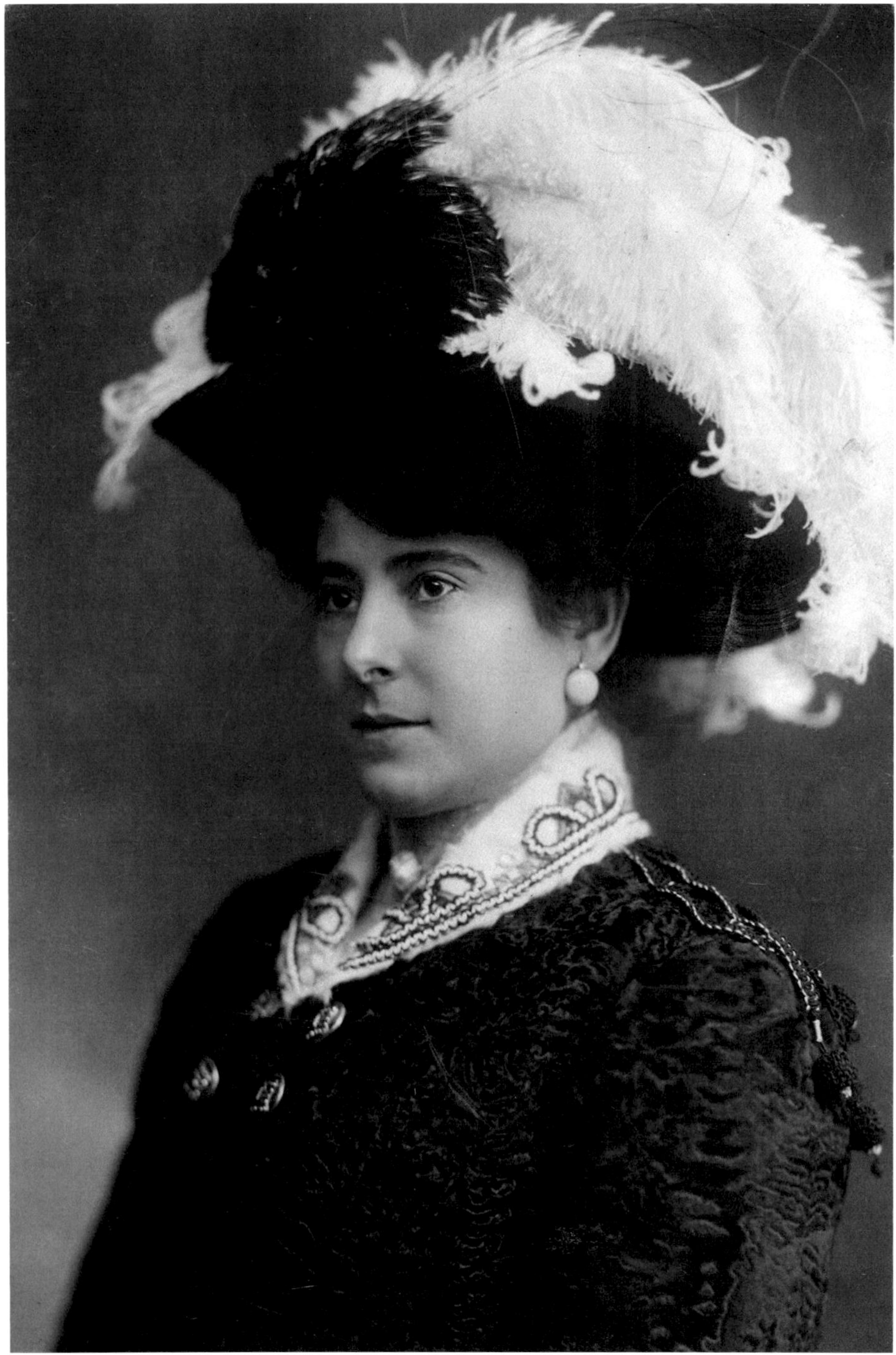

The young Helena in a formal portrait taken in Vienna before she left for Australia, wearing an Astrakhan suit and ostrich feathered hat, c. 1893.

the corset as inhibiting the modern, progressive woman.[32] In terms of both dress and makeup, young women were beginning to reject the parochial conventions and social standards that had defined them. Until the late nineteenth century the use of cosmetics—associated with the painted faces of actresses and prostitutes—had been frowned upon by the middle class. The ideal face was "defined by pale skin and blushing cheeks."[33] But by the time Rubinstein came of age toward the end of the century, attitudes were changing. More varied notions of beauty were emerging as women began to discover new ways to enhance their appearance.

No longer was one's sense of social self tied exclusively to class and parentage, or limited by outdated notions of respectability. Young women were contributing mightily to the new economy that was developing around fashion, interior decoration, and art; more and more, culture reflected modern feminine sensibilities. And feminine taste included makeup. While today it is common to think of makeup as a mechanism for the objectification and sexualization of women, it was seen in the early twentieth century as a means of asserting female independence and autonomy. "Makeup contributed to the constitution of women's identity, no longer to its falsification. In the period from 1900 to 1930, making up became one of the tangible ways women in their everyday lives confirmed their identities as women: they *became* women in the application of blusher, mascara, and lipstick. These applications carried various and contested meanings for women."[34]

As women began to adorn their faces, they also ditched the layers of petticoats and corsets that had restricted natural movement. These changes coincided with the entrance of many young women into the workplace. With the emergence of new work, new attitudes, and plentiful choices, women began to define how they would be seen.

The role played by photography in this appreciation for individuality cannot be overstated: it changed the way people saw themselves. At first, the reality of having one's image frozen into an object of scrutiny was startling, but it soon stirred a desire to improve upon one's natural state. The studio portrait lent a family standing within the community. In middle-class families it became a ritual act, "making of oneself over into a social image."[35] Rubinstein instinctively grasped how the photograph altered the self-image—in particular for middle-class women. It was also a leveling device, a medium that could be employed as well as understood by anyone. Throughout her career she understood the power of such images—the force and authority of even casual portraits, photographs, images of the individual face. In this sense, she intuited photography's aspirational alignment with the American Dream: the medium that the photographer Edward Weston thought "peculiarly adapted to the American psyche . . . vital in that it belongs to an epoch, a race in the making, the becoming."[36]

Beauty Is Power

After her time in Vienna, Rubinstein, at about age twenty-four, moved to Australia, where she had relatives and where her Viennese aunt had suggested that her marital prospects might improve. She opened her first beauty salon, Maison de Beauté Valaze, in Melbourne in 1903. At the time the concept barely existed, even in Europe. A storefront location in a town where women—not necessarily affluent—could go to have specialized beauty treatments for the skin and hair was a new idea. Rubinstein was among the first to found beauty salons for the public. She had raised some capital and began to produce a skin cream called Valaze, which she

32 Conversely, aristocratic styles of dress were often a reactionary protest against social egalitarianism. See, for example, Aileen Ribeiro, "On Englishness of Dress," in Christopher Breward, Becky Conekin, and Caroline Cox, eds., *The Englishness of English Dress* (Oxford, UK: Berg, 2002), 15–28.

33 Peiss, *Hope in a Jar*, 39.

34 Kathy Peiss, "Making Up Making Over: Cosmetics, Consumer Culture, and Women's Identity," in Victoria de Grazia, ed., with Ellen Furlough, *The Sex of Things: Gender and Consumption in Historical Perspective* (Berkeley: University of California Press, 1996), 330–31.

35 Alan Trachtenberg, *Reading American Photographs* (New York: Hill & Wang, 1989), 66, quoted in Peiss, *Hope in a Jar*, 46.

36 Edward Weston, *The Daybooks of Edward Weston*, vol. 2, *California*, 262; quoted in John Raeburn, *A Staggering Revolution: A Cultural History of Thirties Photography* (Urbana, IL: University of Illinois Press, 2006), 249.

marketed with remarkable ease to tough colonial women with pale English complexions that suffered greatly in the harsh climate and relentless sunshine of Australia.[37]

The name of the product was invented. It may have been concocted because it sounded French, but more likely it alluded to the work of a Hungarian chemist, Dr. Jacob Lykuski, whom Rubinstein later claimed was the creator of a cream that her mother had used in Poland.[38] *Válasz*, in fact, means "answer" in Hungarian, and the tonic certainly proved to be that for the young entrepreneur. It was her first commercial beauty product, and it was a hit. Australian country women bought the cream and visited the salon in droves. "Beauty Is Power. Dr. Lykuski's Valaze Will Make You Beautiful," an early advertisement proclaimed. " 'VALAZE' is guaranteed to improve the worst of skin in one Month" (see page 58). Rubinstein's own skin was porcelain fair, and served as an effective advertisement—a lesson she took to heart.

After establishing successful salons in Melbourne and Sydney, Rubinstein decided in 1905 to make the first of several tours of Europe, to acquire as much knowledge as possible about spas and the general status of beauty salons on the Continent, as well as to meet experts in the field of dermatology in Berlin and Vienna.[39] She opened a successful salon in Wellington, New Zealand, in about 1906, and then set her sights on the European market. She settled in London and was soon visited by Edward Titus, who had begun a romance with her in Australia.

Titus, a Polish-born American journalist with literary aspirations, had a knack for copywriting. Under his influence she began to use a sophisticated, text-based advertising that emphasized a more worldly woman. He was instrumental in the development of the company's advertising campaigns and taught Rubinstein much about public relations. She was a good listener and knew how to formulate the ideas of others into products of her own—traits that distinguished her business acumen early on.

She and Titus were married in 1908.[40] Edward immediately became a sort of cultural attaché for his wife, introducing her to London's intellectual elite, dandified writers such as Somerset Maugham, Max Beerbohm, and George Bernard Shaw. Although their long marriage was beset by difficulties, he was not only socially adept, but perspicacious, advising his wife on matters of business. She planned to open a salon in London and he suggested that she launch it "not with extravagant advertising claims about fantasy aristocratic clients, but by giving free treatments to genuine aristocratic clientele."[41]

To succeed in London meant achieving a certain social standing, tricky for an immigrant Jew. Rubinstein demonstrated her publicity savvy when she commissioned a portrait of herself, a set of etchings by Paul César Helleu, in 1908. Some seven years later she used one of them in an early advertising campaign to emphasize her European lineage and thereby distinguish her first American salon from its competitors (see page 58). Portraits were to be an enduring passion and an integral element of her marketing.

The years before World War I were good to Madame. She established successful beauty salons in London in 1908 and on the chic rue du Faubourg St.-Honoré in Paris in 1909. Edward continued to mentor and shrewdly promote his wife's business. He was a bibliophile and publisher in his own right, an important member of the Surrealist circle and supporter of expatriate writers in Paris. His influence on Rubinstein was multifaceted, and she made use of his talents and his connections.

37 For more on Rubinstein's early time in Australia, and the founding of her first salon in Melbourne, see Woodhead, *War Paint*, 36ff.

38 Rubinstein, *My Life for Beauty*, 27–28. It is worth noting, too, that Australia's sheep industry made lanolin, a key ingredient, plentiful.

39 Between 1905 and 1908 she traveled to Europe several times. In Vienna, her old starting place, she opened her first European factory. According to one biographer, she met with one of her consultants, a countess who is said to have invented her waterproof mascara. See Patrick O'Higgins, *Madame: An Intimate Biography of Helena Rubinstein* (New York: Viking Press, 1971), 144.

40 Rubinstein was thirty-six years old, Edward thirty-eight. Edward presumably did not know her actual age, since she had often blithely misrepresented it. On her Australian naturalization papers, filed in 1907, she listed her age as twenty-seven when she was actually thirty-five. See Woodhead, *War Paint*, 48. Rubinstein claimed that the marriage took place in London, but Woodhead suggests that it may have occurred in Australia; see 77.

41 Woodhead, *War Paint*, 80.

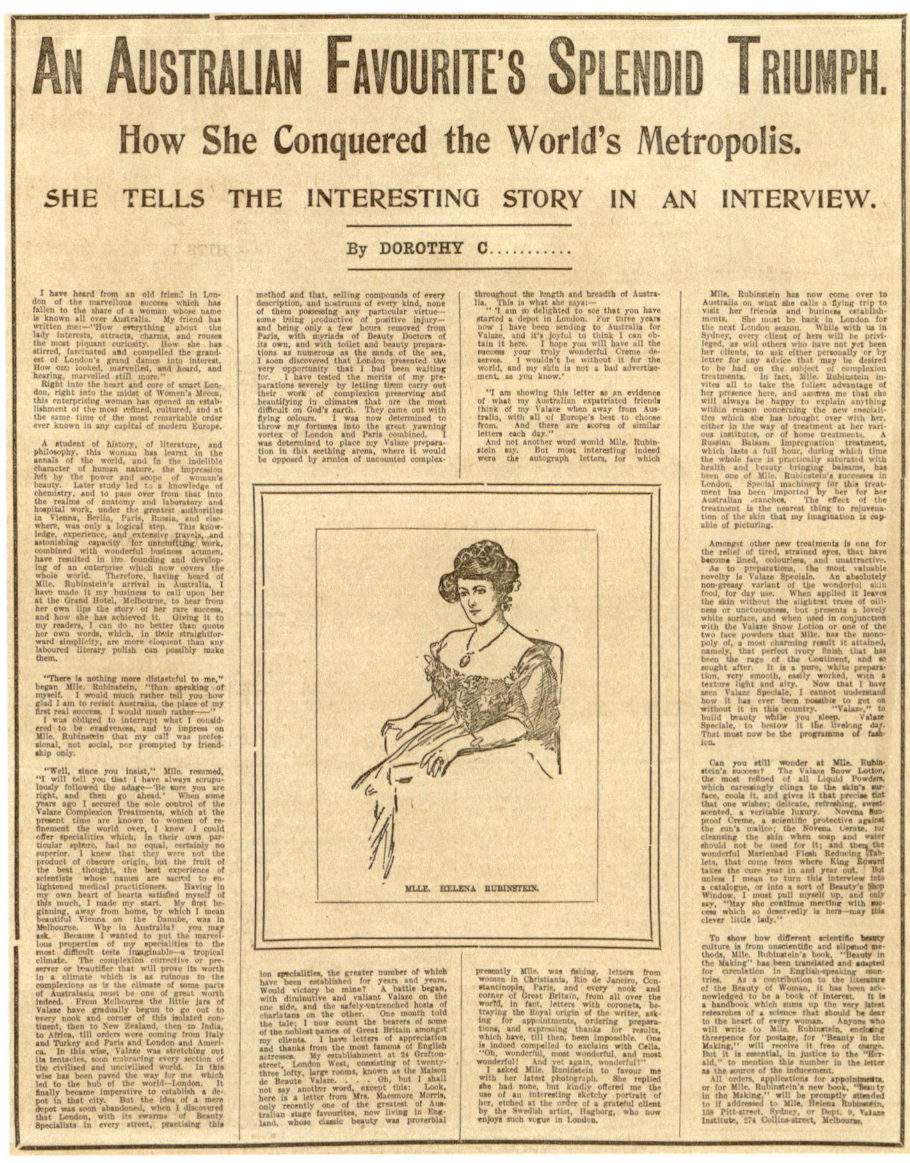

AN AUSTRALIAN FAVOURITE'S SPLENDID TRIUMPH.

How She Conquered the World's Metropolis.

SHE TELLS THE INTERESTING STORY IN AN INTERVIEW.

By DOROTHY C...........

I have heard from an old friend in London of the marvellous success which has fallen to the share of a woman whose name is known all over Australia. My friend has written me:—"How everything about the lady interests, attracts, charms, and rouses the most piquant curiosity. How she has stirred, fascinated and compelled the grandest of London's grand dames into interest. How one looked, marvelled, and heard, and hearing, marvelled still more."

Right into the heart and core of smart London, right into the midst of Women's Mecca, this enterprising woman has opened an establishment of the most refined, cultured, and at the same time of the most remarkable order ever known in any capital of modern Europe.

A student of history, of literature, and philosophy, this woman has learnt in the annals of the world, and in the indelible character of human nature, the impression left by the power and scope of woman's beauty. Later study led to a knowledge of chemistry, and to pass over from that into the realms of anatomy and laboratory and hospital work, under the greatest authorities in Vienna, Berlin, Paris, Russia, and elsewhere, was only a logical step. This knowledge, experience, and extensive travels, and astonishing capacity for unremitting work, combined with wonderful business acumen, have resulted in the founding and developing of an enterprise which now covers the whole world. Therefore, having heard of Mlle. Rubinstein's arrival in Australia, I have made it my business to call upon her at the Grand Hotel, Melbourne, to hear from her own lips the story of her rare success, and how she has achieved it. Giving it to my readers, I can do no better than quote her own words, which, in their straightforward simplicity, are more eloquent than any laboured literary polish can possibly make them.

"There is nothing more distasteful to me," began Mlle. Rubinstein, "than speaking of myself. I would much rather tell you how glad I am to revisit Australia, the place of my first real success. I would much rather——"

I was obliged to interrupt what I considered to be evasiveness, and to impress on Mlle. Rubinstein that my call was professional, not social, nor prompted by friendship only.

"Well, since you insist," Mlle. resumed, "I will tell you that I have always scrupulously followed the adage—'Be sure you are right, and then go ahead.' When some years ago I secured the sole control of the Valaze Complexion Treatments, which at the present time are known to women of refinement the world over, I knew I could offer specialities which, in their own particular sphere, had no equal, certainly no superior. I knew that they were not the product of obscure origin, but the fruit of the best thought, the best experience of scientists whose names are sacred to enlightened medical practitioners. Having in my own heart of hearts satisfied myself of this much, I made my start. My first beginning, away from home, by which I mean beautiful Vienna on the Danube, was in Melbourne. Why in Australia? you may ask. Because I wanted to put the marvellous properties of my specialities to the most difficult tests imaginable—a tropical climate. The complexion corrective or preserver or beautifier that will prove its worth in a climate which is as ruinous to the complexions as is the climate of some parts of Australasia must be one of great worth indeed. From Melbourne the little jars of Valaze have gradually begun to go out to every nook and corner of this isolated continent, then to New Zealand, then to India, to Africa, till orders were coming from Italy and Turkey and Paris and London and America. In this wise, Valaze was stretching out its tentacles, soon embracing every section of the civilised and uncivilised world. In this wise has been paved the way for me which led to the hub of the world—London. It finally became imperative to establish a depot in that city. But the idea of a mere depot was soon abandoned, when I discovered that London, with its swarms of Beauty Specialists in every street, practising this method and that, selling compounds of every description, and nostrums of every kind, none of them possessing any particular virtue—some being productive of positive injury—and being only a few hours removed from Paris, with myriads of Beauty Doctors of its own, and with toilet and beauty preparations as numerous as the sands of the sea, I soon discovered that London presented the very opportunity that I had been waiting for. I have tested the merits of my preparations severely by letting them carry out their work of complexion preserving and beautifying in climates that are the most difficult on God's earth. They came out with flying colours. I was now determined to throw my fortunes into the great yawning vortex of London and Paris combined. I was determined to place my Valaze preparation in this seething arena, where it would be opposed by armies of uncounted complexion specialities, the greater number of which have been established for years and years. Would victory be mine? A battle began, with diminutive and valiant Valaze on the one side, and the safely-entrenched hosts of charlatans on the other. One month told the tale; I now count the bearers of some of the noblest names of Great Britain amongst my clients. I have letters of appreciation and thanks from the most famous of English actresses. My establishment at 24 Grafton-street, London West, consisting of twenty-three lofty, large rooms, known as the Maison de Beaute Valaze. . . . Oh, but I shall not say another word, except this: Look, here is a letter from Mrs. Maesmore Morris, only recently one of the greatest of Australian stage favourites, now living in England, whose classic beauty was proverbial throughout the length and breadth of Australia. This is what she says:—

" 'I am so delighted to see that you have started a depot in London. For three years now I have been sending to Australia for Valaze, and it's joyful to think I can obtain it here. I hope you will have all the success your truly wonderful Creme deserves. I wouldn't be without it for the world, and my skin is not a bad advertisement, as you know.'

"I am showing this letter as an evidence of what my Australian expatriated friends think of my Valaze when away from Australia, with all of Europe's best to choose from. And there are scores of similar letters each day."

And not another word would Mlle. Rubinstein say. But most interesting indeed were the autograph letters, for which presently Mlle. was fishing, letters from women in Christiania, Rio de Janeiro, Constantinople, Paris, and every nook and corner of Great Britain, from all over the world, in fact, letters with coronets, betraying the Royal origin of the writer, asking for appointments, ordering preparations, and expressing thanks for results, which have, till then, been impossible. One is indeed compelled to exclaim with Celia, "Oh, wonderful, most wonderful, and most wonderful! And yet again, wonderful!"

I asked Mlle. Rubinstein to favour me with her latest photograph. She replied she had none, but kindly offered me the use of an interesting sketchy portrait of her, etched at the order of a grateful client by the Swedish artist, Hagborg, who now enjoys such vogue in London.

MLLE. HELENA RUBINSTEIN.

Mlle. Rubinstein has now come over to Australia on what she calls a flying trip to visit her friends and business establishments. She must be back in London for the next London season. While with us in Sydney, every client of hers will be privileged, as will others who have not yet been her clients, to ask either personally or by letter for any advice that may be desired to be had on the subject of complexion treatments. In fact, Mlle. Rubinstein invites all to take the fullest advantage of her presence here, and assures me that she will always be happy to explain anything within reason concerning the new specialities which she has brought over with her, either in the way of treatment at her various institutes, or of home treatments. A Russian Balsam Impregnation treatment, which lasts a full hour, during which time the whole face is practically saturated with health and beauty bringing balsams, has been one of Mlle. Rubinstein's successes in London. Special machinery for this treatment has been imported by her for her Australian branches. The effect of the treatment is the nearest thing to rejuvenation of the skin that my imagination is capable of picturing.

Amongst other new treatments is one for the relief of tired, strained eyes, that have become lined, colourless, and unattractive. As to preparations, the most valuable novelty is Valaze Speciale. An absolutely non-greasy variant of the wonderful skin food, for day use. When applied it leaves the skin without the slightest traces of oiliness or unctuousness, but presents a lovely white surface, and when used in conjunction with the Valaze Snow Lotion or one of the two face powders that Mlle. has the monopoly of, a most charming result it attained, namely, that perfect ivory finish that has been the rage of the Continent, and so sought after. It is a pure, white preparation, very smooth, easily worked, with a texture light and airy. Now that I have seen Valaze Speciale, I cannot understand how it has ever been possible to get on without it in this country. "Valaze," to build beauty while you sleep. Valaze Speciale, to bestow it the livelong day. That must now be the programme of fashion.

Can you still wonder at Mlle. Rubinstein's success? The Valaze Snow Lotion, the most refined of all Liquid Powders, which caressingly clings to the skin's surface, cools it, and gives it that precise tint that one wishes; delicate, refreshing, sweet-scented, a veritable luxury. Novena Sunproof Creme, a scientific protective against the sun's malice; the Novena Cerate, for cleansing the skin when soap and water should not be used for it; and then the wonderful Marienbad Flesh Reducing Tablets, that come from where King Edward takes the cure year in and year out. But unless I mean to turn this interview into a catalogue, or into a sort of Beauty's Shop Window, I must pull myself up, and only say, "May she continue meeting with success which so deservedly is hers—may this clever little lady."

To show how different scientific beauty culture is from unscientific and slipshod methods, Mlle. Rubinstein's book, "Beauty in the Making" has been translated and adapted for circulation in English-speaking countries. As a contribution to the literature of the Beauty of Woman, it has been acknowledged to be a book of interest. It is a handbook which sums up the very latest researches of a science that should be dear to the heart of every woman. Anyone who will write to Mlle. Rubinstein, enclosing threepence for postage, for "Beauty in the Making," will receive it free of charge. But it is essential, in justice to the "Herald," to mention this number in the letter as the source of the inducement.

All orders, applications for appointments, or for Mlle. Rubinstein's new book, "Beauty in the Making," will be promptly attended to if addressed to Mlle. Helena Rubinstein, 158 Pitt-street, Sydney, or Dept. 9, Valaze Institute, 274 Collins-street, Melbourne.

The first commissioned portrait of Helena Rubinstein, drawn by the Swedish artist August Hagborg, appeared in the *Sydney Morning Herald*, January 30, 1909.

BEAUTY IS POWER.

DR. LYKUSKI'S

VALAZE

RUSSIAN SKIN FOOD

WILL MAKE YOU BEAUTIFUL.

"Valaze" Eradicates Freckles, Wrinkles, Sallowness, Sunburn, Blackheads, Acne, Pimples, Roughness, and all Blemishes and Eruptions of the Skin, rendering it soft, white and transparent. "Valaze" is guaranteed to improve the worst skin in one Month.

MISS NELLIE STEWART Says:

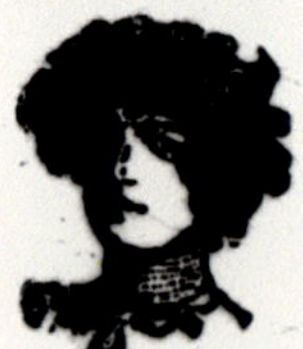

"I have tried face preparations from all parts of the world, and paid fabulous prices for some, and nothing has proved half as good as 'Valaze'. If I run short, and write you from London or America, will you kindly forward it immediately, as I would not be without it no matter what cost. It is absolutely the very best Skin Food I have ever used. I can never praise it enough. It is simply marvellous.

Price 3/6 and 6/-, Posted, 6d. extra.

HELENA RUBINSTEIN & CO., 243 Collins St, Melb.

Send Four 1d. stamps for Illustrated" Guide to Beauty".

Above: "Beauty Is Power," one of the first slogans for Rubinstein's Valaze beauty cream, published in the *Queenslander* newspaper, May 21, 1904, with an early use of celebrity endorsement. *Below*: A 1920 Art Deco advertisement for the cream. *Opposite*: An advertisement that appeared in *Vogue*, May 15, 1915, using a portrait of Rubinstein by Paul César Helleu.

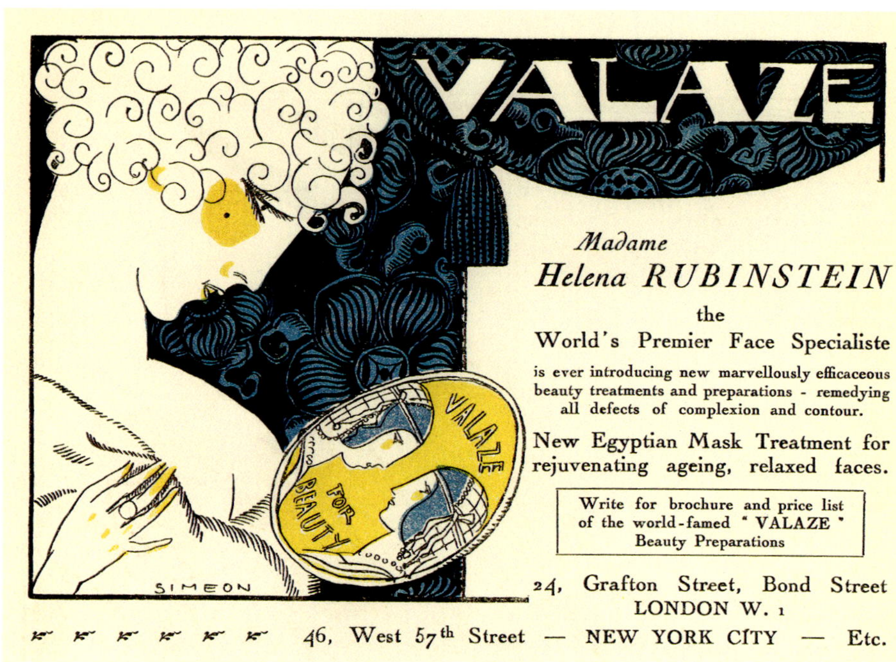

A FAMOUS EUROPEAN "HOUSE OF BEAUTY"

Announces the Opening of its Doors in New York

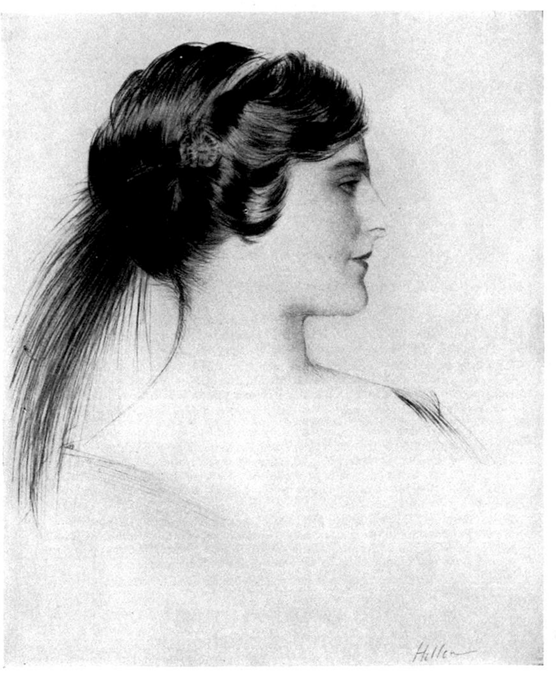

MADAME HELENA RUBINSTEIN
(From etching by Helleu)

MADAME HELENA RUBINSTEIN, who is the accepted adviser in beauty matters to the Royalty, Aristocracy and the great Artistes of Europe; whose position as a scientific Beauty Culturist and whose unique work on exclusive lines have created for her a world-wide fame; whose establishments, the Maison de Beauté Valaze, at 24 Grafton Street, Mayfair, London, and at No. 255 Rue Saint Honoré, Paris, are well-known landmarks in the itinerary of the ladies of high society of both Continents; whose "Valaze" specialties have been found essential to the maintenance of their complexion beauty by the world's most beautiful women announces the opening of her American

MAISON
de BEAUTÉ VALAZE
at No. 15 EAST 49th STREET
NEW YORK CITY

This establishment, equipped in much the same manner as Madame Rubinstein's London and Paris houses, in itself radiates the Spirit of Beauty.

The same famous beauty treatments that have won the admiring gratitude of uncounted numbers of women abroad are now being administered here; and for ladies who, owing to distance or other reasons, find it inconvenient or impossible to come to see her in person, carefully individualized home-treatments will be devised by Madame Rubinstein herself.

While Madame Rubinstein would naturally prefer to meet her clients face to face, yet she wishes to impress upon all those who are prevented from calling on her, that by writing to her freely on the needs and condition of their complexions they will not be calling in vain upon the fund of her great experience.

Madame Rubinstein does not pretend to "wizardry" in her beauty-work—this being the charming compliment paid her by one of the most beautiful women of now so unhappy France, Madame Jeanne Faber of the Comédie Française—but she *does* know the ins and outs of a woman's beauty requirements. And what is more to the point, she can fully satisfy these requirements in her own uniquely unfailing way.

Madame Rubinstein's knowledge and unequalled expertness are now at the disposal of the women of New York and sister cities.

A visit to her sanctum or an inquiry by letter solves many a little heartache that may be due to some shortcoming in appearance.

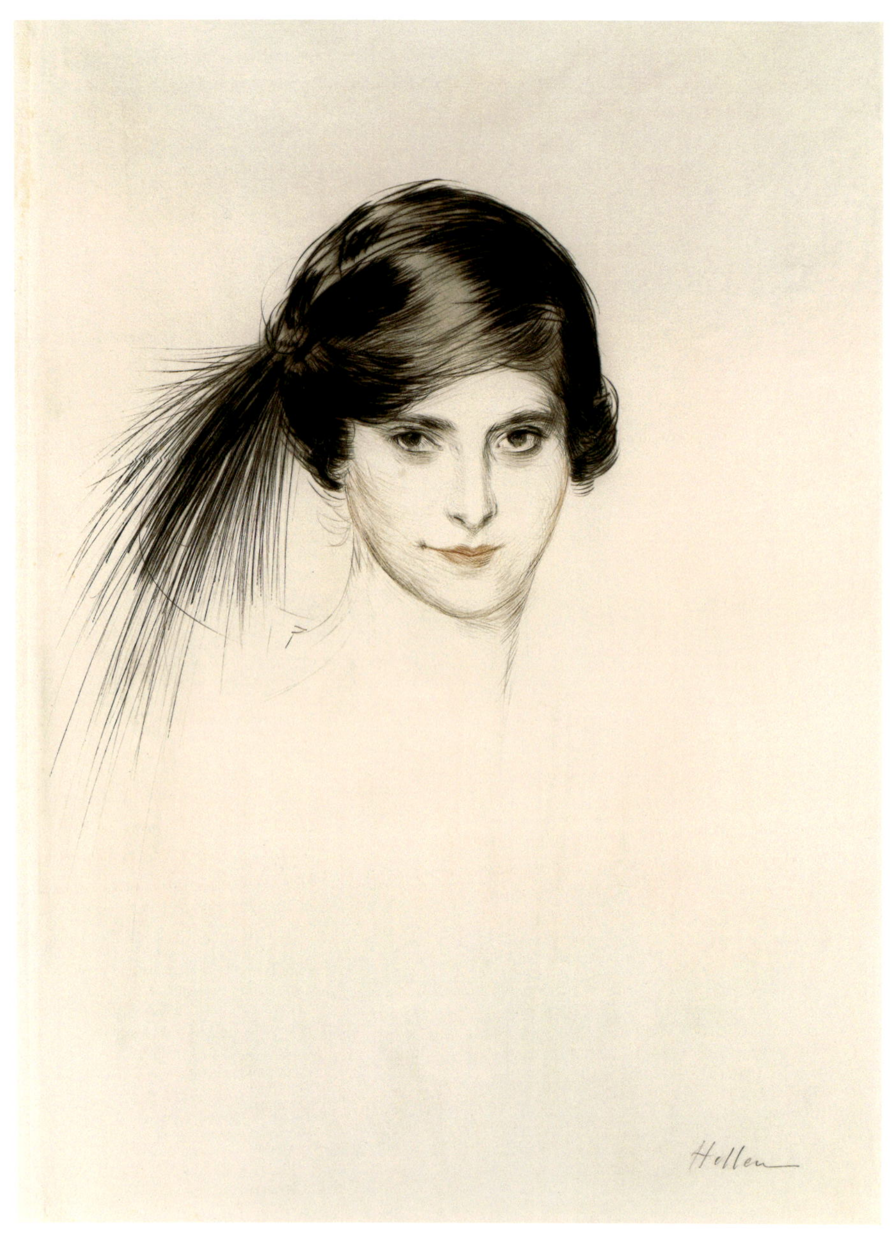

Paul César Helleu
Portrait of Helena Rubinstein with Egret Feathers, c. 1908
Etching on paper, 28 × 21¼ in. (71.1 × 54 cm)
National Portrait Gallery, Smithsonian Institution, Washington, DC, acquired through the generosity of the Abraham and Virginia Weiss Charitable Trust, Amy and Marc Meadows

But she had little interest in his world, and the marriage began to wither quite soon. By the onset of the war they were living largely separate lives. During these years they had two sons, Roy and Horace. While Edward helped his wife enter the artistic vanguard, his philandering eventually became insufferable, and they divorced in 1937.[42]

As the marriage deteriorated, Rubinstein sought savvy counsel elsewhere, and found it in Baroness Catherine d'Erlanger, who helped her navigate the intricate hierarchy of London society and cultivate her artistic sensibilities.[43] Called Flame for her red hair, the baroness patronized all kinds of artists, including the risqué. A supporter of Sergei Diaghilev and the Ballets Russes, she was a social fixture among musicians and writers for decades, in both Europe and the United States. Flame was a model of idiosyncrasy for the arriviste Helena, with whom she shared a fervor for scrounging at flea markets. There, according to the baroness's friend, the society photographer Cecil Beaton (no slouch himself when it came to style), she and Helena dawdled in search of beautiful things, "an eclectic display of shell-flowers, witch-balls and mother-of-pearl furniture, all picked up for a song" (see page 65).[44]

The other social figure to help Rubinstein and Titus make their way through the Parisian *haute bohème* was the legendary *salonnière* Misia Sert, a talented Polish-born pianist known as the muse of the Belle Epoque. Although they were the same age, by the time Rubinstein opened her Paris beauty salon, Misia was already twice married and was the cultural arbiter of Paris; her home had been the turn-of-the-century meeting place for the city's artistic intelligentsia. She was, the writer Paul Morand once said, "a collector of geniuses, all of them in love with her."[45] Such role models as Flame and Misia appealed to Madame as women who were interested in "what people are, not in who they are," as she stressed in her memoir. "This is the accepted attitude today among all thinking people, but there was a time when it was considered quite daring. . . . d'Erlanger was one of the first sophisticated originals who lived on an international scale . . . truly avant-garde, and her taste and complete confidence in it and herself permitted her to create about her an atmosphere of rare excitement."[46]

Rubinstein claimed to have known of Misia through mutual friends in Poland. When she and Edward moved to Paris in 1909, the two women met. Rubinstein credited Misia with boosting her confidence, since she was not yet conversant in French, and encouraging her to socialize, telling her, "I always received guests on Thursdays; you must give your parties on Sundays. But to do it regularly—that is the secret of being a good hostess." "Our common interest in art became an immediate link," Helena recalled, "and our husbands . . . became friends." Misia was famous in the art and fashion worlds, a close friend of Coco Chanel, then an emerging modiste. As such, she provided the best public relations Helena could have wished for, guiding her through elite circles, "even making lists of the guests I was to invite to my first Paris 'At Home.'" Many of these became regulars at her beauty salon, clients "whose names read like pages out of a fashion magazine. The leading members of the aristocracy, the stage and the arts." Such mentorship contributed immeasurably to the swift success of her Paris establishment, and helped to shape her self-image. It was in Paris more than anywhere else that Madame learned to express her distinct sense of taste and to present herself as a sharply defined, authoritative figure.[47] As she once told her assistant, Patrick O'Higgins, "Misia was some meshuggenah, an eccentric . . . but when I first came to Paris—pfft! more than forty years ago—she was a Queen. Rich. Social, artistic . . . Polish! I was green. I didn't know about society. I had to make my own way. Someone had

42 Titus's literary ambitions were subsidized by his wife. In Paris in 1924 he opened a bookshop called At the Sign of the Black Manikin, which became a gathering place for expatriate writers from Ernest Hemingway to D. H. Lawrence. He founded the Black Manikin Press, producing some twenty-five books, including a reprint of *Lady Chatterley's Lover* in 1929. He was also editor of the literary magazine *This Quarter* for a time. Neither the press nor the magazine lasted beyond 1932.

43 For more on Rubinstein's early years in London and her business relationship with Titus, see Woodhead, *War Paint*, 80ff.

44 Woodhead, *War Paint*, 80; O'Higgins, *Madame*, 91.

45 Edmonde Charles-Roux, *Chanel and her World: Friends, Fashion, Fame* (London: Hachette-Vendome, 1981), 157. At this time Misia had already married and divorced Thadée Natanson, publisher of the influential arts magazine *La Revue blanche*, and was about to divorce her wealthy second husband to marry the Spanish painter José-Maria Sert.

46 Rubinstein, *My Life for Beauty*, 44.

47 Rubinstein, *My Life for Beauty*, 54–55.

to show me, to guide me. That's where Misia came in." One of the more harmless habits of Misia that Madame emulated was to have her portrait painted by artists of her circle. "Misia's only interest was for antiques, for writers, and for artists. She collected them all. Many of the good artists painted her portrait—Renoir, Bonnard, Vuillard. It was through her Helleu and Dufy did things of me."[48]

She was now ensconced among the most fashionably elite of London and Paris, an experience that helped spark her extravagant tastes for art and haute couture. It was during this time that the mold for Rubinstein's eccentric persona and dreamlike world was cast. As a young, independent woman, she had learned many lessons: how to survive, to trust her instincts, to listen to experts—the many brilliant, madcap figures she met in London and Paris who delighted in flouting conventions of behavior and taste. It was a period of extraordinary cross-pollination within the avant-garde, when standards could be irreverently challenged in myriad ways, from the social to the sartorial, on stage or at the dinner table.

At the turn of the twentieth century two fashion houses dominated Paris couture, the House of Worth and that of Jacques Doucet. The former had been founded by the so-called father of haute couture, Charles Worth, clothier to the French Empress Eugénie during the fashion-conscious Second Empire. Worth dressed many celebrated women throughout the Continent, including such luminaries of the stage as Sarah Bernhardt and the operatic soprano Dame Nellie Melba. By the end of the nineteenth century, the House of Worth was world famous, its founder having revolutionized dressmaking and ushered in the modern concept of couture, presenting his collection four times a year.[49]

Rubinstein wore Worth's dresses, but it was the designer Paul Poiret, who had worked for Doucet, who captivated her in the years around World War I. Having already traveled widely and acquired a penchant for exoticism, she was drawn to Poiret's free-flowing, Orientalist clothes and his modernized versions of historical costumes borrowed loosely from the Middle and Far East. No less alluring were the designer's sweeping tunics that liberated their wearers from the constraints of the nineteenth century's corseted silhouette. Rubinstein, like Poiret, had fallen under the theatrical spell of Diaghilev's Ballets Russes, with their stirring colors and set designs.

Poiret was more than a designer or couturier; he was a diviner of style, a performative artist who thought in terms of theatricality and helped to establish modernism's inherent relationship between art and fashion. His impact on Rubinstein and her extravagant decor is undeniable. As Madame admitted later in life,

> *Whenever I was in Paris I would make it a point to visit Poiret, not only to see his newest collection but to enjoy his outspoken opinions on everything and everybody and to call on him at his extraordinary flat. . . . He was strongly influenced by Asiatic art, and he lived in crowded, lamp-lit rooms filled with innumerable Chinese screens, rococo furniture, and Venetian mirrors. . . . Frankly an exotic, it pleased Poiret to receive his personal friends (at least those who dared come) with live panthers chained in the entrance hall, each one attended by a six-foot Negro stripped to the waist, a bejeweled turban around his head, and his bare torso oiled to resemble statuary.*[50]

One need only look at images of Madame's Surrealism-inspired rooms to see how influenced she was by Poiret, pragmatically eschewing his

48 O'Higgins, *Madame*, 92–93.

49 The Australian Melba became a client of Madame's at her first salon in Melbourne. Prior to Worth's advances in dressmaking, clients would choose fabrics and designs and have clothes made to order, rather than have those decisions determined for them. On Worth see Jacqueline C. Kent, "Charles Frederick Worth: The Father of Haute Couture," in *Business Builders in Fashion* (Minneapolis: Oliver Press, 2003), 21–37.

50 "Poiret was an idealist, a dreamer," Madame recalled, "but he was also a fashion tyrant. He was the first man to wage war on the corset." "Like all revolutions, he said, "mine is in the name of Liberty. . . . I hereby free the bosom and the waistline." Rubinstein, *My Life for Beauty*, 48.

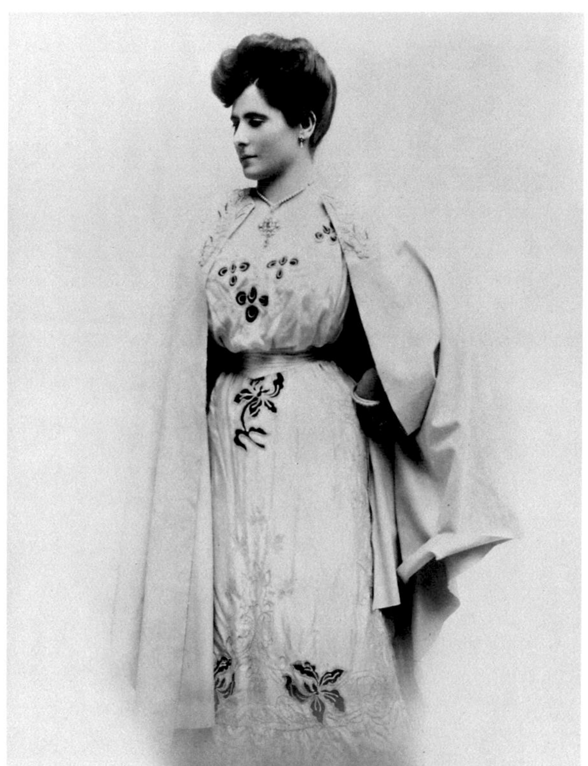

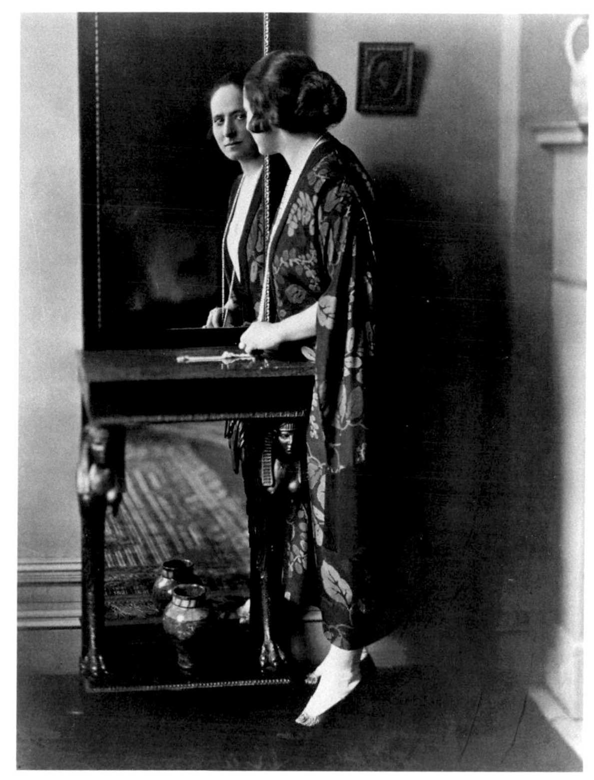

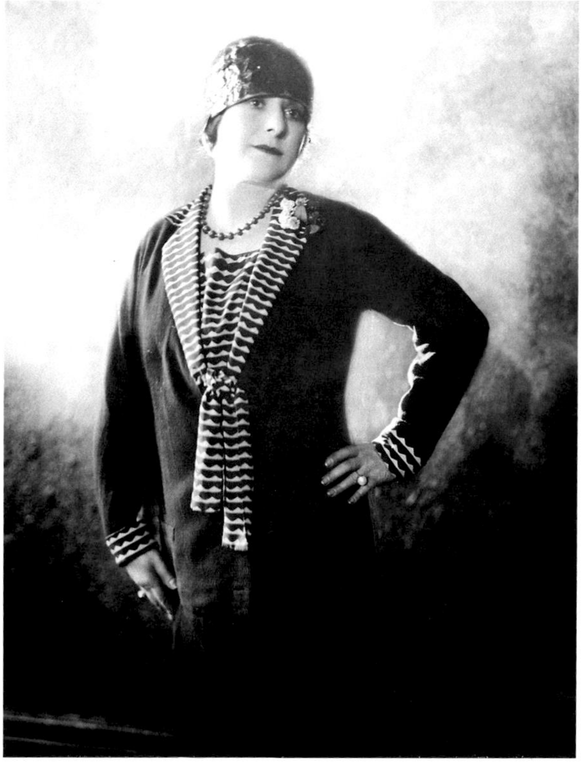

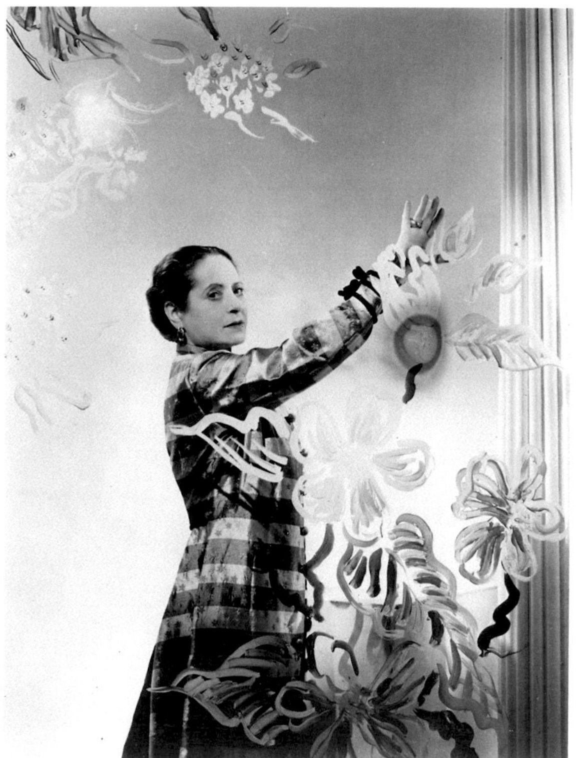

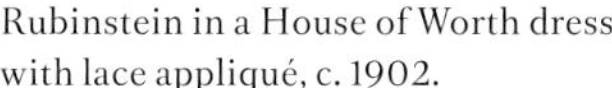

Rubinstein in a House of Worth dress with lace appliqué, c. 1902.

A Coco Chanel suit, late 1920s; Madame was influenced by Chanel, who designed for the modern working woman and encouraged the creative use of affordable accessories, from costume jewelry to scarves.

A Jacques Doucet tea gown, early 1920s; Doucet, a progressive connoisseur of modern art, was a leading couturier of Paris in the Jazz Age.

A Schiaparelli housecoat, in a 1939 photograph by Cecil Beaton, who also painted the glass through which Rubinstein is seen.

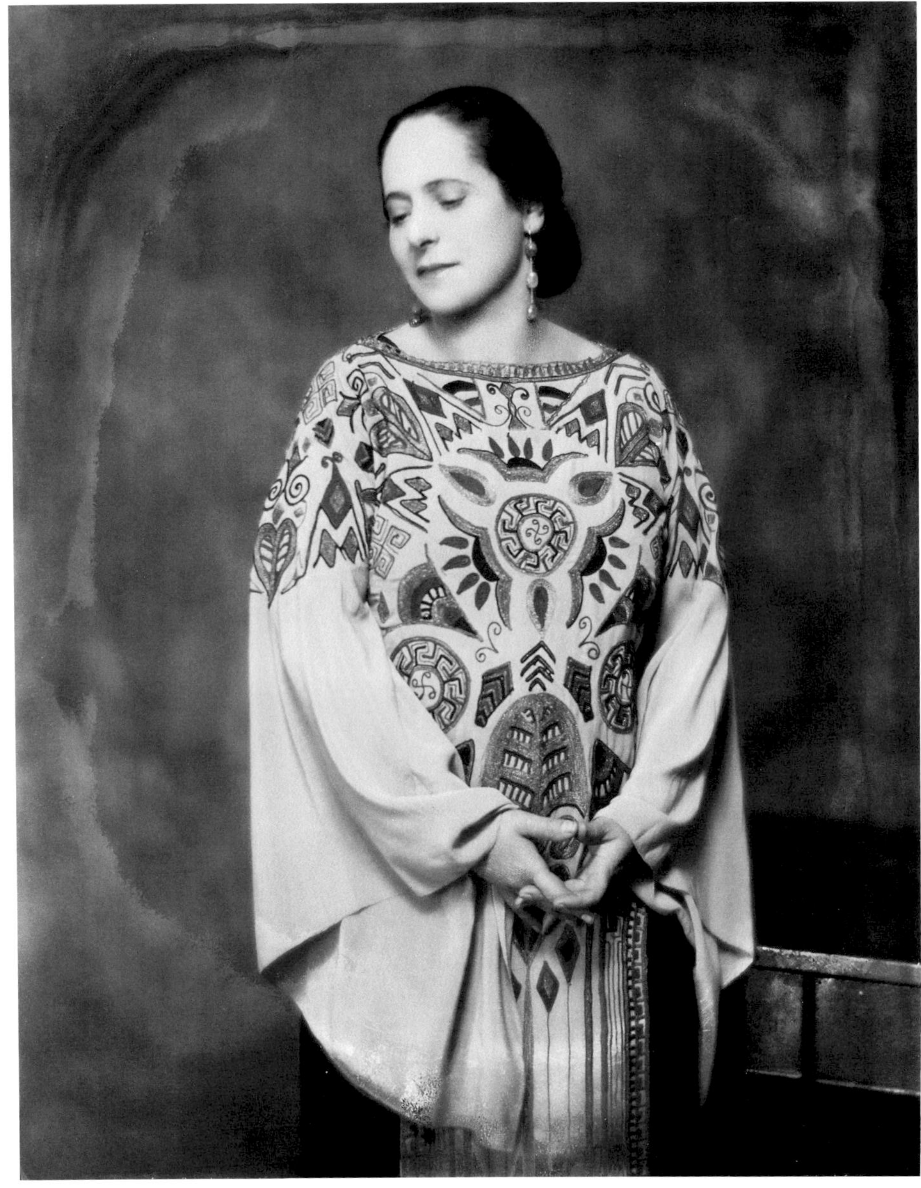

Rubinstein wearing a 1923 Paul Poiret dress, photographed by Nickolas Muray, c. 1924
George Eastman House, International Museum of Photography and Film.

Hand-tinted photograph of the master bedroom in Rubinstein's Paris apartment in the mid-1950s. The gold satin bed is set within an ivory quilted satin alcove, which matches the two similarly treated doors. According to Madame's longtime assistant, Patrick O'Higgins, the mother-of-pearl furniture had belonged to a relative of Napoleon.

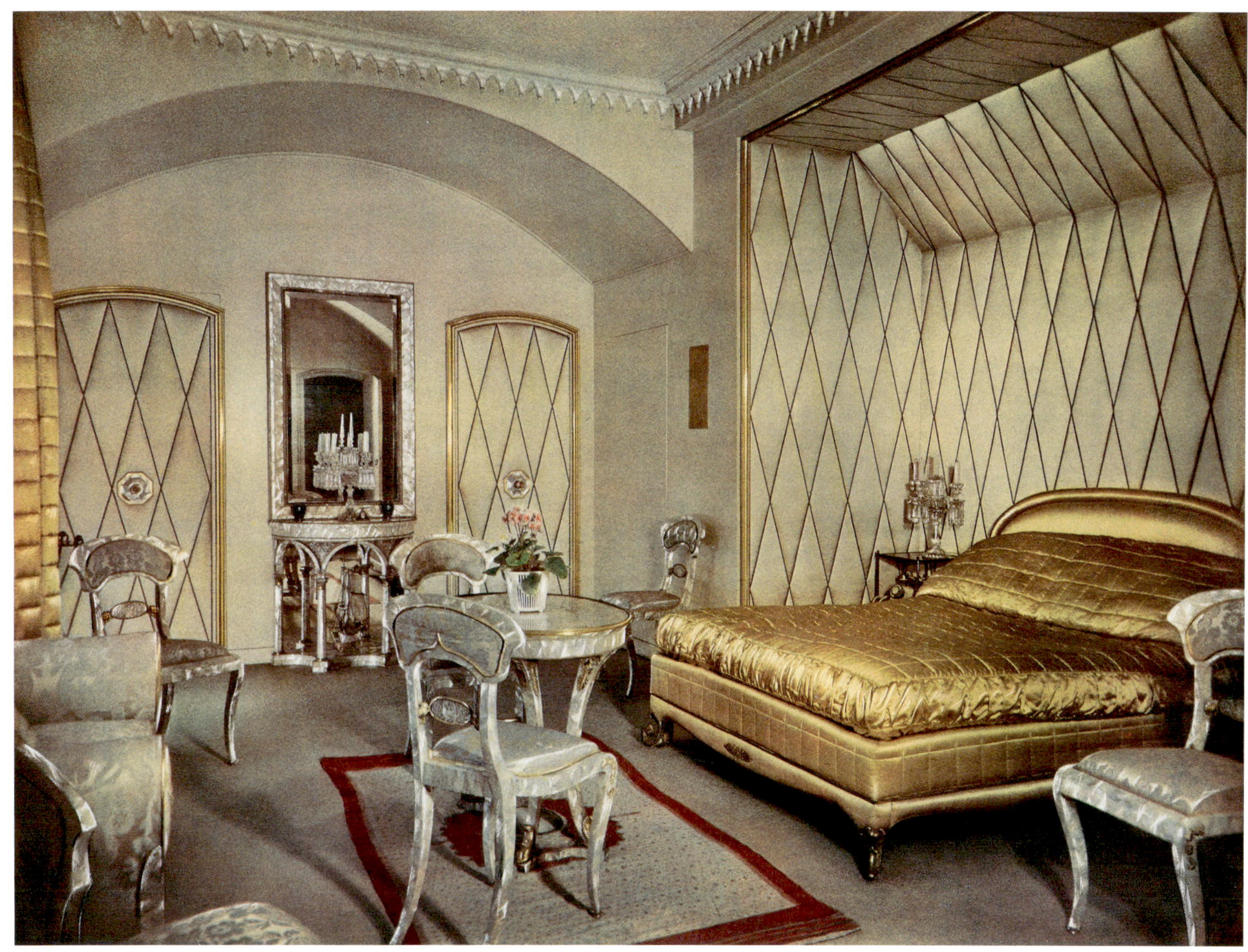

panthers but retaining the Venetian mirrors, Moorish figures, and Rococo furniture, and adding such outlandish touches as padded cellophane-covered walls and a Lucite bed with internal fluorescent lighting (see pages 47, 68, and 69).

Titus encouraged her to draw on such sources for inspiration in her beauty salons. He had been underwhelmed by the white brocade curtains she had chosen for her London salon, and took her to the Ballets Russes "to see what's really new." She was stunned by the set designs of Léon Bakst and Alexandre Benois, as she later recalled:

> *Accustomed as I was to the sweet-pea pastel stage sets of the times, the electric combinations of purple and magenta, orange and yellow, black and gold, excited me beyond measure!... After the ballet, late as it was, I went straight back to the salon and tore down my white brocade curtains. Next day I gave orders for them to be replaced with the brilliant color schemes I had fallen in love with the night before, and over the years they have been seen in Rubinstein salons everywhere.*[51]

And, of course, in her homes.

Triumph in America

With the onset of World War I Madame determined to launch her business in America. This decision was, of course, colored by events in Europe, especially the German advance toward Paris in the fall of 1914. She left her two young sons with Titus in England and sailed alone to New York, with the help of her husband's American passport. There, in the spring of 1915 she opened her first beauty salon, at 15 East 49th Street, just off Fifth Avenue.

Titus, ever skilled in advertising, masterminded the ad in *Vogue* magazine that announced the opening of "A Famous European 'House of Beauty'" (see page 59). It is, iconographically, a striking piece of work. The headline is blazoned in a large font, more prominent than the salon's name, the Maison de Beauté Valaze, or its address. An Helleu etching of "Madame Helena Rubinstein" in elegant profile, wearing a stylish aigrette, or headband of feathers, commands more than half the ad's space. Madame is introduced as "the accepted adviser in beauty matters to the Royalty, Aristocracy and the great Artistes of Europe," and her salons are billed as "well-known landmarks in the itinerary of the ladies of high society of both Continents." But after associating her in word and manner with fairy-tale royalty, the text goes on to address more common subjects: "While Madame would naturally prefer to meet her clients face to face, yet she wishes to impress upon all those who are prevented from calling on her, that by writing to her freely on the needs and condition of their complexions they will not be calling in vain upon the fund of her great experience." While the phrase "calling on her" suggests aristocratic protocol, it is made clear that Madame wished to make herself available to as great a number as she humbly could, welcoming all not to a mere commercial establishment, but to a "sanctum," which "itself radiates the Spirit of Beauty."[52] This brilliantly conflates the defining components of the prevailing zeitgeist that elevated Madame herself and her salon to another level, rendering it a modernist sanctuary in which the new aesthetics of design and art blended indistinguishably with the commercial world of cosmetics and fashion.

51 *My Life for Beauty*, 38–39.

52 Advertisement for Helena Rubinstein's New York salon, *Vogue* 45 (May 15, 1915), 82.

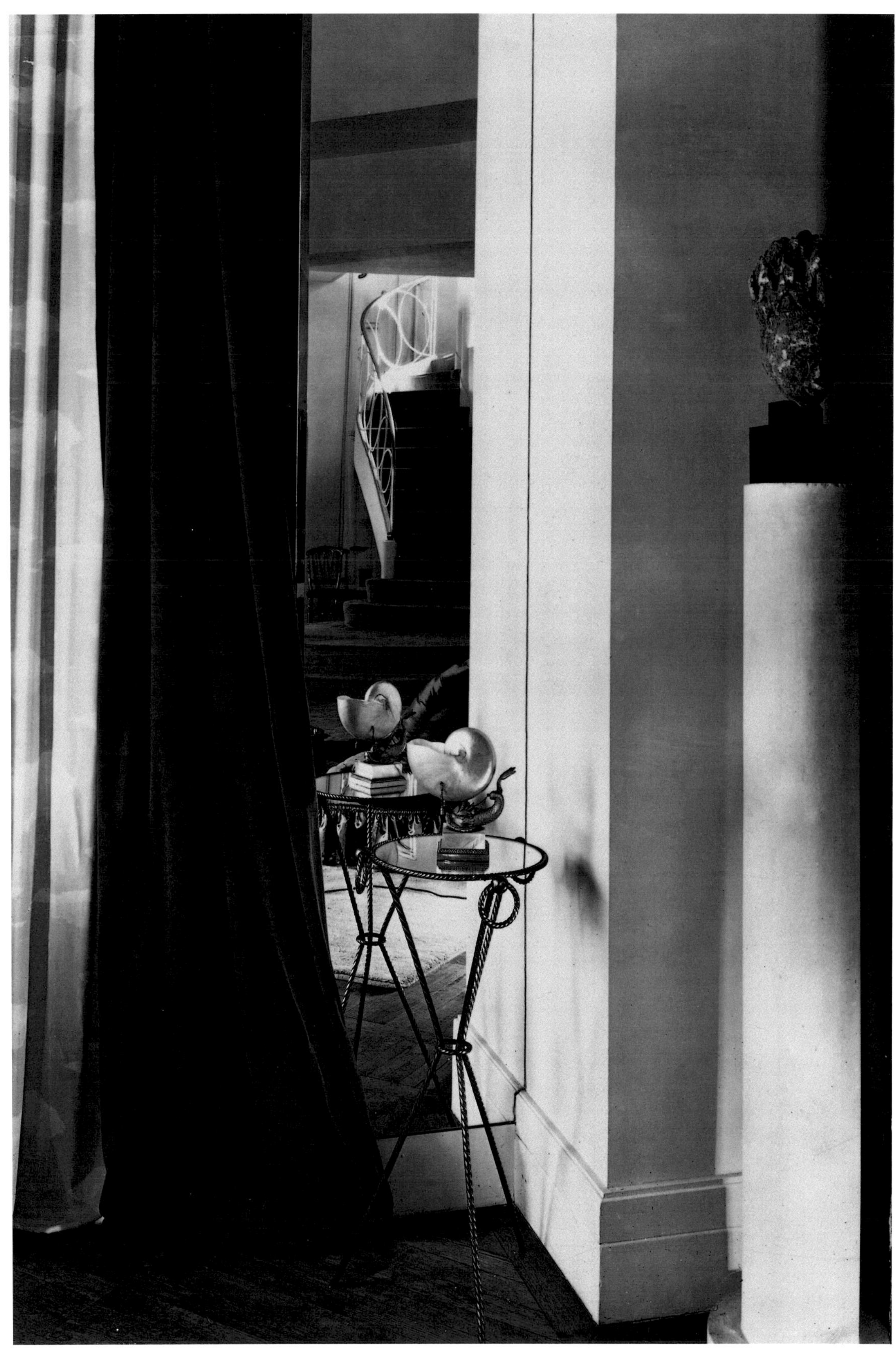

Rubinstein's extravagant apartment on the Ile St.-Louis in Paris, photographed by the French Surrealist Dora Maar, c. 1937. Reflected in a plate mirror is a staircase designed by the Art Deco architect Louis Süe, with a banister of overlapping loops. Madame's love of mirrors and reflected or doubled images appears in both her home decor and her product advertisements and labels.

Madame Rubinstein reads by the fluorescent lighting that suffuses the head and foot of her Lucite bed, designed by Ladislas Medgyes and produced by Rohm & Haas in the late 1930s.

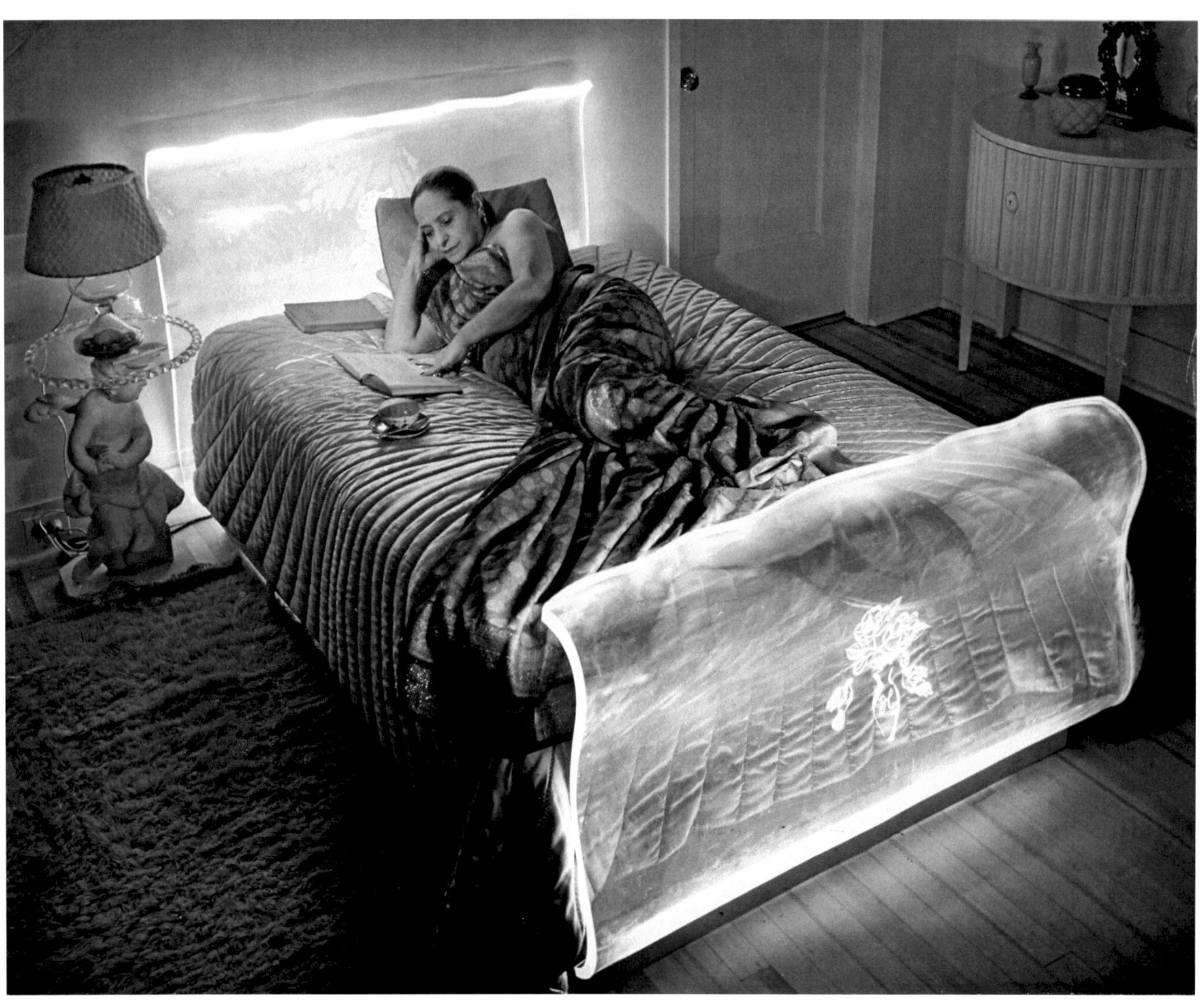

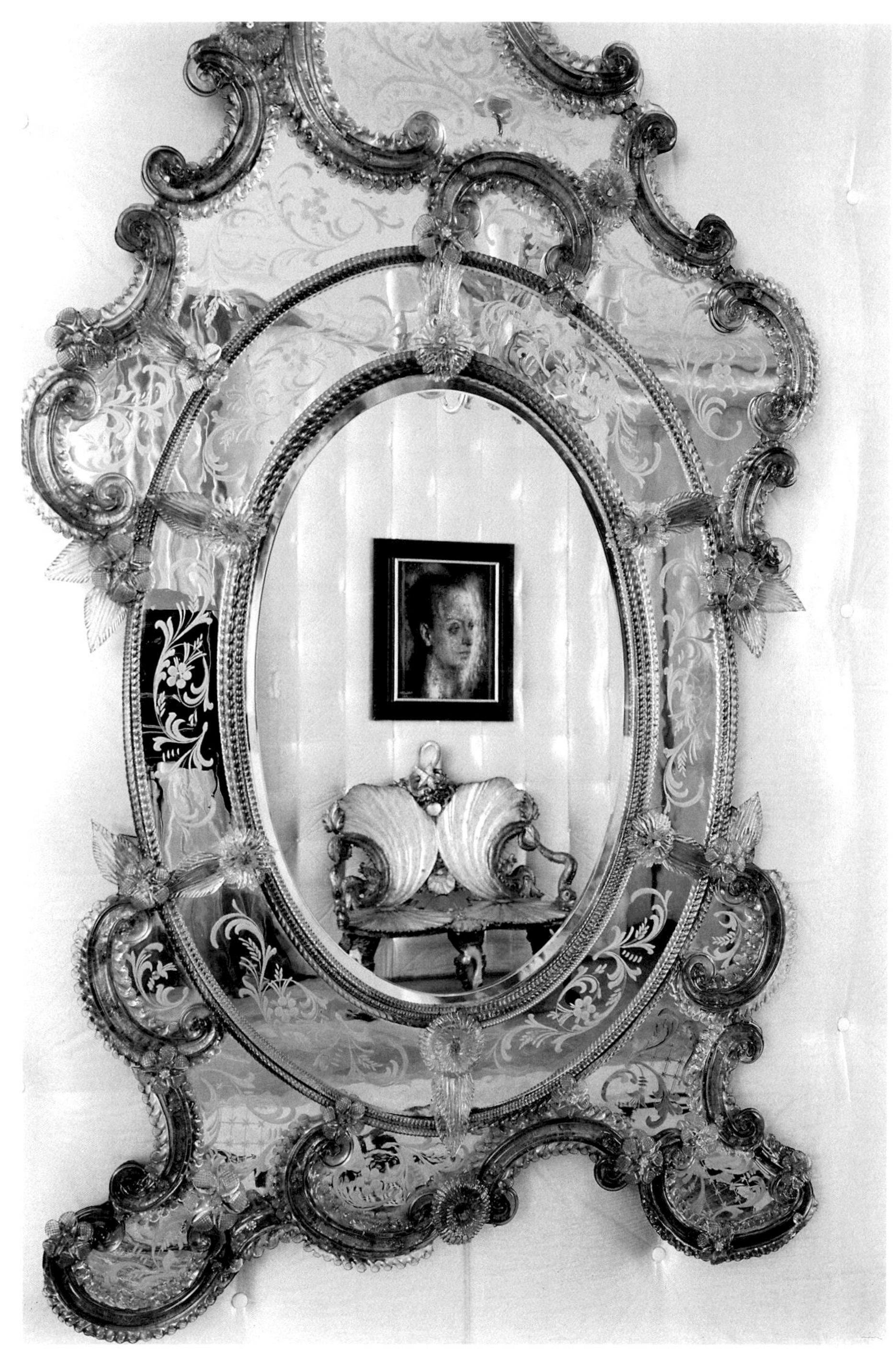

Rubinstein's apartment at 895 Park Avenue, 1938. Reflected in a Venetian mirror are Pavel Tchelitchew's *Head of Helena Rubinstein Encrusted with Sequins*, 1934, and a Venetian Rococo settee of fanciful design.

Titus, as a journalist, would have been familiar with the American tradition of confidence tricksters, charlatans who hawk miracle wares, and with yellow journalism, the exaggerated claims and unabashed self-promotion associated with popular newspapers of the time. Hence the copy's assurance that Madame Rubinstein "does not pretend to 'wizardry' in her beauty-work." Ultimately, however, what so strongly compels attention in the ad is the image by Helleu, a French painter best known for his portraits of fashionable women of the Gilded Age. Rubinstein used her own beauty and charisma, and the skills of a contemporary artist, to promote her business. She is shown as radiantly youthful, her dark hair highlighting the pallor of her skin, in an artwork already seven years old.

By the time she settled in New York, Rubinstein was forty-two and had matured as both a businesswoman and a social figure. So it was a sophisticated, culturally conversant Madame Helena Rubinstein who set up shop on New York's fashionable East Side. The only serious competitor in town was Elizabeth Arden, who had soon relocated her Salon d'Oro, a suite of five rooms at 509 Fifth Avenue and 42nd Street, to 673 Fifth Avenue, as if she felt her turf had been intruded upon.[53] The fanfare that accompanied Madame's debut was considerable, with the press focusing more on her collection of art and *objets*, her European imprimatur, and the chic decor than on her beauty expertise. *Vogue* wrote: "The walls are covered with dark blue cloth, the skirting boards are deep rose pink, period mahogany furniture is upholstered in rose silk; and the sculptures are the work of a Russian, much praised in Paris."[54] The sculptures were actually those of Elie Nadelman, an expatriate Pole whose move to New York the previous year had been sponsored by Rubinstein.[55] Although her gesture was no doubt generous, she had also decided that her connection to the art world was to be part of the promotional plan for her salons.

Titus encouraged this, continuing to write ad copy for his wife, give her useful advice, and make connections for her to the Greenwich Village art world. Nevertheless, although Rubinstein depended heavily on her family to help run her expanding empire, their relationship was strained. Certainly she did not place her sons and their father above her work. That she was aware of the effects of her workaholism on her family she amply acknowledged in a letter to Titus:

> *I have had such a long siege of it, working like mad since I was eighteen, having to be in a dozen places at one time, always on guard to keep above water and seldom ever a resting time. I'm so weary of it all, yet what does the future hold for me but work? Perhaps I don't know how to play any more. I wonder if the boys will answer my need for consideration and understanding. Life hasn't held a great deal for me this far, but responsibility and work.*[56]

Madame's business, on the other hand, was proving to be anything but a failure. The bold decorative scheme of her salon, with its prominently featured art, contrasted vividly with the sedate decorating standards maintained by Arden, whose "sumptuous serenade" to the old money of Fifth Avenue continued in the same key. A photograph of Madame's 49th Street salon shows all the trappings of an inviting home—dining table and chairs, fireplace and mantel, even a window seat. The intersection of beauty, art, and design within a feminine, domestic environment was Rubinstein's signature (see page 73).

She had met Elie Nadelman four years earlier, in London, and had realized then that he would be the perfect artist to show in her salons.

53 After coming to New York in 1907, Elizabeth Graham became partners with Elizabeth Hubbard in 1909—a partnership that lasted only nine months. The facts surrounding their separation are unknown, but Graham soon changed her surname to Arden, and removed Hubbard's name from the shop.

54 "On Her Dressing Table," *Vogue* 45 (June 1915), 82, 84.

55 Press release for the exhibition "Elie Nadelman: Sculptor of Modern Life," Whitney Museum of American Art, New York, 2003.

56 Woodhead refers to the family as a "bizarre bunch," among whom tensions ran high: "Horace, for example, didn't see eye-to-eye with his brother Roy, and simply loathed his cousin Oscar, a feeling which was mutual. Madame on the other hand liked Oscar very much. Roy cared little for his brother, and even less for his mother, from whom he was virtually estranged, seeking solace in the company of his wives; his mother apparently liked neither daughter-in-law one, two, three *or* four very much. Roy hardly spoke to his father or his stepmother; Horace did, but Helena of course did not. As far as her sisters were concerned, Helena was not particularly close to Erna, was virtually estranged from Manka, constantly at loggerheads with Stella, and was irritated by Ceska. All of the sisters were terrified of Helena. Various cousins kept their heads down and got on with their work." Woodhead, *War Paint*, 158, 246.

A sculptor concerned above all with style, Nadelman claimed for his new work a modernist ethos, "a new life which had nothing to do with nature."[57] Yet it had a quality that Madame found fascinating: a stylishness that was timeless but abstract enough to be called modern. Nadelman specialized in a mannered interpretation of classical Greek sculpture—heads, figures, and horses—expressing a historicism tweaked by a twentieth-century sensibility informed by irony and humor. The mix sparked Madame's enthusiasm; in 1911 she had bought his entire show at Paterson's Gallery in London (see page 74). Perhaps she saw in his amalgam of sources—from classical to Asian to Egyptian to American folk art—a nonhierarchical aesthetic interpretation of the blended styles that she aimed to integrate into her homes and salons.

With Nadelman's bas-relief *Two Nudes* prominently mounted above the fireplace and his bronze *Reclining Nude* providing contrapuntal balance on the mantelpiece, it was not just "the dark blue fabric on the walls and deep-rose painted baseboards" that created an atmosphere of luxurious taste, but the integration of art into the environment. The expressive use of color and design was no less important than the rouge and powder applied to women's faces in the salon. In 1921 Madame reprinted her initial ad, her portrait by Helleu now filling nearly half a page in *Vogue* and captioned thus: "The image here reproduced is that of Madame Helena Rubinstein by the great Parisian artist, Helleu, now visiting the country. The portrait was made several years ago in Madame Rubinstein's world-famous salon in Paris."[58]

Almost from the beginning, Rubinstein's salons offered more than hairdressing or a manicure, with treatments for the skin, hair, eyes, and body, as well as classes in deportment. They were often large establishments, with a variety of facilities. A 1928 advertisement for the opening of Maisons de Beauté in New York and Chicago boasted, "Here, in treatment alcoves, rest rooms, and gymnasiums, superlatively hygienic and exotically beautiful, you will find every service for cultivating beauty of face, gracefulness of form and charm of hands and hair."[59]

By the 1930s, the Rubinstein salon experience had become even more lavish. She developed a concept of total indulgence called "A Day of Beauty," luxurious but affordable. This devotion of an entire "rapturous" day chez Helena Rubinstein began with a physical examination by a resident doctor to determine "just where your figure needs reducing, where building up." Then, if desired, one was brought breakfast, followed by a "custom-made" workout, made bearable by a subsequent "made-to-measure massage on the Sana-Therm table." Next, one was off to the Sun-Ray Clinique for a sun bath on a bed of sand under a shimmering ceiling of ultraviolet rays, with a cool drink in hand. A Beautylift Masque, "made of specially treated pink silk, [is] dipped in a special lotion, then fitted to the basic muscle structure of the face and throat. As it dries, the masque braces the contours, tightens and firms flabby spots. An adjustable nose piece helps to smooth out expression lines under the eyes." The morning phase concluded in a "foamy" Pasteurized Milk Bath, in which "compressed air forced into a milk preparation provides the bubbles and makes the bathwater ripple. The mask is a special device for restoring youthful contours."

Luncheon was then provided in the salon's Zurich Room, where Madame's "matière vivante," or menu of energizing orchard fruit and garden vegetables was presented. Such a healthy and delicious dietetic array was intended to inspire. Following this beauty break, serious attention was given to one's face and hair; after a shampoo and scalp massage, hair

57 Nadelman had prepared a statement to accompany an exhibition of his drawings at Alfred Stieglitz's gallery 291 in New York. The drawings had to be sent back to London for an exhibition at Paterson's Gallery in April 1911. Stieglitz, however, published Nadelman's text in *Camera Work* 32 (October 1910), 41.

58 *Vogue* 57 (May 1921): 107. Marie Clifford expressed it well: "It let Rubinstein's customers know that the artist rendered the picture in the beautician's Paris salon, effectively transposing her beauty parlor with the artist's studio"; see her "Helena Rubinstein's Beauty Salons, Fashion, and Modernist Display," *Winterthur Portfolio* 38, no. 2/3 (Summer–Autumn 2003): 88.

59 Advertisement, *Vogue* 71, no. 2 (January 15, 1928): 99.

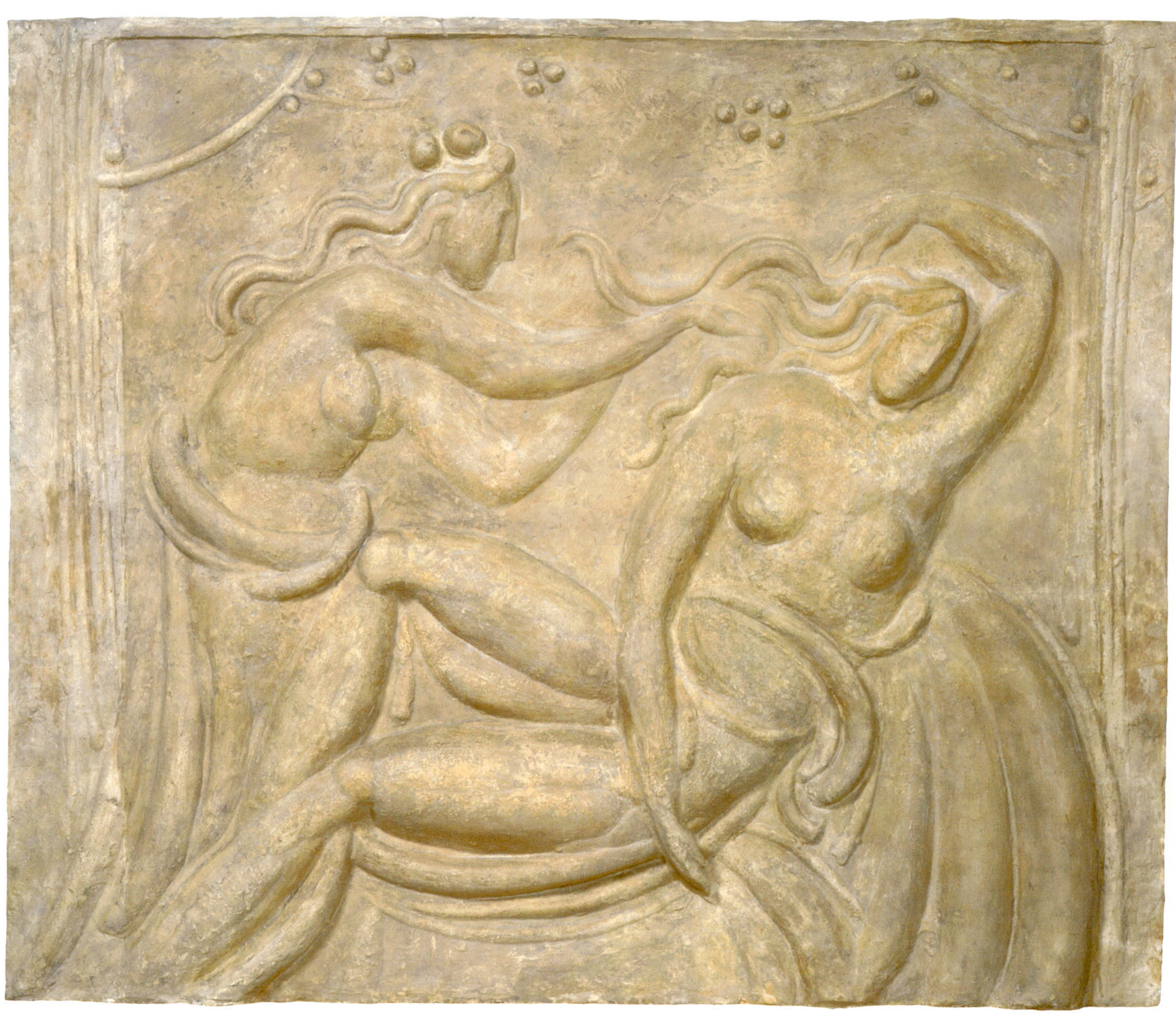

Elie Nadelman
Two Nudes, c. 1911
Plaster, 47⅞ × 58¾ × 3¾ in. (121.6 × 149.2 × 9.5 cm)
National Gallery of Art, Washington, DC
Gift of Robert P. and Arlene R. Kogod

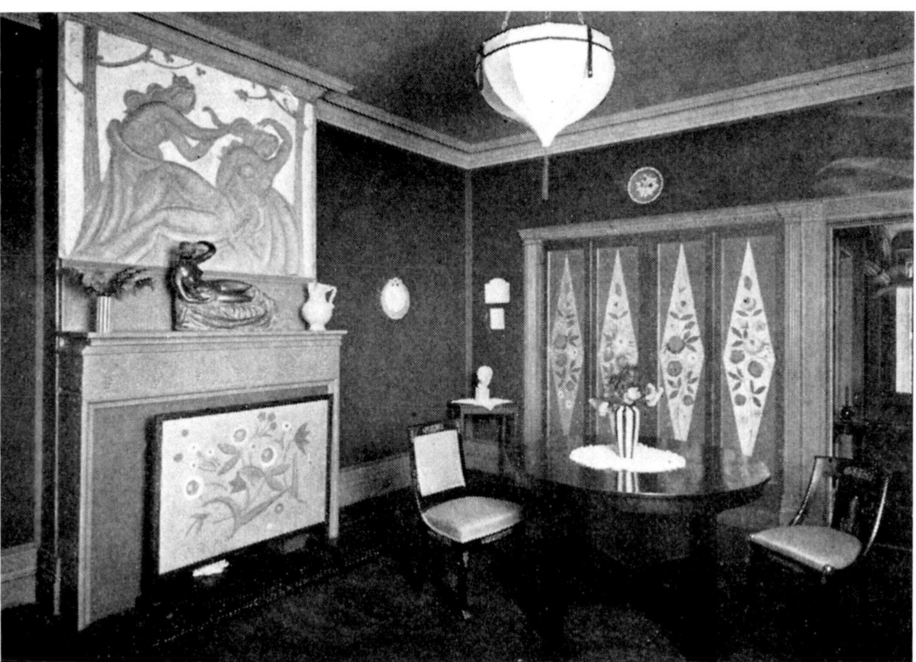

Helena Rubinstein's first New York salon, the Maison de Beauté Valaze, at 15 East 49th Street, in a photograph published in "Beauty Bought and Paid For," *Vogue*, November 15, 1915. Above the mantel is Elie Nadelman's plaster frieze *Two Nudes*, which Rubinstein moved to many different locations over the years. *Below*: In a class in the library at the 715 Fifth Avenue salon (established in 1936), Rubinstein's niece Mala demonstrates how to massage around the eyes to avoid crow's feet. Nadelman's frieze is mounted on the wall.

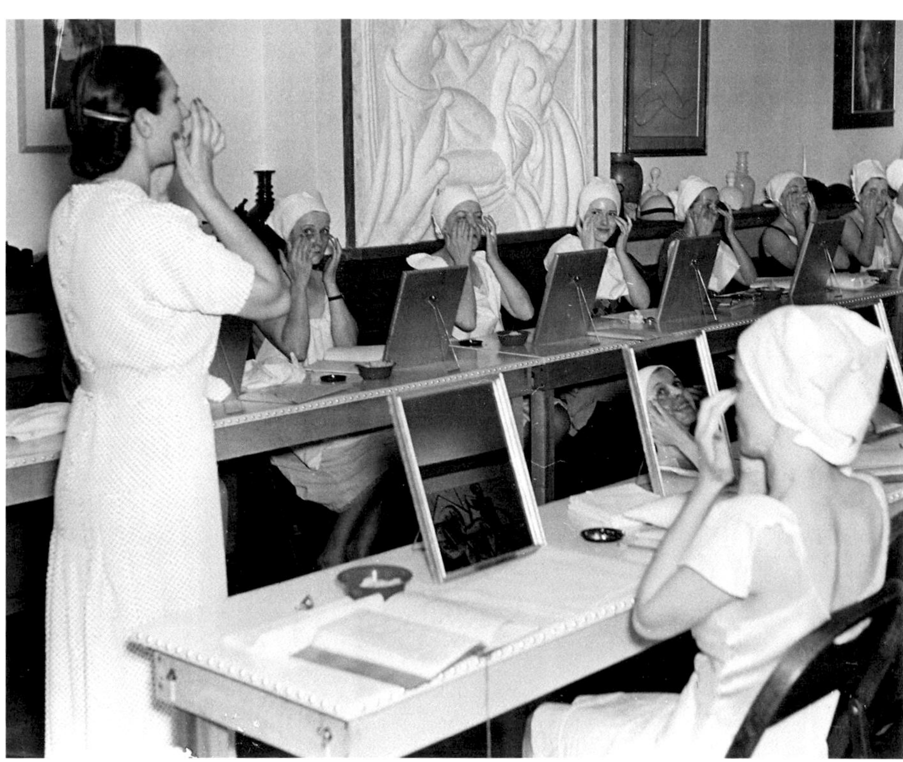

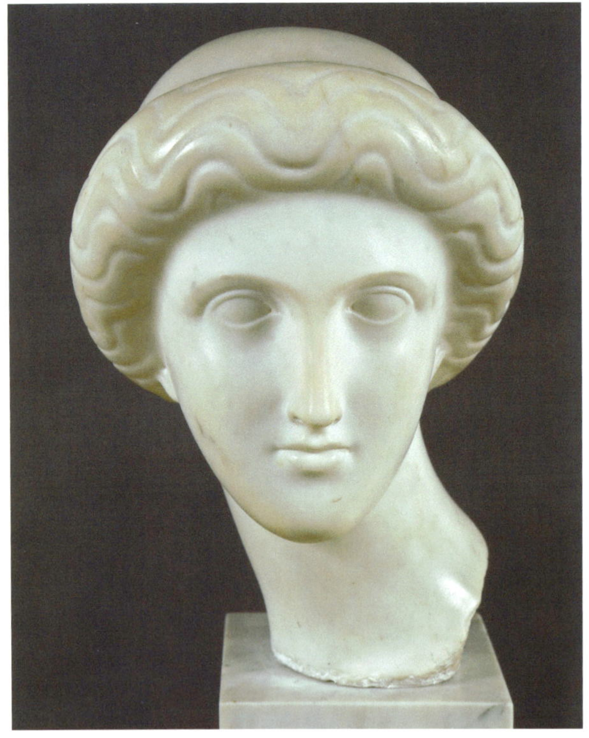

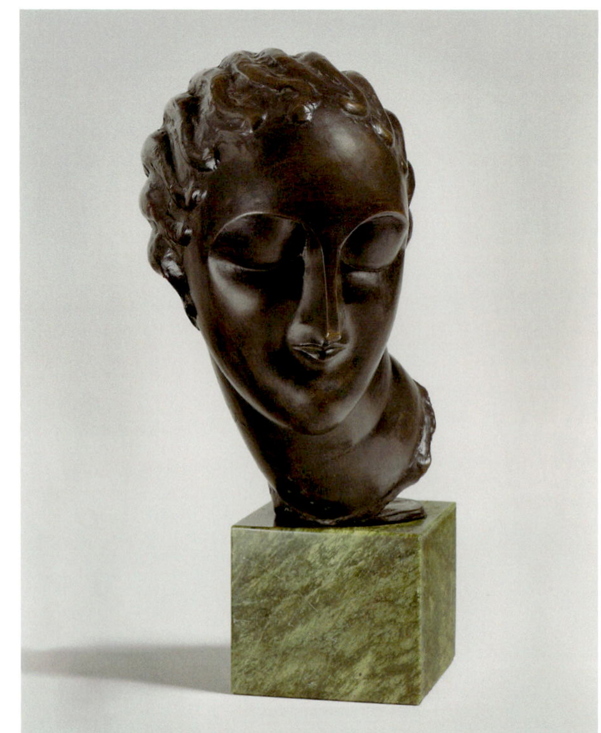

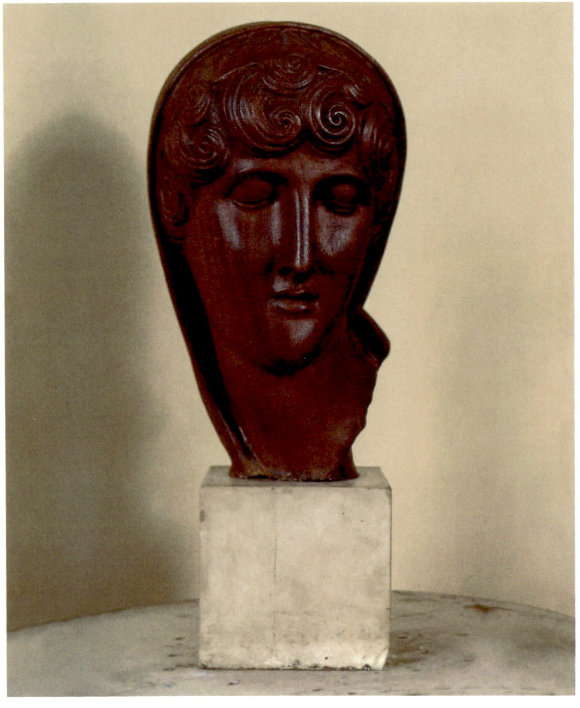

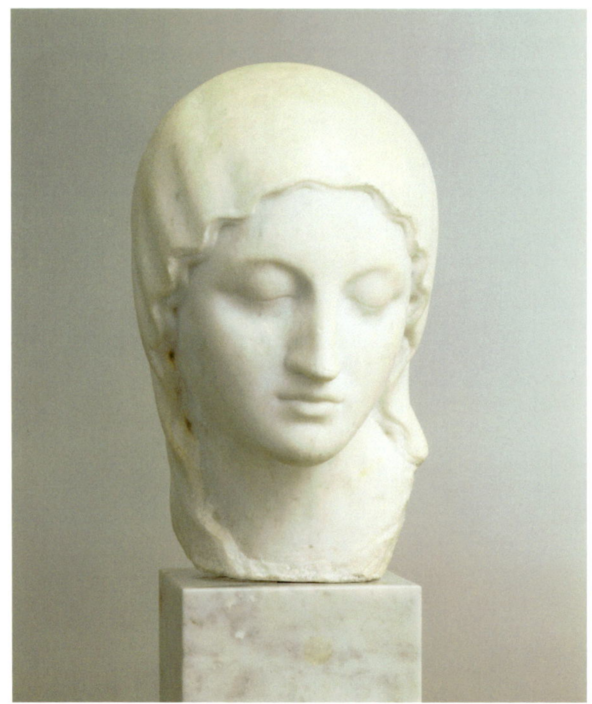

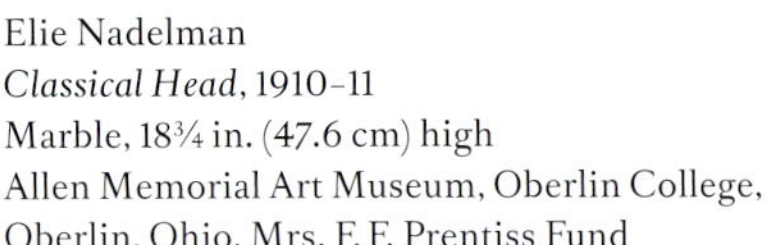

Elie Nadelman
Classical Head, 1910–11
Marble, 18¾ in. (47.6 cm) high
Allen Memorial Art Museum, Oberlin College, Oberlin, Ohio, Mrs. F. F. Prentiss Fund

Elie Nadelman
Hooded Head of a Woman, c. 1916–17
Wood, 15½ in. (39.4 cm) high
Collection of Suzanne Slesin and Michael Steinberg

Elie Nadelman
Head of a Woman, c. 1907–8
Bronze on marble base, 13½ in. (34.3 cm) high
Hirshhorn Museum and Sculpture Garden, Smithsonian Institution, Washington, DC, Gift of Joseph H. Hirshhorn, 1966

Elie Nadelman
Head of a Girl, c. 1909
Marble, 14 in. (35.6 cm) high
Daniel Wolf and Mathew D. Wolf in memory of Diane R. Wolf

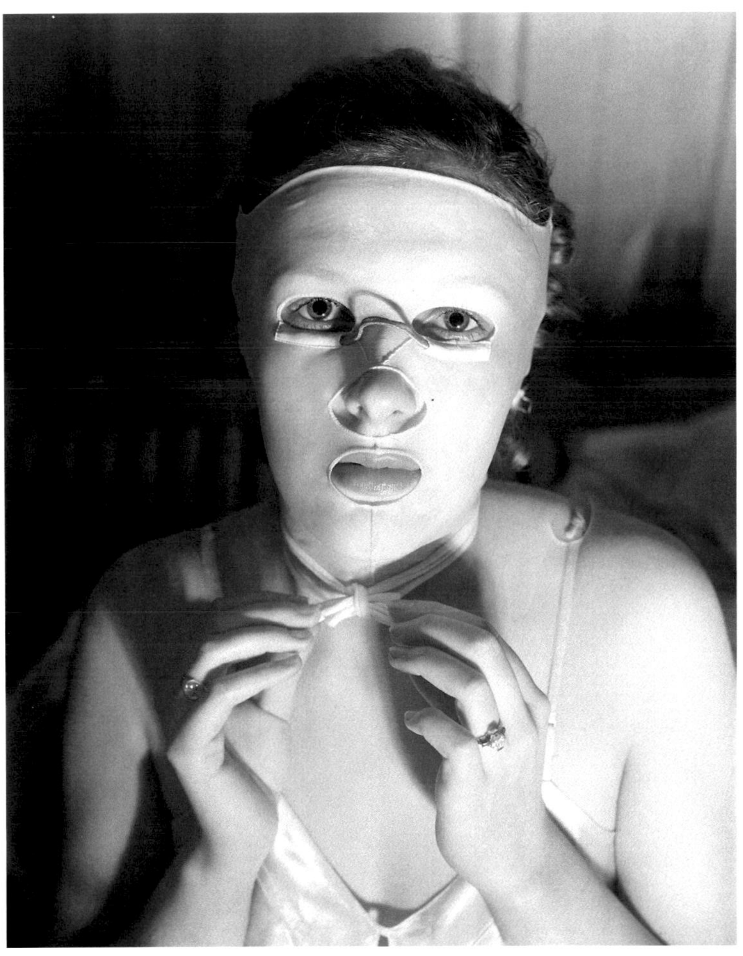

Occasionally, Rubinstein's publicity images bordered on the bizarre. The Beautylift Masque, one of her invented treatments, was "designed to lift sagging, relaxed contours upward and youthward."

was cut and styled, while a manicure and pedicure were administered, with more soothing massage. One was then ready for the famous customized Face Treatment with Rubinstein's celebrated creams, and the final rapture was achieved by a talented makeup artist who brought out the best in one's face, providing the "end of the line and a new lease on self-esteem."[60]

For those not near a salon, the products were always available in shops and sometimes by mail. The Rubinstein print advertisements made a point of proffering guidance to any and all women, and often struck a distinctive personal note. Whether it was Madame's image, presented as a work of art (see page 59), or her signature at the bottom of the page, there was always the sense that she was addressing the reader directly. (One ad showed her on the back of a camel, visiting North Africa, supposedly to study how the "science of the West" could learn from the "secrets of the East"; see page 80.) Many of her ads were didactic, offering advice on self-improvement and inviting the reader to correspond with questions—all such inquiries would be readily answered. With a provincial earnestness, some told stories.

Over time, the advertisements became more modern and designed. In about 1928 Rubinstein commissioned the Bauhaus artist Herbert Bayer to create a striking ad for her Clinique de Beauté in Paris. He produced a futuristic image of a disembodied woman's face with an intent stare emerging from a geometric Art Moderne ground. By the 1950s the image said it all: a 1957 ad for Circulotion Mask shows a woman holding a surreal mask of her own transformed face with eyes askance. In a sixties ad for the scent Emotion, dizzying swirls of black and white speak equally of romance, high fashion, and Op art. Perhaps most arresting is a 1953 ad for a perfume called Fourth Dimension, featuring two paintings from Rubinstein's personal art collection, Joan Miró's *Portrait*, 1927, and Willem de Kooning's *Elegy*, 1939. In the foreground modernist bottles with radical mid-century shapes echo the sensuous physicality of the chic "high key, exciting" couple in the background (see pages 81–86).

Commissioning Modernism

Always ready to listen to good advice, Madame had hired an old acquaintance of Nadelman's from Paris, the Hungarian Jewish designer Paul T. Frankl, who had studied architecture in Vienna and Berlin, to design the interiors of her 49th Street salon. While the new salon had caught the fancy of critics, she had requested that it remain traditional.[61] As a businesswoman, she was shrewd enough to know that her innovative "maison de beauté," her "foreign" cachet, and her introduction of art into such a

60 "Along the Line in a Glamor Factory," March 2, 1937, photograph caption, Acme / Corbis.

61 Christopher Long, *Paul T. Frankl and Modern American Design* (New Haven: Yale University Press, 2007), 31.

Rubinstein's salons offered an array of beauty and health treatments, including the Derma-Lens skin treatment, ultraviolet sun bath, foaming milk bath, and Hormone Heat Masque. Classes were available for both clients and sales staff from department stores throughout the United States and Canada. The photographs on these pages and page 78 are from 1935–41.

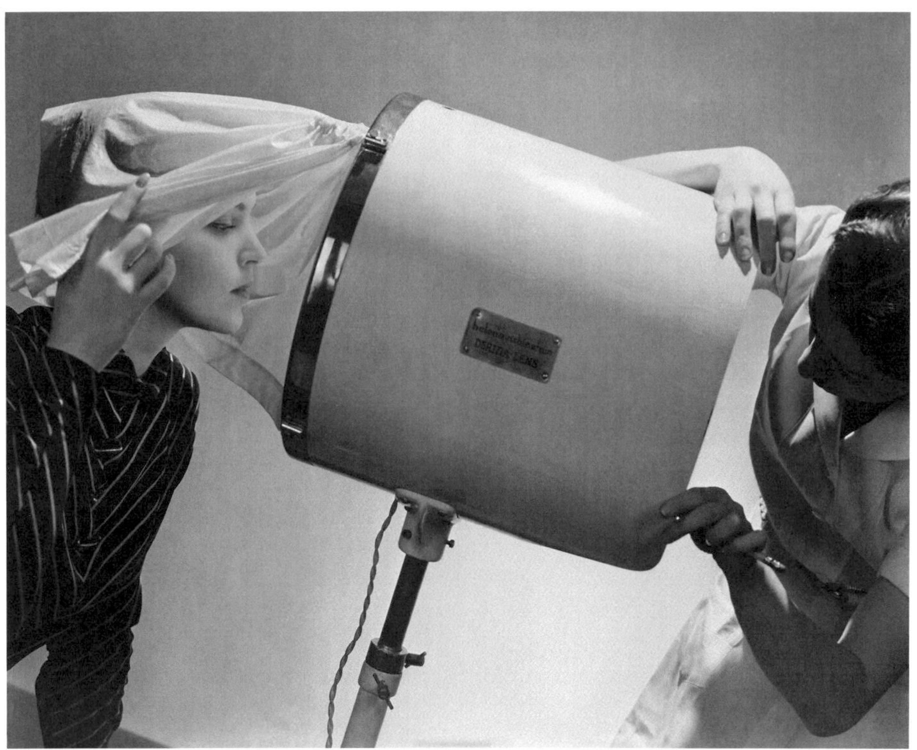

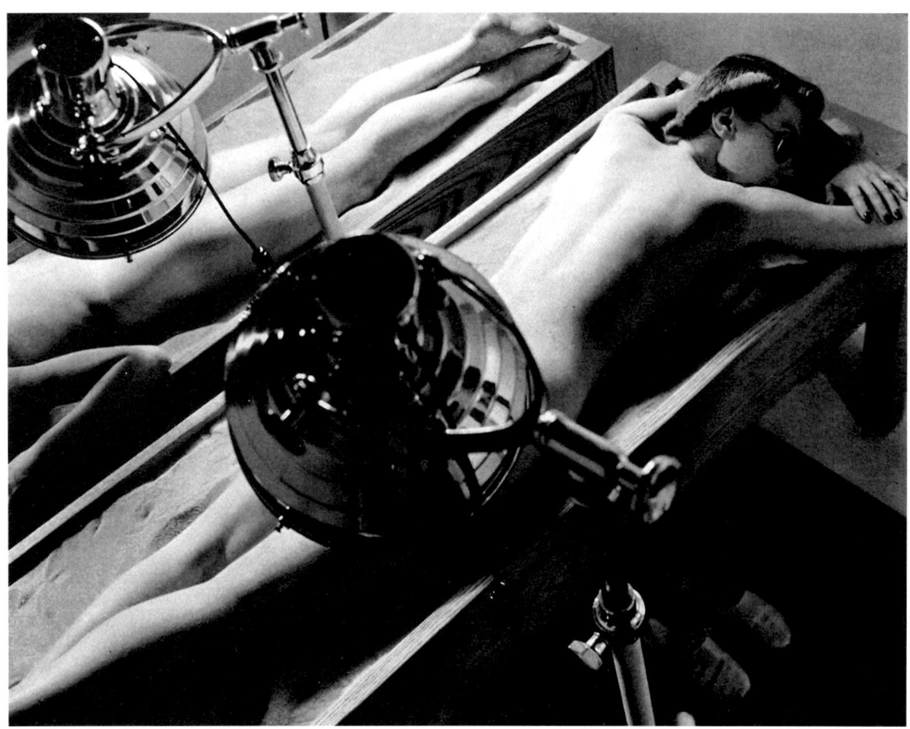

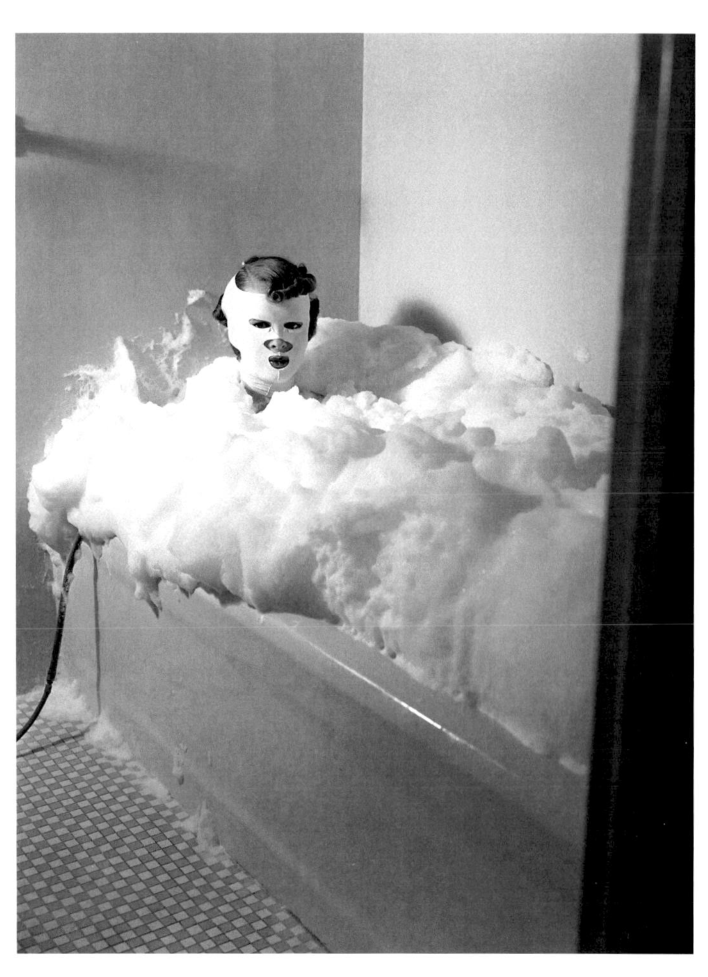

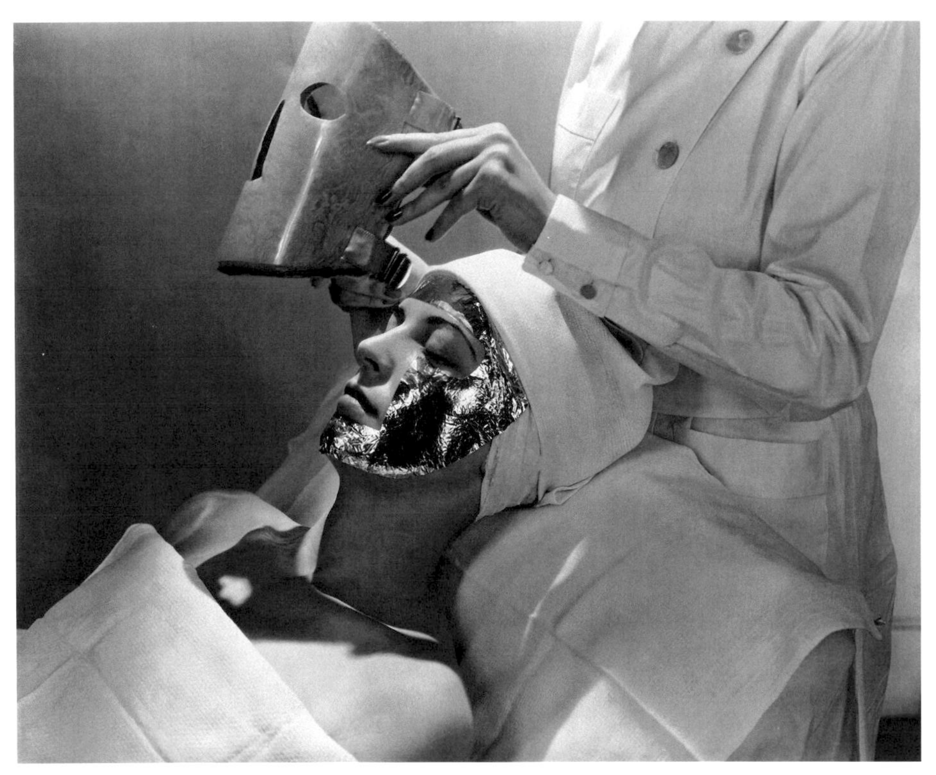

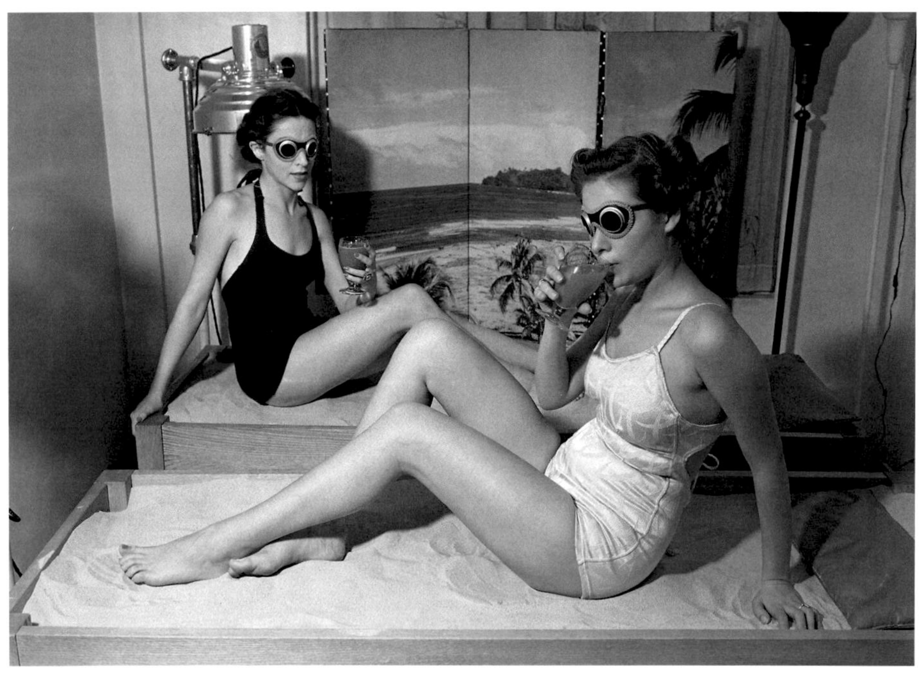

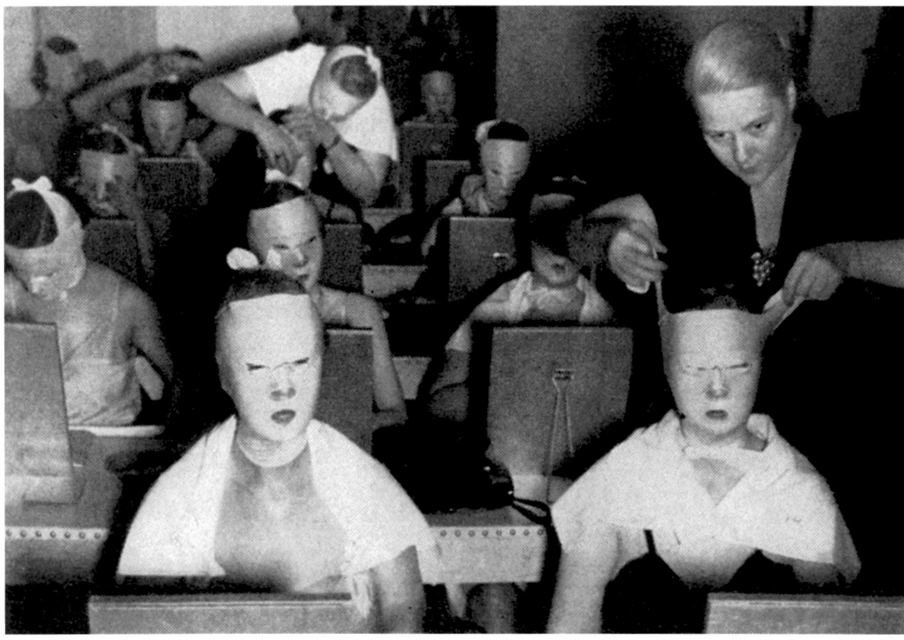

Opposite: "Beauty as a Duty," a 1918 advertisement, published during World War I, suggests that beauty culture serves the war effort. The Valaze label was taken from an Italian Renaissance portrait of a lady by Ambrogio de Predis, which Rubinstein has doubled, so that two women look at each other, or a woman looks at herself. Over the years the image was revised numerous times (see page 127).

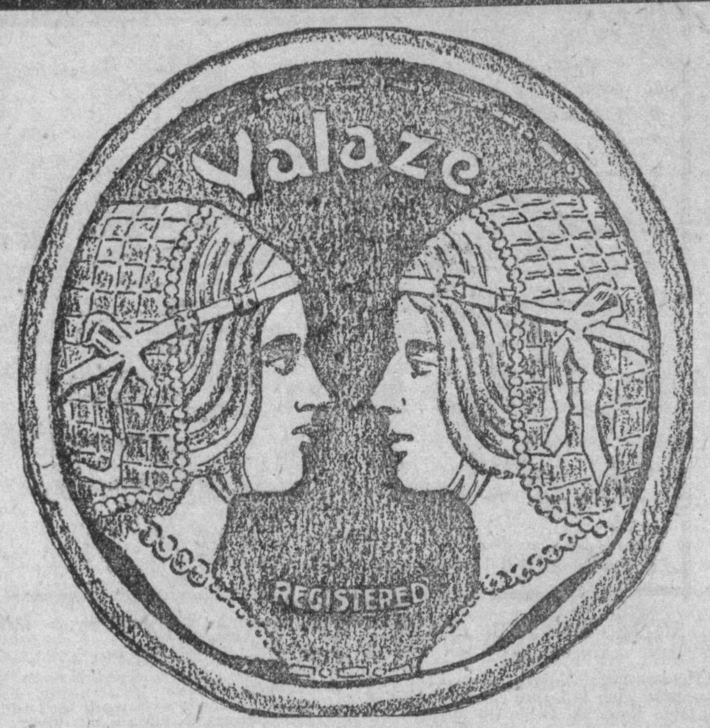

Beauty as a Duty

It is a woman's duty at the present time to further the cause of the Allies. There is another duty, however, which is sometimes classed as an extravagance. It is the duty of Beauty. The husband, brother, or friend, after the horrors of war, deserves to be surrounded with brightness and beauty, which cheers and heartens—not by depressing unattractiveness.

The woman who seeks to "make the best of herself" should make certain that her Beauty Culture combines EFFICACY and ECONOMY. For these two virtues Madame Rubinstein's Valaze Complexion Remedies are world-famed. Full particulars and descriptive lists will be sent on application. No charge is made for consultations or advice by post.

Mme. Rubinstein recommends the following Home Treatments:—

To Refine and Whiten a Coarse Skin. Those whose skin is coarse and greasy should take immediate steps to remedy it, for such a skin is always susceptible to other blemishes, such as blackheads and open pores. The Face should be washed with Valaze Beauty Grains, 2/10 posted, the very latest discovery for refining and whitening the skin, and these may be alternated with Valaze Blackhead and Open Pore Cure, 2/10 posted. The use of these two specialities and an application of Valaze Skinfood every night, 3/6, posted 6d., will keep the face fresh and clear, and entirely free from any appearance of coarseness or greasiness.

A Flabby, Wrinkled Skin. This state of the skin will gradually yield to judicious treatment, particularly when begun in time, and it is most important that it should be taken in time, as nothing is more ageing. The wonderful Eau Qui Pique should be applied to the face. Eau Qui Pique, as its name implies, gives a prickling, tingling sensation to the skin, and is the most effective astringent preparation of the day. It banishes puffiness, flabbiness, and moderates wrinkles, restoring at the same time freshness and colour to the skin. Price 5/6, 10/6, and 21/.

Have You a Smooth, White Neck? This is really essential to most women, especially just now when fashion demands that we should all wear low-necked dresses. The skin of the neck is exceedingly apt to turn brown and to show signs of discoloration, due chiefly to the friction of collars and furs. To remove this resource must be had to the Extra Strong Valaze, one of Madam Rubinstein's latest remedies. The Extra Strong Valaze will clear the skin and make it clear from this blemish. The price is 11/ posted.

For Redness of Nose and Cheeks. For home treatment, the use of the Novena Red Nose Ointment and Powder, as well as Valaze Liquidine, are recommended as the first resort. In the more advanced stages of the trouble, when small vein-like vessels become noticeable, home treatment is more difficult, and more radical treatment should be taken at the Valaze Massage Institute. The price of the Novena Red Nose Ointment and Powder is 8/6, postage 6d., and the Liquidine is 5/, 8/6, postage 6d.

Beauty Massage. If there is anything in the whole of Beauty Culture which one can truthfully say that is a "natural remedy" it is massage. The Valaze Massagette is a new, wonderful invention for home use. It improves the appearance of the skin; it overcomes blemishes of the complexion; it sets up a greater activity of the tissues; it increases the circulation, and produces fresh colour. The price of the Massagette is 21/ and 25/. VALAZE MASSAGE ROLLERS form a very simple remedy for the removal of wrinkles, double chin, and excess of the flesh about the face. Used with Valaze or Novena Cerate, the benefit that accrues is most marked. Prices, Single Roller, 8/6; Set of Two, in case, 18/6; Set of Three, in case, 25/.

Care of the Hair. The most frequent cause of loss of hair is excessive activity of the scalp's fat-secreting glands. One of the consequences of this condition is dandruff. Profuse falling out and thinning of the hair, fragility, and lack of lustre, discoloration, and dandruff are now very common affections amongst women. By the use of Dr. Lykuski's Hair Tonic the care of the hair is made at once pleasant and effective. It goes to the root of all hair troubles, produces natural growth where the process is sluggish. Price of the tonic is 4/ posted.

A Pretty, Natural Colour may be imparted to cheeks that have become drab and pallid by the use of the Valaze Crushed Rose Leaves, a new and delightful colouring for the face, composed of the pulp of roses. This preparation reproduces natural tints to perfection, and does not betray even the slightest trace of artificiality. To lips that have become dull and lifeless, Valaze Lip Lustre will restore the full and rich lip colour. Valaze Lip Lustre protects the delicate outer membrane of the lip from cracks and chaps, and is the best cure for such afflictions. Price 2/6, Special 4/. The price of the Valaze Crushed Rose Leaves is 5/6, 10/6, and postage 3d.

Protection from Cold and Wind, Before going out a little Baume Verte should be applied to the face and powder dusted over it. This will protect the skin from the ill-effects of the weather. The Baume Verte is 5/6, 10/6, postage 6d.; the Valaze Powder is 2/, 3/, and 5/6, postage 3d.

Beauty in the Making. Mme. Helena Rubinstein's clever treatise on the scientific care of the complexion and hair will be read with interest by every woman who has her appearance at heart. A copy will be sent to any address on receipt of 3d. for postage.

Pause Before Powdering. Use discrimination when buying powders or complexion-ruin will follow. If your skin is greasy, over-moist, or shiny, use Valaze Complexion Powder; if it is dry or normal, use Novena Poudre, these preparations being specially prepared to suit the different conditions. They are famous the world over, and are not only beautifying, but protective. Prices, each 2/, 3/, and 5/6, postage 3d.

VALAZE PREPARATIONS Obtainable all Chemists or direct from

HELENA RUBINSTEIN Pty. Ltd., Dept. T.

274 Collins Street, Melbourne
24 Grafton Street, London, W.
255 Rue St. Honore, Paris
15 East 49th Street, New York.

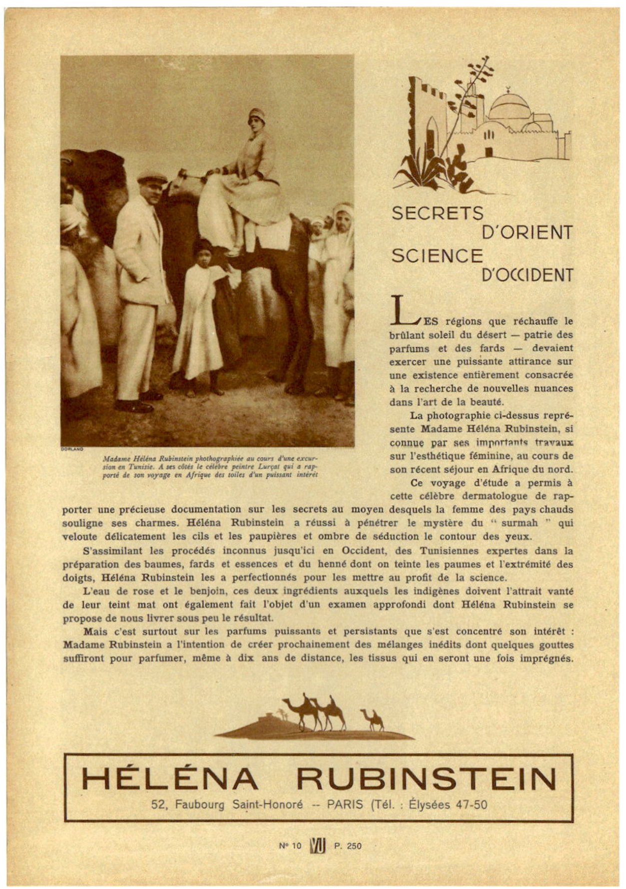

In an advertisement from c. 1921 Rubinstein presents herself as "entirely dedicated to searching for new nuances in the art of beauty." She has made a research trip to North Africa, "land of perfumes and cosmetics," accompanied by the artist Jean Lurçat. There she has discovered "the secrets used by women in hot climates to emphasize their charms. Helena Rubinstein has succeeded in penetrating the mystery of the 'Surma'"; Tunisian women are "experts in the preparation of balms, cosmetics, and essences," which she "has perfected for the benefit of science."

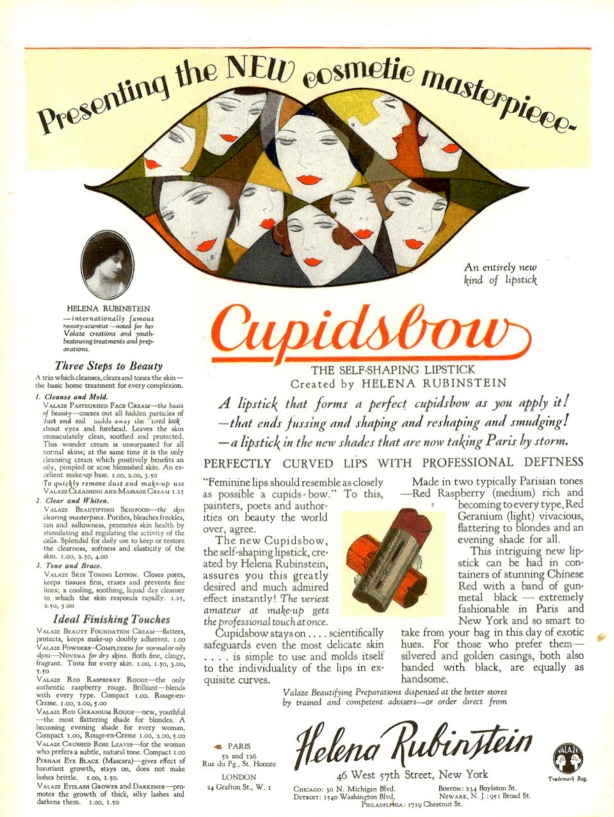

By 1926, when this advertisement appeared in *Harper's Bazaar*, lipstick was no longer scandalous, and bright red shades were in vogue. Using the language of the art connoisseur, Rubinstein produced a "new cosmetic masterpiece": the Cupidsbow "self-shaping" lipstick. Shaped like a tiny pair of lips, it was designed to be pressed to the pursed mouth in a single deft gesture.

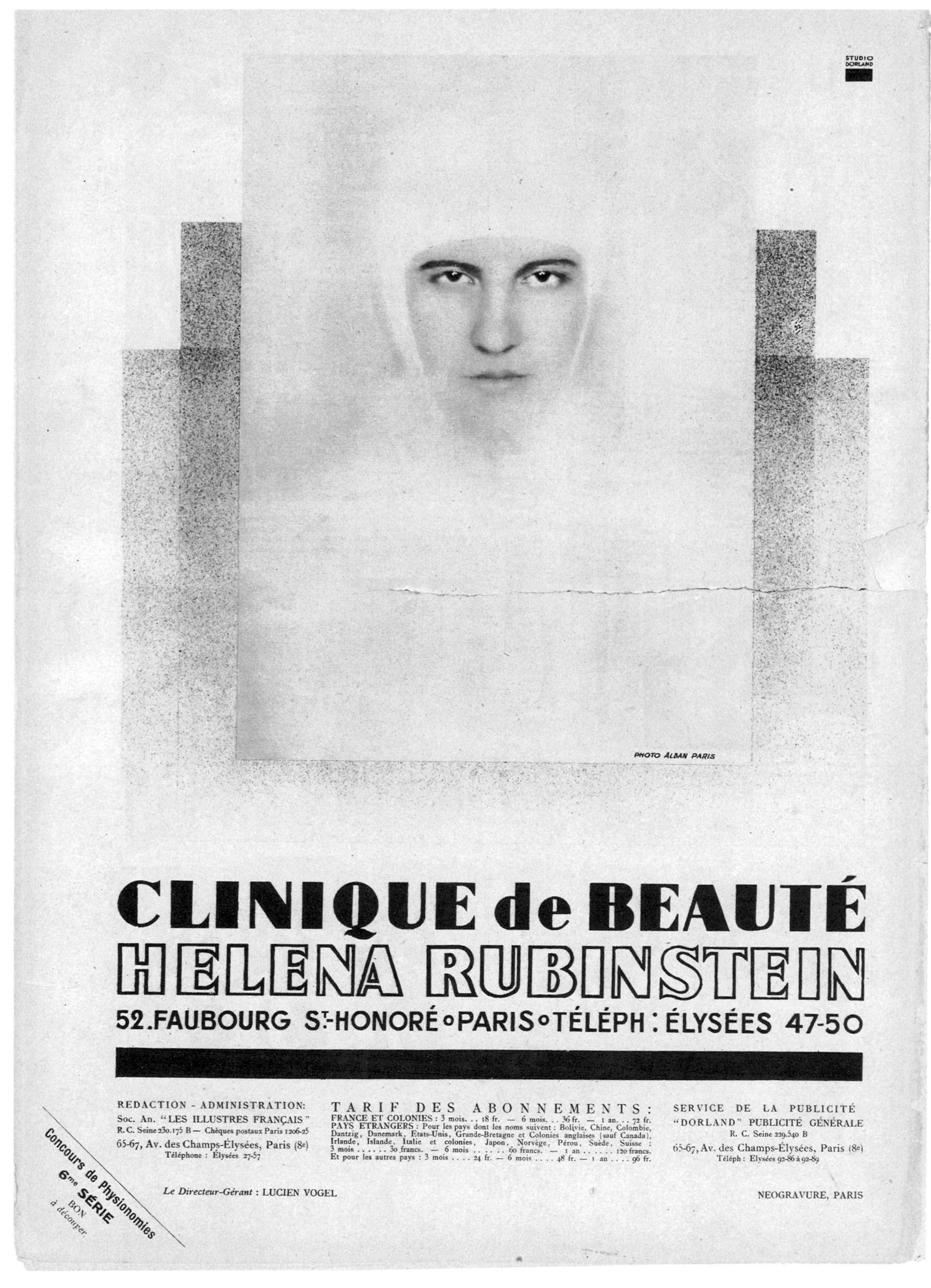

In 1928 Studio Dorland, a well-established advertising agency, hired the Bauhaus designer Herbert Bayer as artistic director. Bayer introduced an aesthetic attuned equally to industry and art, and developed a visual commercial language that emphasized new technologies, such as the photomontage seen here. This medically swathed and isolated face presciently anticipates the extremes to which future women would go to change their appearance.

Overleaf: An advertisement from 1930 displays a suite of Art Deco products, including the square "Cubist Lipstick."

ENCHANTING NEW of PARISIAN CHIC

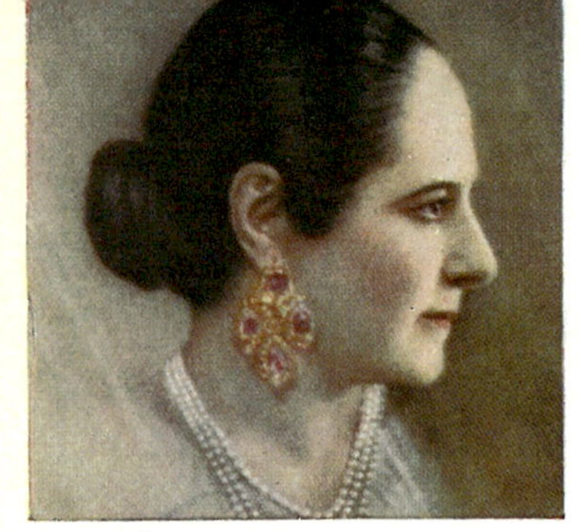

MADAME HELENA RUBINSTEIN
World Famous Beauty Authority

SOFT, clinging powders . . . brilliant rouges . . . lipsticks provocatively gay . . . all born of the genius of Helena Rubinstein! And how fitting their exquisite new cases—cases as patrician as the slim, tapering fingers which are destined to hold them.

Each enchanting cosmetic seems to crystalize the rare talent of the world's foremost beauty specialist! Smart enough to accompany the newest ensemble, distinctive enough to grace the most fastidious handbag! And the colors, the lovely glowing colors . . . now blending, now daring to contrast . . . are as young, as blithe, as romantic as Spring!

Once you have seen these Parisian cosmetics for yourself, you will realize that the greatest values in all beautydom are here for your choosing! Certainly no one else in the world could so startlingly combine chic with moderate cost! But Helena Rubinstein is constantly on the qui vive for new ideas . . . originations . . . variations of beauty's theme. And in these exquisite new items created for the beauty-loving women of Europe and America, she reaches new heights of brilliant achievement!

The same artistry . . . the same scientific skill . . . the same background of experience which have made possible her remarkable creams and lotions, go into the making of Helena Rubinstein's delightful cosmetics to render them not only flattering but pure and safe for you!

As your own cherished possessions, as fascinating gifts or prizes, these newest creations leave nothing to be desired! For the pleasure and assurance of correctness which one derives from gowns by Lanvin or inimitable little hats by Carolyn Reboux . . . one gains in like measure from these enchanting cosmetics by Helena Rubinstein.

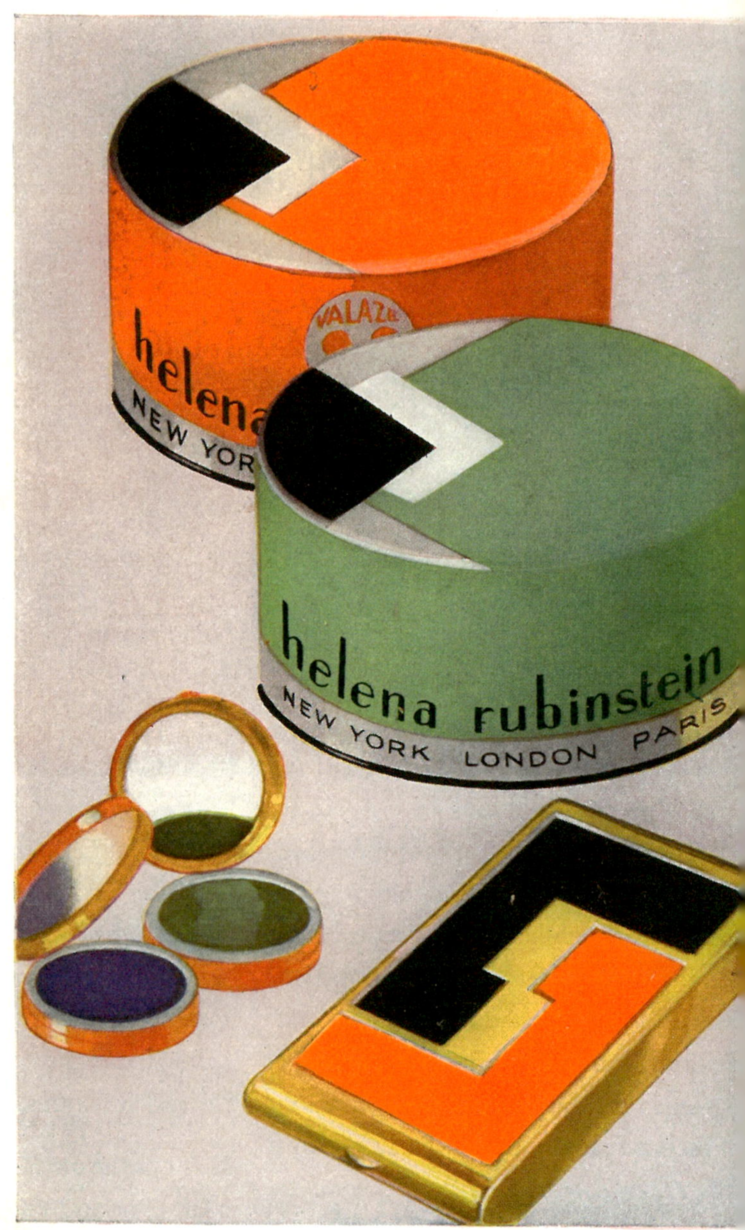

Exquisite New Valaze Face Powders

These vivid new powder boxes will lend distinction to smartest dressing-table. And the minute you lift off the c you will be captivated by the subtle fragrance of the lo Valaze powder within! So delicate . . . yet it will cling for h to your skin in a fragrant, invisible film! In the *jade* box, Nov powder for dry skin . . . in the *vermillion*, Complexion pov for normal or oily skins. Featuring a complete color rang blend with every type—from the palest Nordic to the dee sun-bronzed skin. $1.00 . . . without question the most sig cant value in exquisite face powders ever offered!

COSMETICS . . . TRIUMPHS . . . by HELENA RUBINSTEIN

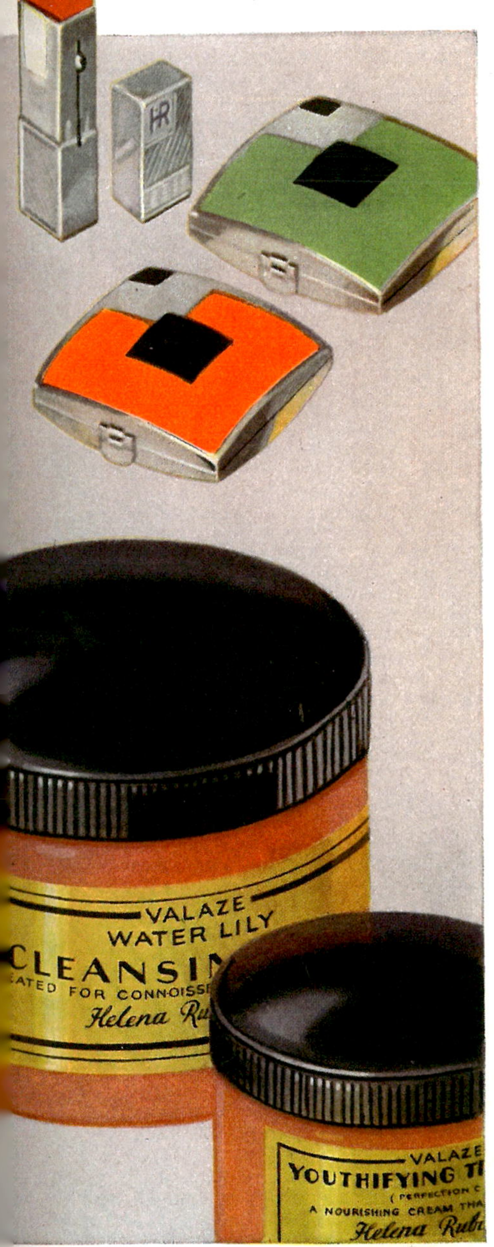

harming New ouge Compacts

n *vermillion* or *jade* vith intriguing modern motif . . . (beside he silver lipstick) . . . adorably designed o match the new powder boxes! And hese gay rouge compacts in their slim, win cases contain the desired shade of elena Rubinstein's famous rouges to omplement one's natural coloring, the ccasion and the costume . . . $1.25 each!

The Modern Triple Vanity

With its smart, exotic modern design, this colorful expression of Helena Rubinstein's art is really enchanting enough for a princess . . . and its price a source of amazement to every woman who has seen it! Containing the most wanted shades of powder and rouge . . . a lipstick, too, cunningly concealed in the hinge . . . but 2.50 complete!

The Newest French Lipstick

At last, the superlative in lipsticks, ENCHANTÉ in its stunning silver case! Vivid as a crimson flower. Indelible, of course, and fragrant as a memory! Vivante, blonde or brunette—3.50.

The CUBIST LIPSTICK—for those who prefer a lipstick exceedingly smart but less expensive —in black or gold colored case . . . as trim and enticing as the gay debutantes who choose it! Non-drying, indelible, in lovely day or evening shades. Every purse will welcome its smartness and appreciate its price—1.00.

The Chic Enchanté Compact

. . . is more than a compact! For it comes in a box which boasts six tiny packages of Helena Rubinstein powder in six delightfully varying shades. The compact itself contains compact rouge and a loose powder compartment so that one may fill it with powder in the shade which suits one's ensemble for any occasion 3.00—complete.

Eye Enhancements

VALAZE EYE SHADOW en crème, smoothed over your eyelids, will deepen the color of your eyes and make them more alluring, more softly mysterious than you ever dreamed they could be! In blue, brown, blue-green, green or black to correspond with the shade of your eyes. The little Chinese red cases will slip into the smallest handbag yet the 1.00 size will last and last!

PERSIAN EYEBLACK *(Mascara)* will make your eyelashes appear silky and luxuriant. This does not make the lashes brittle and will stay on as long as you want it to. Leather-like cases, as smart as they are practical, in Chinese red or jet black—tiny brush and all—1.50.

Two Favorite Creams

WATER LILY CLEANSING CREAM, Helena Rubinstein's luxury cleanser, presents itself in all the elegance of its new rose-and-black jar! Rare herbs and the youth-renewing essence of water lily buds are the precious ingredients in this rejuvenating cream—2.50, 4.00, 7.50.

YOUTHIFYING TISSUE CREAM, a remarkable new preparation which is already causing a sensation on two continents! A richly nourishing cream, so beauty-bestowing, no woman over twenty can afford to be without it—2.00, 3.50, 6.00.

Fashion's Last Word

To be chic in every detail, one's face, arms and legs should harmonize in a vibrant health glow for the active months to come! So Helena Rubinstein chose four enchanting "Sunplexion" shades of powder for the outdoor woman (Mauresque for pale or medium blondes, Gypsy Tan for golden blondes, Ochre for medium brunettes, Dixie Tan for dark brunettes) . . . which Onyx, leading stocking manufacturers, have correlated in lovely gossamer-sheer hosiery. A sample of Helena Rubinstein powder is enclosed with each pair of Sunplexion Hosiery.

Consultation and Expert Advice

Helena Rubinstein's famous Salons de Beauté strategically located in metropolitan centers, are the rendezvous of smart women everywhere.

Regardless of where you buy your preparations, you are cordially invited to visit the Salons for expert advice and written instructions designating the correct preparations for you to purchase at your favorite store.

Helena Rubinstein takes a personal interest in the individual problems of those who seek her advice through correspondence.

Helena Rubinstein

8 EAST 57th STREET NEW YORK

PARIS · LONDON · TORONTO · CHICAGO
PHILADELPHIA · BOSTON · DETROIT

Helena Rubinstein's world-famous beauty preparations are obtainable at the better department and drug stores in U. S., Canada and Europe.

"DON'T GUESS – KNOW – YOUR BEST COLORS!"

RED VELVET
PINK CHAMPAGNE
RED RASPBERRY
COCHINELLE
PINK CHAMPAGNE
ORCHID RED
APPLE RED
RED VELVET

...and now, Helena Rubinstein, far-famed color and beauty authority, tells you how to wear colors, in make-up and fashions—with the assurance that they are *right* for *you*.

In the light of actual scientific relationships, she has evolved individual COLOR-SPECTROGRAPHS, to call forth all the beauty of the blonde, brunette, redhead, medium-brown and silver-gray types.

Write Helena Rubinstein, 715 Fifth Ave., Dept. 5, for your personal COLOR-SPECTROGRAPH, which actually places in your hands 32 timely fashion colors and the perfect lipstick and make-up shades for you. Merely specify your hair-type.

Fabrics shown in this advertisement, courtesy of The Forstmann Woolen Co.

Helena Rubinstein

Copyright 1945, Helena Rubinstein, Inc.

An advertisement from 1945 invites a woman to choose her color palette as if decorating an interior with sample fabric swatches.

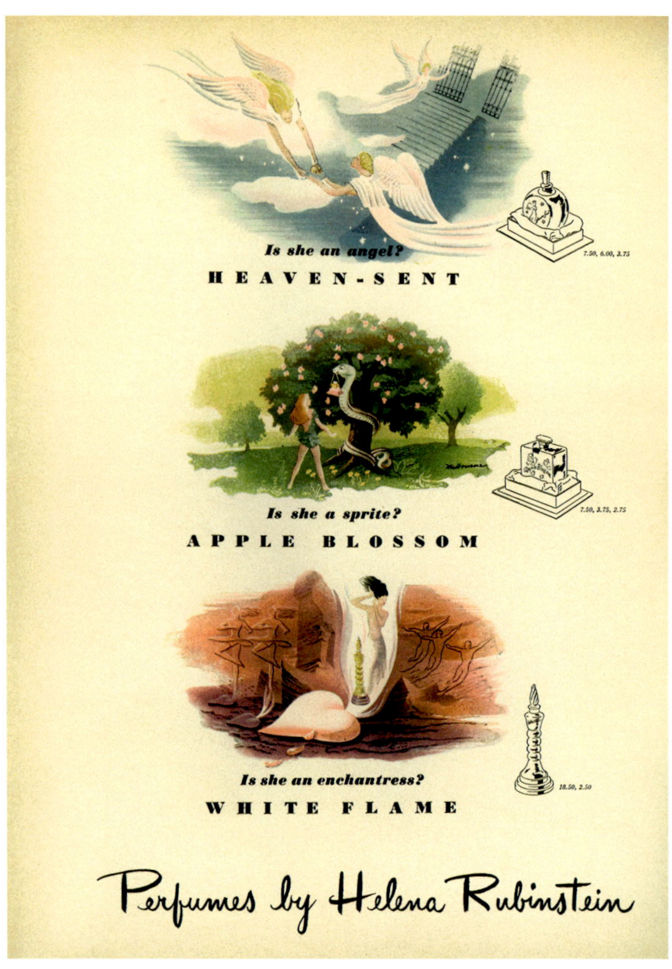

Is she an angel?
HEAVEN-SENT
7.50, 6.00, 3.75
Is she a sprite?
APPLE BLOSSOM
7.50, 3.75, 2.75
Is she an enchantress?
WHITE FLAME
18.50, 2.50
Perfumes by Helena Rubinstein

An advertisement from the 1940s for three of Rubinstein's popular perfumes identifies categories of female personality.

In addition to collecting masks as works of art, Rubinstein also used them in her "scientific" beauty regimens and products. A mask applied to the face produced a refreshed appearance. The final step in a woman's health and beauty routine was the application of makeup, another kind of mask. The idea of self-invention, using such tools to determine one's own identity, was fundamental in her life and work; her goal was to provide women with the means to control how they were seen. In this 1957 advertisement, Rubinstein's fascination with masks reaches its most Surrealist expression: the image converts a liquid skin mask into a literal second face. A woman has a double presence: she gazes confidently outward, while her seductive second self looks slyly to the side.

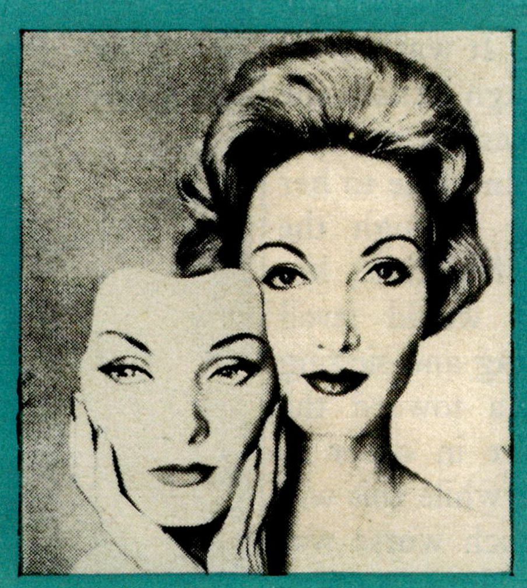

CIRCULOTION MASK is a fine, transparent film of animating herbs. Give it twenty minutes, no matter how weary the face, and see a beauty miracle! A years-younger look. A complexion glowing, refreshed, radiant. Don't deny yourself Circulotion Mask, one of Helena Rubinstein's revolutionary Tree of Life* developments. 30 treatments, $7.50 plus tax *T. M.

HELENA RUBINSTEIN®
TREE OF LIFE

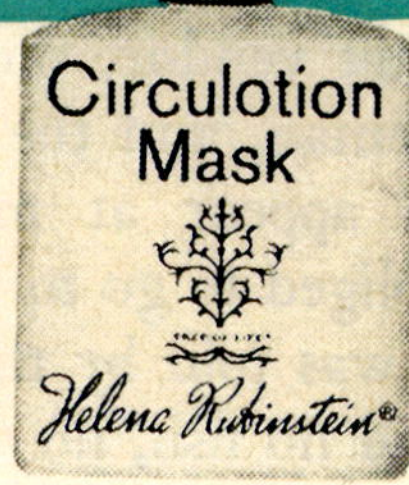

All she wants is a little Emotion
(a lot of it if she's daring!)

Emotion... the new perfume
born in France...
translated in America
into Spray Mist, Eau de Parfum
and everything for her bath
3.00 to 17.50
EMOTION® by Helena Rubinstein

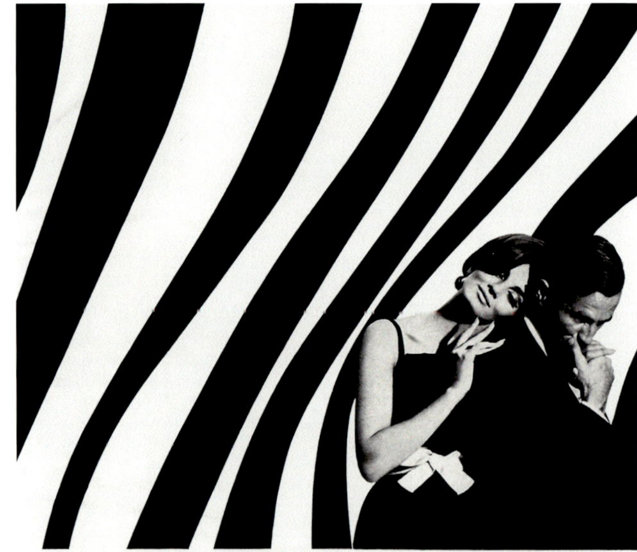

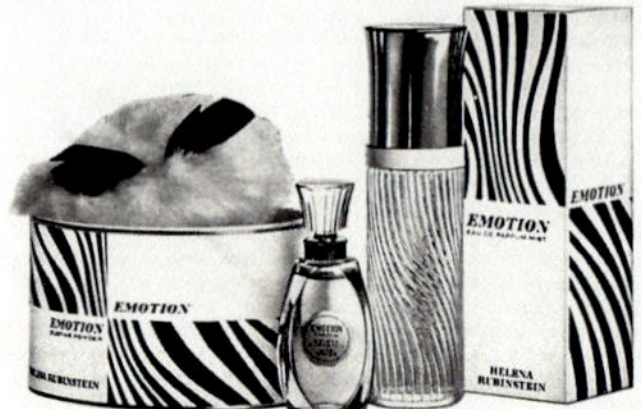

Op art and Space Age style infuse advertisements from 1965 (*above*) and 1953 (*below*), reflecting changes in art as well as fashion. Rubinstein now includes men in her advertisements, openly emphasizing romance and sexuality.

Gourielli presents FOURTH DIMENSION –a perfume for moderns... complex, high key, exciting
Keyed to contemporary living–new concepts of space, freedom of motion, and freedom of *spirit*–Gourielli's new FOURTH DIMENSION is definitely the perfume for today's woman–agelessly young, and unlimited in possibilities!
FOURTH DIMENSION opens new horizons in emotional living. Try it. It is a new note in fragrance–subtly and mysteriously different from any perfume you have ever used before. Wearing an aura of FOURTH DIMENSION around you will be a rich and rewarding experience.
You'll applaud the House of Gourielli for having conceived and created it–and for presenting it in this inspired new assortment of flacons, a delight to the eye, and a joy to use. Perfume, 3.50 to 45.00. Toilet Water, 5.50. Cologne, 3.50. At all the better stores.
HOUSE OF GOURIELLI, 16 E. 55 Street, New York 22, N.Y.

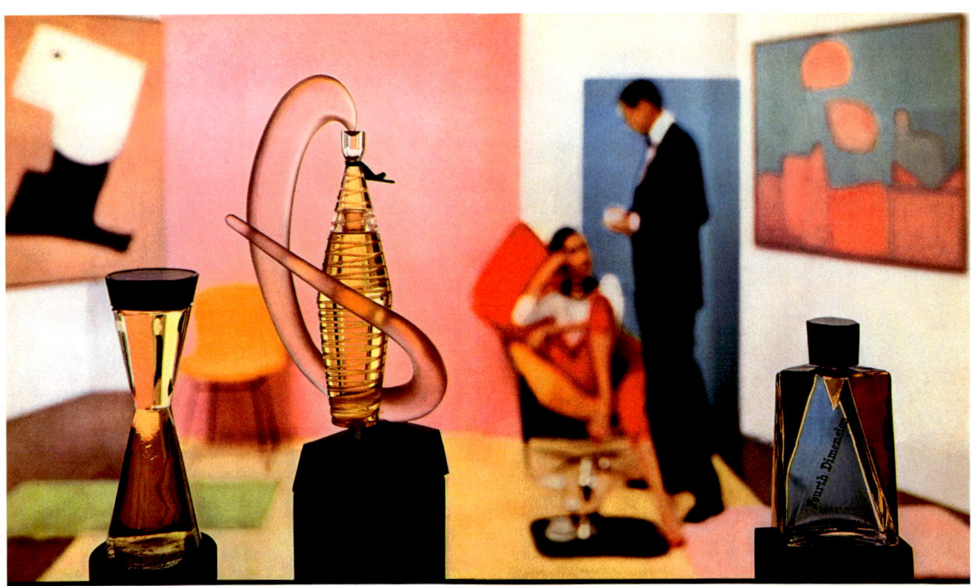

context were as far as she could reasonably go. After all, she wanted the average woman to feel welcome, not intimidated. Frankl, along with the Polish-born painter and book illustrator Witold Gordon, may have wanted to be more experimental, but Madame reined them in. Nevertheless, they welcomed the opportunity to introduce some of their modernist ideas, and enjoyed the upbeat press the beauty parlor received as "the first completely modern commission of importance on American soil." Elizabeth Arden, not to be outdone, immediately asked Frankl to redo some rooms in her salon. Both Frankl and Gordon continued to work on Rubinstein projects throughout the next decade: Frankl designed salons throughout the United States, usually juxtaposing his modernist furniture with his friend Nadelman's marble sculptures.[62]

Rubinstein by this point was becoming quite the decorator, and seems to have enjoyed every moment of it. And critics were noticing:

> *I can't begin to tell you of the infinite details that have been worked out for this wonderful place. All by Madame Rubinstein herself. For weeks she has had in the house—it is an old one remodeled—a retinue of carpenters, painters, marble polishers, sewing women, whom she has overseen and directed with untiring energy. If she had not been the artist in the particular line that she is she could have made her reputation twice over as an interior decorator. Offers, in fact, were made her in Paris to embark on interior decorating of such unusual artistic distinction was her establishment there, with its collection of furniture and pictures and statuary. These, by the way, are all being brought from the other side to take their place in the big reception room on the third floor and Mme. Rubinstein's own living apartments.*[63]

By the mid-1920s, modernism was establishing itself in Europe, shocking some with its pared-down design. Madame refurbished her Paris home in an Art Deco style after visiting the Exposition Internationale des Art Décoratifs et Industriels in 1925. Astutely, she decided in 1926 to redo her Grafton Street salon in London as well. Emboldened by her success in New York, she hired two novice designers to give it a more contemporary look. She chose Ernö Goldfinger, a young Hungarian émigré architect, still a student at the Ecole des Beaux-Arts in Paris, and his partner, András Szivessy (who later changed his name to André Sive).

Goldfinger was a distinctive figure, an iconoclast with a passion for the new. The combination of his imperious youth—he came from a wealthy family—his uncompromising idealism, and his aversion to anything that smacked of unnecessary ornamentation proved too rebelliously modernist even for her. Influenced by the flawless austerity of Adolf Loos, he proposed to create a glass facade for the shop that would contrast starkly with the Georgian style of the building and its neighbors. That, Madame could accept. He also wanted to run Madame's name in a repeated illuminated band over each floor, a detail she vetoed as being in bad taste. The interior he envisioned was unadorned, largely stripped of architectural detail or decoration. While she thought certain aspects of the design attractive, she found it both too much and too little; it had "just a slight appearance of an operating theatre." When client and designers reached an impasse, she called in the architect Ashley Benjamin, who helped complete the interior; over Rubinstein's objections, he retained many of Goldfinger's ideas. The walls were overlaid, floor to ceiling, with black metal and plate glass; lighting was indirect; and the carpet, which Rubinstein despised, was gray pile.[64] Goldfinger had to go to court to get paid, but in 1927 the completed

62 See Christopher Long, in Slesin, *Over the Top*, 38. The story goes that Nadelman worried that Rubinstein might acquire paintings for her new salon, rather than commission more of his sculpture. So Frankl decided to make the rooms round or oval to minimize the opportunity to hang pictures. As Frankl recalled years later, the budget precluded such remodeling. Modernist designs were to be found in the first New York salon at 15 East 49th Street, and the one at 46 West 57th Street, in 1918, where Gordon painted the walls with murals and decorated various architectural features. In 1928 Frankl teamed with Donald Deskey at 8 East 57th Street.

63 "The Vanity Box," *Theatre Magazine*, 28 no. 214 (December 1918): 376, reviewing the new 57th Street salon.

64 Slesin, *Over the Top*, 44.

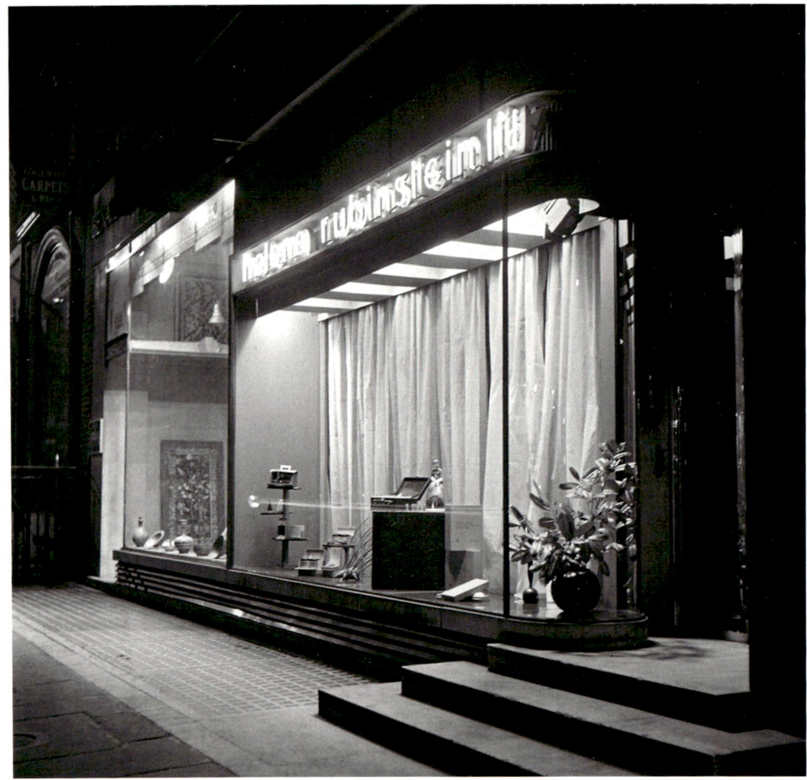

Night view of the Helena Rubinstein salon, 26 Grafton Street, Mayfair, London, with exterior design by Erno Goldfinger, c. 1927.

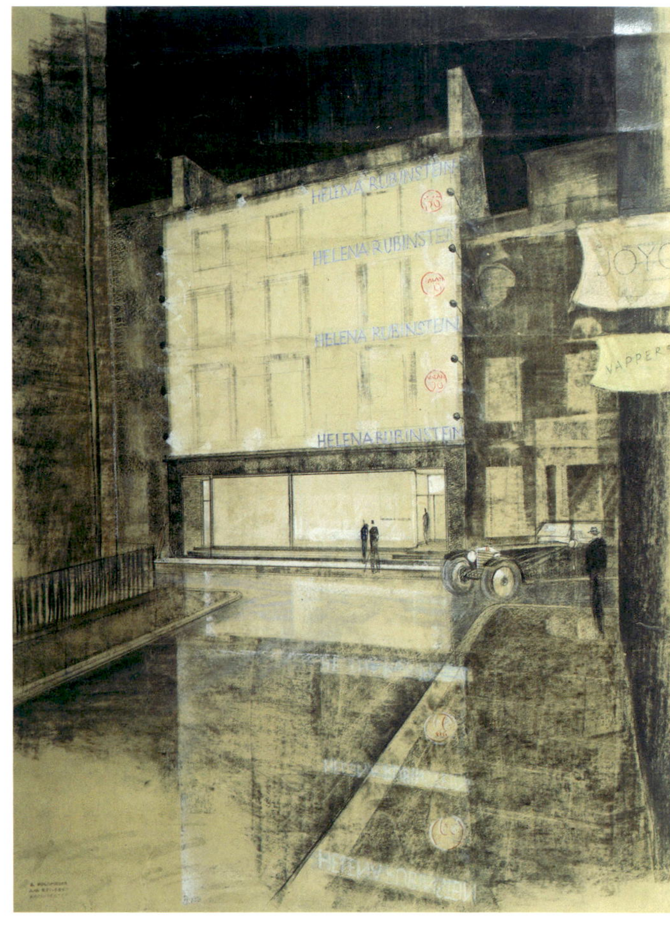

Design by Ernö Goldfinger for a salon for Helena Rubinstein, 26 Grafton Street, Mayfair, London, 1926.

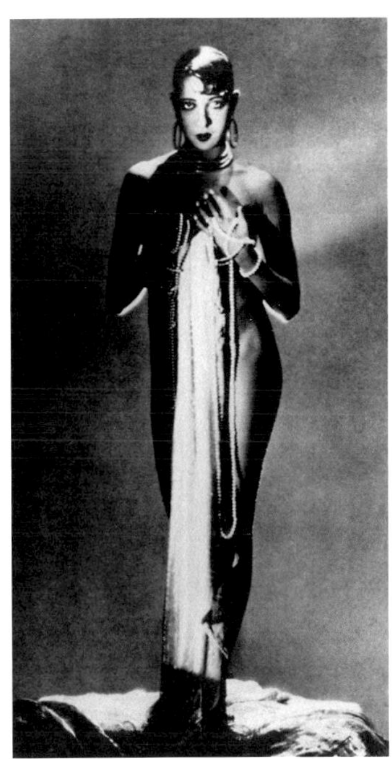

Josephine Baker, c. 1925.

and updated Helena Rubinstein salon became the first modernist shop front in London.[65]

What Rubinstein learned from working with Goldfinger was that she had to assert her will with her partners, to be more actively engaged in her collaborations with architects and designers. She also realized from these early critical experiences that her strength lay in knowing just how far to go aesthetically—namely, understanding what her clients were ready for.

In Paris the 1920s saw a boom not only in art and design but also in fashion and cosmetics. The trend was toward a thin, glamorized mannequin look, with a shorter, crisper hairdo and a face made deliberately artificial through the application of lipstick, eye shadow, kohl liner, and rouge. Accompanying these shifts and the growth of a modernist aesthetic came an efflorescence of night culture, reverberating with the new music emerging from the Harlem Renaissance. From her own fluid French-American perch, Madame took part in a burgeoning fashion for "aesthetic primitivism," an appropriation of Negro culture. The taste for African and African American music, design, and fashion arose first in the Parisian avant-garde but became increasingly fashionable, especially in the United States. This culminated in the spectacle of the young African American singer and dancer Josephine Baker.

When Baker began performing "La Revue Nègre" in 1925, many from the art and literary world were on hand. The pollination of Paris with American cultural idioms like black jazz music and dance was unprecedented. Its cultural impact was manifold, though the reception was mixed. While many on the right regarded such a blatant display of negritude as symptomatic of cultural decadence, her admirers adored Baker. She became a craze and was quickly signed to appear at the Folies-Bergère night club, with songs commissioned by Irving Berlin and others.

For that revue, "La Folie du Jour," Baker altered her image, exaggerating her features so as to make an ethnographic spectacle, a masquerade of otherness. She used Helena Rubinstein's makeup to accentuate her eyes with black kohl, a Rubinstein foundation called Crème Gypsy toned her skin to a "distinctive ochre-brown color, her lips were made fuller with a dark lipstick, her teeth whitened for contrast, and her hair brilliantined, and her forehead adorned with a kiss curl."[66] Baker may have embodied a Parisian fascination with racy exoticism, but there is no question that she was also seen as beautiful; Rubinstein understood that unconventional beauty like Baker's embodied an idea with staying power.

The marketing of Baker was carefully staged to exploit the negrophilia that had caught on in Paris. African chic grew as African and Oceanic art continued to influence contemporary Western painting and photography, most significantly in the hands of Man Ray (see page 31). In this convergence of experimental modernism, primitivism, and ethnography, Baker stands as a pivotal figure. But her success was short-lived. By the end of the decade a growing xenophobia had altered the cultural atmosphere. When Baker attempted to transform her image, aspiring to broaden her career as a chanteuse, her act was not successful.[67] As politics grew more polarized, it became clear to Rubinstein that the cultural diversity that was intrinsic to her world view was not tenable in Europe.

Artists in Paris were responding to the Jazz Age interest in exotic otherness and nonwhite images of beauty. Constantin Brancusi's 1923 sculpture *White Negress I* was reportedly inspired by an African woman whom he had seen in Marseilles the year before, but it is not hard to imagine that the second version, *White Negress II*, carved in 1928, was inflected

65 This is the judgment of the architectural historian Sir Charles Herbert Reilly, cited in Nigel Warburton, *Ernö Goldfinger: The Life of an Architect* (London: Routledge, 2004), 42.

66 For more on the period's negritude and on Baker, see Jon Kear, "Josephine Baker and the Parisian Music-hall," *Parisian Fields* (London: Reaktion Books, 1996), 46–70; for the makeup quotation, see 59.

67 She left Paris and went on tour. From Vienna to Berlin to Zagreb to Budapest, however, she was met with violent protest, a swelling tide of nationalism and racism, driven by economic depression and unemployment. Upon her return to Paris in 1928, she managed, nonetheless, to transform herself from a curiosity into a bona fide chanteuse. See Kear, "Josephine Baker," 67–68.

by the tumult ignited by Baker's meteoric celebrity. Brancusi's oxymoronic title may be read as an undertone of the decade's charged racial conflict, which Baker ignited in Paris and elsewhere in Europe.[68] Rubinstein purchased the sculpture around 1931. She displayed it in her Paris home, but may also have put it in the window of her Paris salon at one time.[69] For her, *White Negress II* synthesized the confluence of exoticism and modernism. It embodied her overarching dual enterprise: to establish a correspondence between modern art and cosmetics, both of which she felt should be subjectively engaged. That is, just as modern art must be understood as departing from nature and existing in its own creative realm, so too the new woman creates herself on her own terms, rather than in accordance with a standard of beauty. It was Rubinstein's genius to see this, and to sense instinctively that there was a connection between these two modernist phenomena.

Rubinstein had a sweeping interest in the female face as an icon—hence her lifelong interest in commissioning and collecting portraits. Here, as elsewhere, her taste was expansive. She owned painted or carved figures from innumerable periods and cultures, and collected African and Oceanic art extensively. She had begun buying African sculptures before World War I, advised by the sculptor Jacob Epstein, whom she had met when she first was in London.[70] Unsurprisingly, a significant number of the sculptures were female heads and figures, a further mark of Madame's inclusive sense of beauty.

Her passionate collecting began during a period when African and Oceanic art was for the most part housed in the Musée d'Ethnographie, where the Parisian avant-garde flocked to see it. It was during this time that Western art, principally with the development of Cubism, began to seriously address and sanction such work within a positive aesthetic. This trend culminated in the "negrophilia" mania of the 1920s in Paris, heavily influenced by the Harlem Renaissance in New York. Throughout this period, racist ethnic stereotypes began to yield to positive connotations of a liberatory and timeless source of inspiration, which was also seen as "an access to true modernity."[71]

Rubinstein was scarcely concerned with countering the tendency, common at the time, to interpret African art in conventional Western art-historical terms. Nevertheless, her keen identification with non-Western art and her interest in multicultural diversity were based on an effort to elevate such work to a "fine art" context. Further, she employed that art to reflect her unusual openness to ethnicity. Meanwhile, Rubinstein, ever responsive to the cultural moment, was selling her cosmetics at a furious rate. She has been called "the woman who invented beauty," but as one contemplates her life and influence it becomes clear that she was not interested in a concept of ideal beauty, but its implied opposite, the imperfections of a nature that could be refashioned.[72]

As the twenties roared on, Paris grew glitzier, its fashions more brazen; women's makeup was heavy and widely used: not a natural face was to be seen on the street. Such a spectacle would have intrigued the nineteenth-century poet and critic Charles Baudelaire, who had poetically invoked the concept of the redemptive, modernist potential of cosmetics, a chance to make nature right. He implored individuals, artists no less, to reject "laziness; for it is much easier to decide" that something is ugly "than to devote oneself to the task of distilling from it the mysterious element of beauty that it may contain."[73]

"The ideal," Baudelaire declared, "is not that vague thing, that boring and impalpable dream—which we see floating on the ceilings of

Opposite: In a photograph from the 1930s, Rubinstein poses with *White Negress II*, her cherished marble by Brancusi.

68 Brancusi referred to a "woman at the fair" (presumably the Marseilles Exposition Coloniale of 1922); quoted in Flora Merrill, "Brancusi, the Sculptor of the Spirit, Would Build 'Infinite Column' in Park," *New York World*, October 3, 1926. See also Pontus Hulten, Natalia Dumitresco, and Alexandre Istrati, *Brancusi* (New York: Harry N. Abrams, 1987), 147.

69 Michèle Fitoussi, *Helena Rubinstein: The Woman Who Invented Beauty* (Sydney: HarperCollins, 2012), 222.

70 The collection was dispersed at auction at Parke-Bernet in 1966 in more than seven hundred lots of objects, and its success propelled the field into a highly competitive market.

71 Beginning with such studies as Carl Einstein's *Negerplastik* in 1915. See also the interdisciplinary scholar James Clifford, "Negrophilia," in Denis Hollier, *A New History of French Literature* (Cambridge, MA: Harvard University Press, 1989), 901.

72 Fitoussi, *Helena Rubinstein: The Woman Who Invented Beauty*.

73 Charles Baudelaire, "IV. Modernity," from "The Painter of Modern Life," in *The Painter of Modern Life and Other Essays*, Jonathan Mayne, trans. and ed. (London: Phaidon Press, 1964), 13.

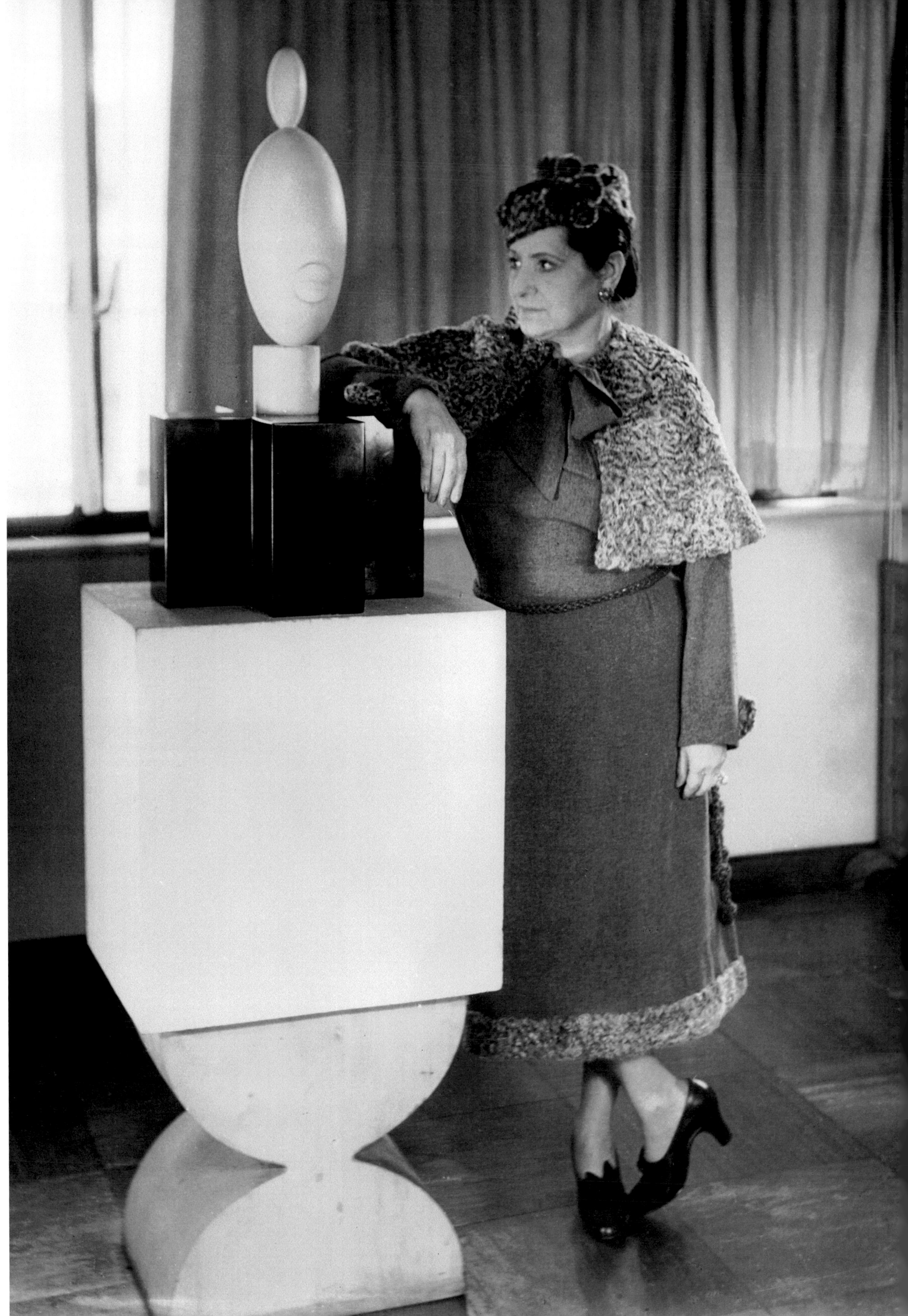

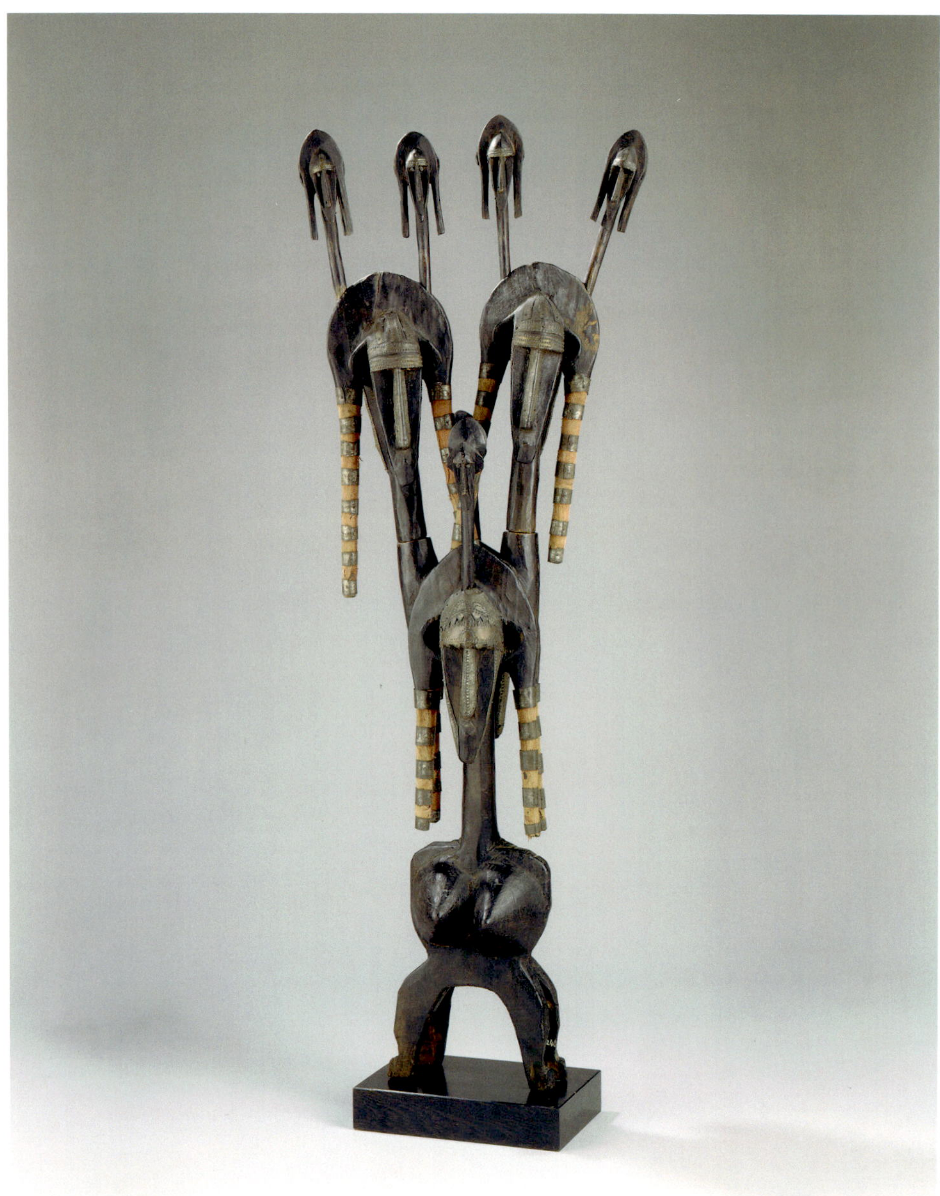

Bamana puppet headdress
Mali, Sela village, early 1930s
Wood, brass, cloth, 57¾ in. (146.7 cm) high
Indiana University Art Museum, Bloomington

Rubinstein's acclaimed collection of African art included works from a broad range of cultures. She was an eclectic buyer, often choosing works for their striking decorative and visual qualities, rather than focusing on one type or tradition. "I have always favored the unusual," she declared. "When I followed such sound advice as Jacob Epstein's, as well as my own 'inner eye,' my purchases were invariably good."

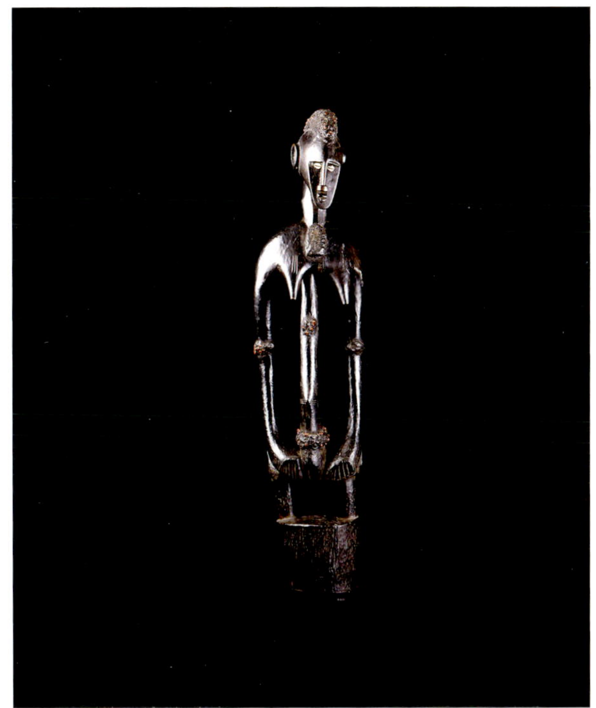

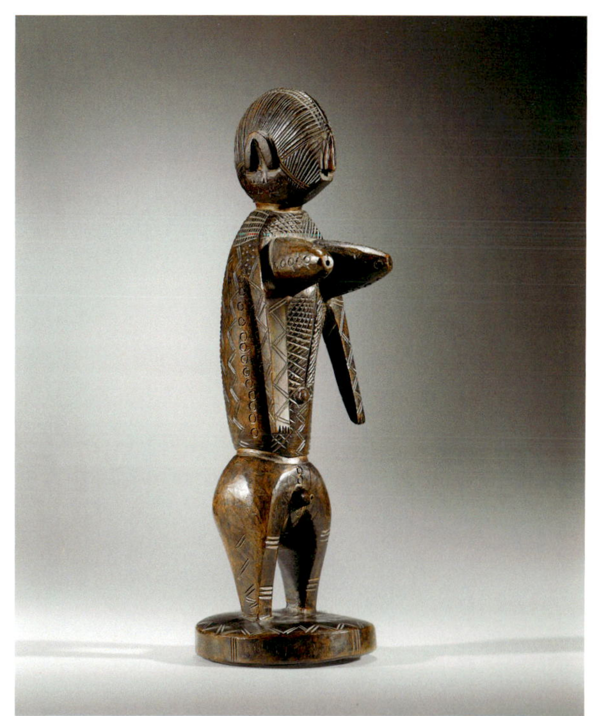

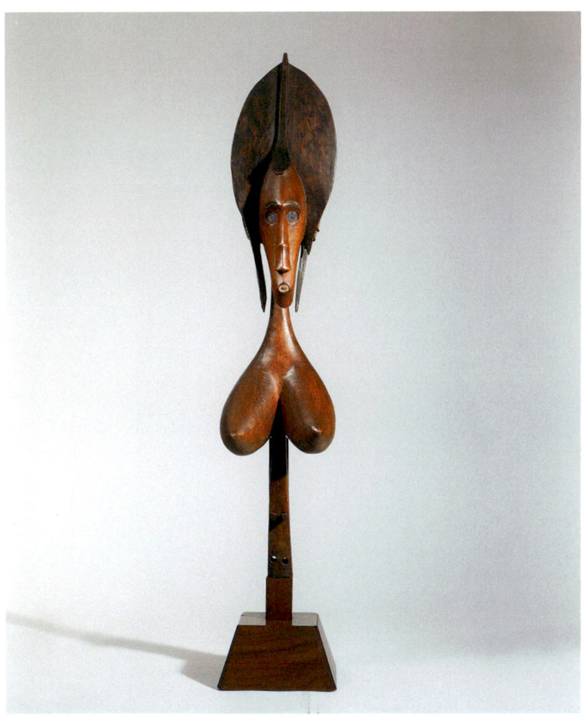

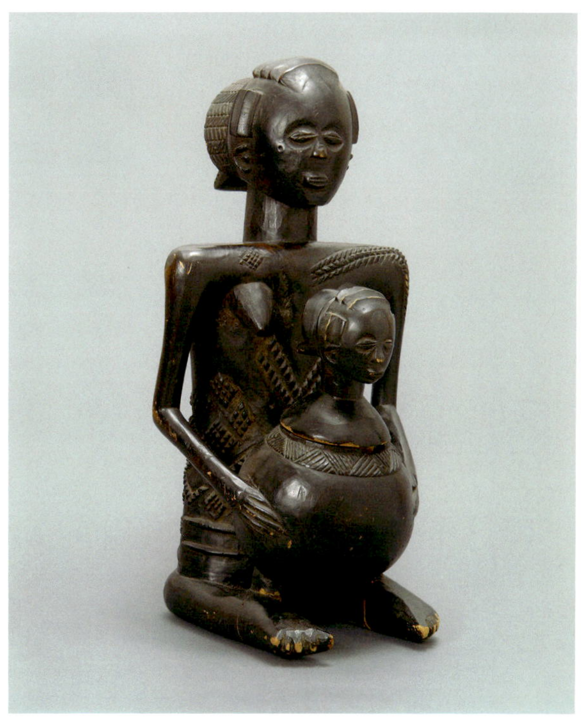

Senufo rhythm pounder (*Pombilele*)
Mali, Sikasso, Folona, nineteenth century
Wood, cowrie shells, seeds, dried red berries, secured with latex, 36 in. (91.4 cm) high
Private collection

Bamana female *Sogo Bo* marionette head
Mali, Ségou region, date unknown
Wood, 31½ in. (80 cm) high
Drs. Daniel and Marian Malcolm, New Jersey

Bamana statue
Mali, Sikasso, c. 1934
Wood, 17¾ in. (45 cm) high
Mr. Celestin Clamra, New York

Luba Shankadi maternity divination figure
Democratic Republic of Congo, Mwanza, late nineteenth–early twentieth century
Wood, 20⅞ in. (53 cm) high
Collection of Valerie Franklin, California

Bete or Guro male and female pair of combs
Ivory Coast, date unknown
Wood, 9¾ in. (24.8 cm) high each
Private collection, New York

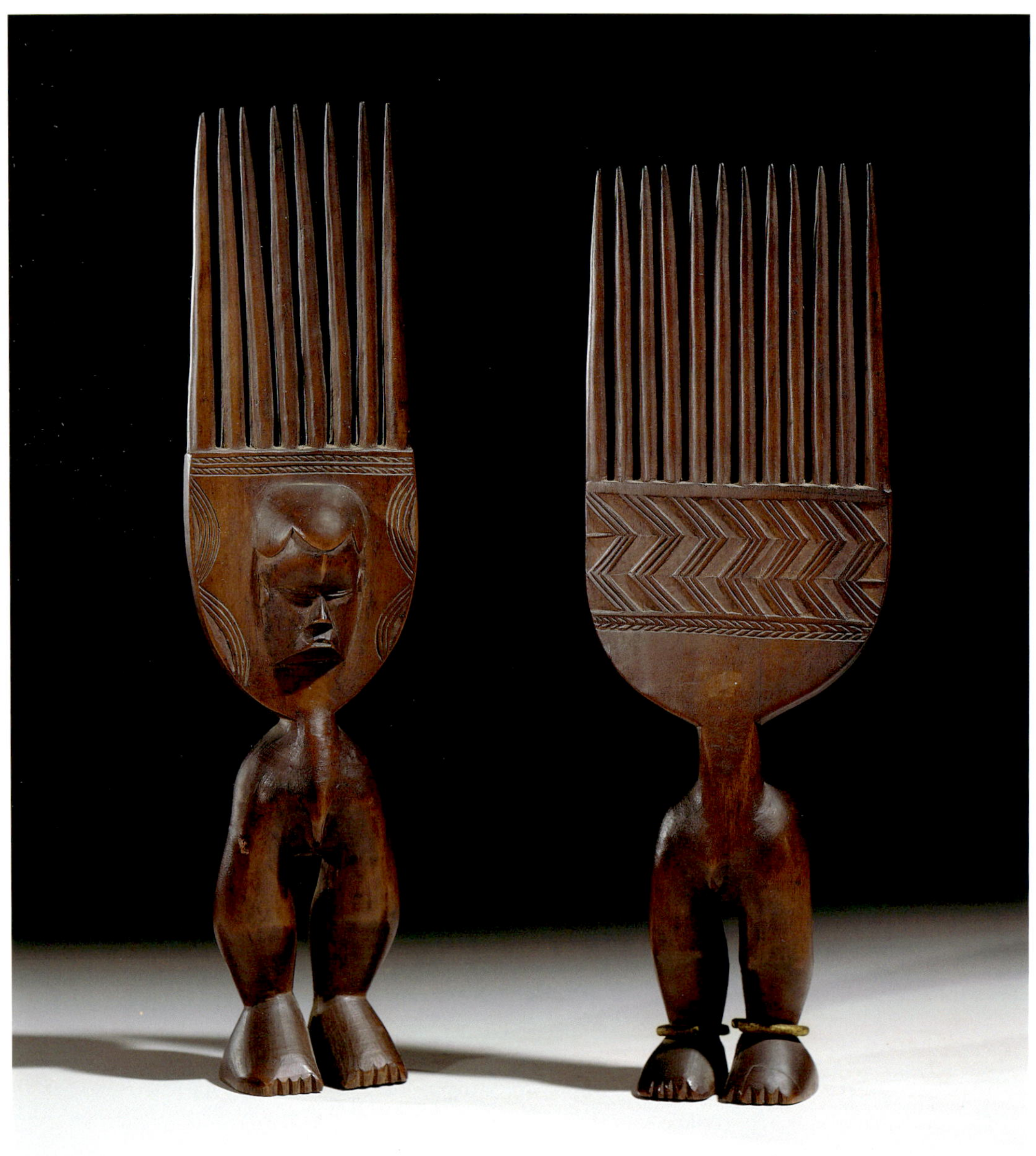

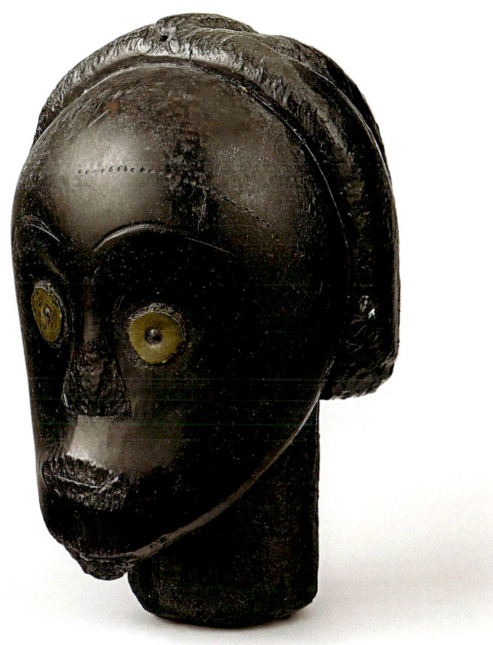

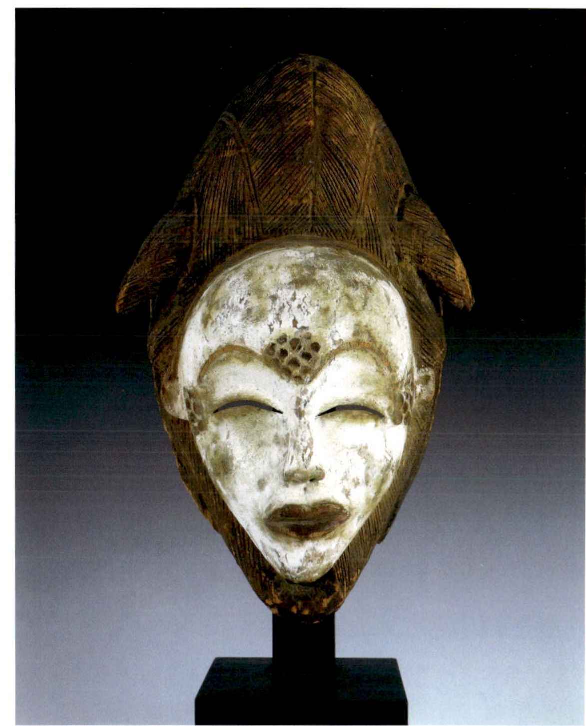

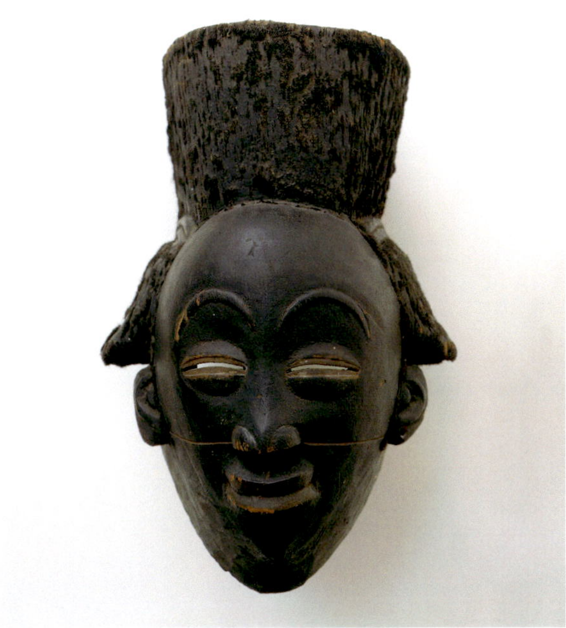

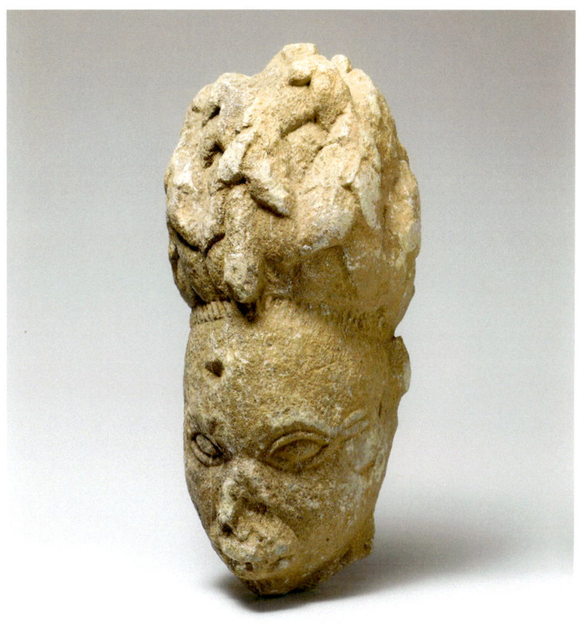

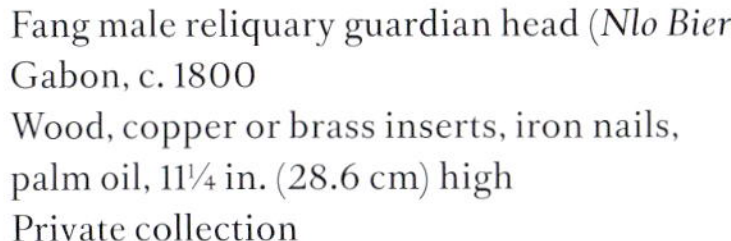

Fang male reliquary guardian head (*Nlo Bieri*)
Gabon, c. 1800
Wood, copper or brass inserts, iron nails, palm oil, 11¼ in. (28.6 cm) high
Private collection

Punu face mask (*Ikwar*)
Gabon, date unknown
Wood, hair, 11¾ in. (29.9 cm) high
The Kreeger Museum, Washington, DC

Punu face mask (*Mukuyi/Okuyi*)
Gabon, date unknown
Wood, kaolin, pigment, 12½ in. (31.8 cm) high
The Kreeger Museum, Washington, DC

Yoruba head
Nigeria, Esie region, Offa, twelfth–fifteenth century
Soapstone, 11¾ in. (29.9 cm) high
Metropolitan Museum of Art, New York,
The Michael C. Rockefeller Memorial Collection,
Bequest of Nelson A. Rockefeller, 1979

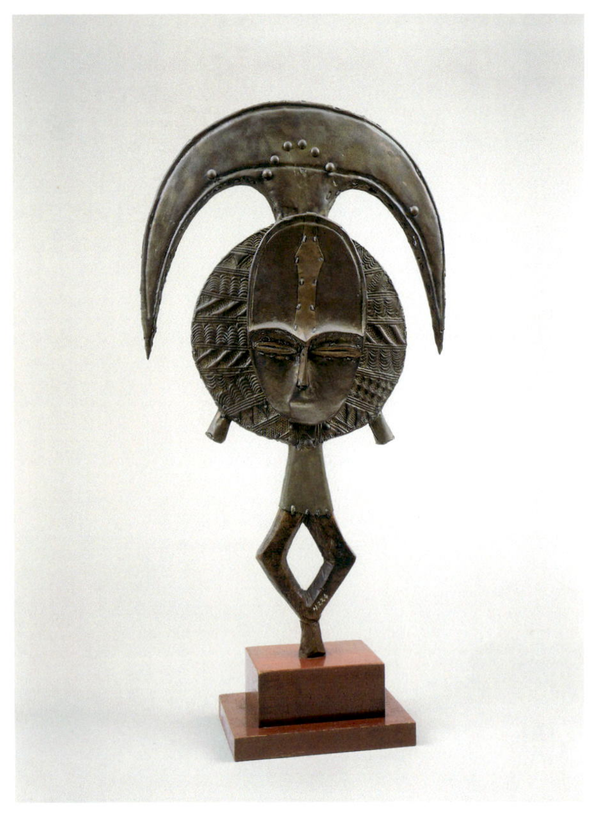

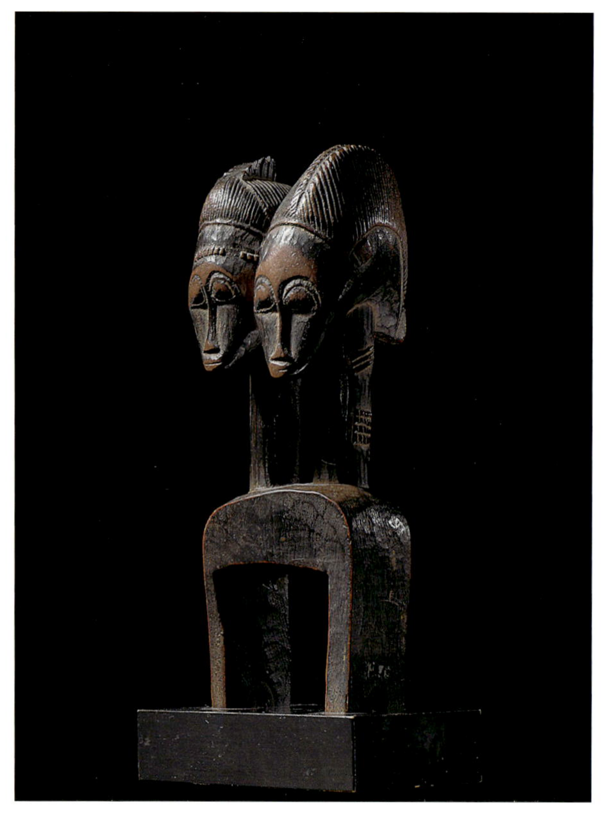

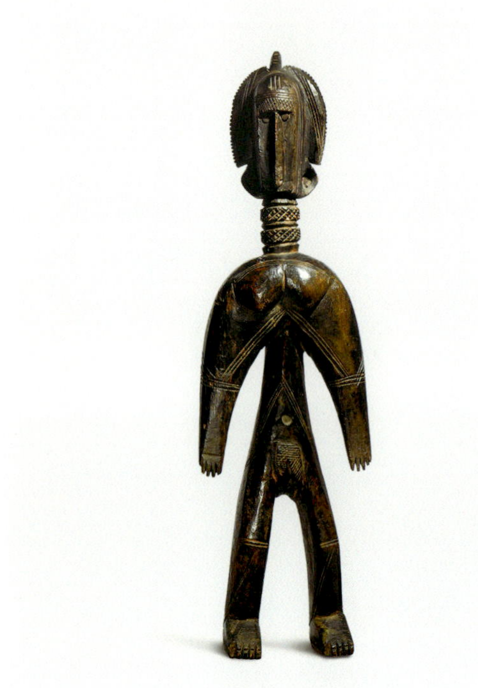

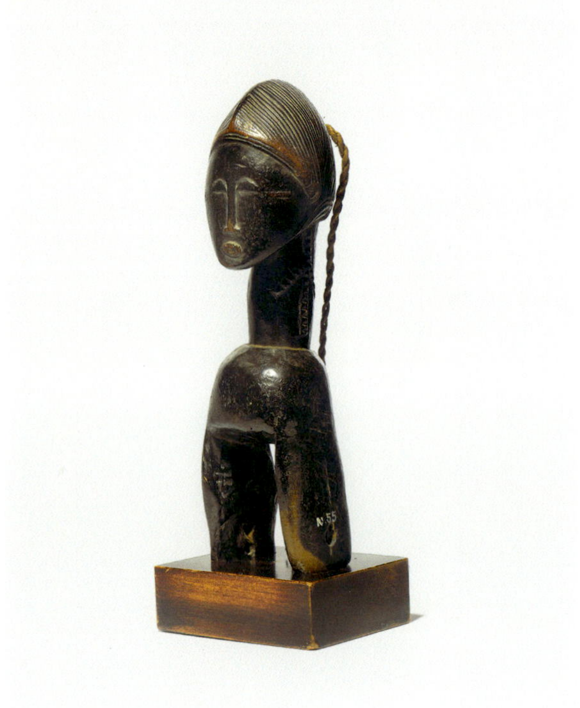

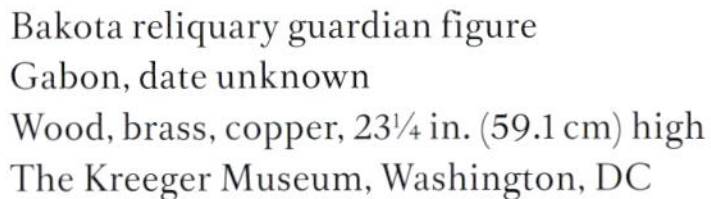

Bakota reliquary guardian figure
Gabon, date unknown
Wood, brass, copper, 23¼ in. (59.1 cm) high
The Kreeger Museum, Washington, DC

Bamana female figure
Mali, Ségou region, date unknown
Wood, 14¾ in. (37.5 cm) high
Collection of Gilbert and Doreen Bassin

Baule double-headed heddle pulley
Ivory Coast, date unknown
Wood, 7 in. (17.8 cm) high
Private collection, New York

Baule heddle pulley
Ivory Coast, date unknown
Wood and fiber cord, 7¼ in. (18.4 cm) high
Private collection, New York

academies; an ideal is an individual put right by an individual, reconstructed and restored by brush or chisel to the dazzling truth of its native harmony." He argued for a conception of beauty that was contingent and mutable, not unique and absolute. He was advocating the transformation of the natural into something "supernatural" through the artifice of art.[74] He exhorted artists not merely to copy nature, producing a sterile imitation, but to render their own vision, their own "ideal." In his essay "In Praise of Cosmetics," he invoked makeup as a means of achieving beauty, equating the artifice of beauty with the elevation of nature to art:

> *Woman is quite within her rights, indeed she is even accomplishing a kind of duty, when she devotes herself to appearing magical and supernatural; she has to astonish and charm us; as an idol, she is obliged to adorn herself in order to be adored. Thus she has to lay all the arts under contribution for the means of lifting herself above Nature, the better to conquer hearts and rivet attention.*[75]

Baudelaire was using the notion of cosmetics and fashion as a metaphor for the "reformation" of nature, as that which "adds to the face of a beautiful woman the mysterious passion of a priestess." Rubinstein, true to form, put it more succinctly: "There are no ugly women, only lazy ones." What she could not tolerate was a lack of effort to maximize creative impact. In effect, Rubinstein literalized Baudelaire's use of cosmetics as a metaphor for modernism's alteration of nature. In advertising campaigns, in the how-to beauty guides she published, in the classes offered at her salons, she emphasized individualism—that every woman should work to discover not just her strengths and faults, her beauty and her flaws, but the potential for self-realization. Rather than follow this or that look, Madame constantly appealed to the female consumer to be creative, to follow "what direction your subconscious is taking. It will help you to develop style—your own instinctive style."[76] When she opened her salon at 8 East 57th Street in 1928, her advertisement read, "These new Maisons de Beauté are the response to an expressed demand: A demand for a type of beauty which is not a type at all, but is a perfection aimed in every detail toward the expression of individuality." Moreover, increasingly aware of the correspondence between art and cosmetics, she referred to her new salons as "perfectly appointed *ateliers*."[77]

And of course Madame lived by her own precepts. Her own particular form of "instinctive style" involved both excess and a clear-eyed realism. Asked about her distinctive, heavy jewelry, she simply wrote:

> *One interesting point about the wearing of jewels is that they reveal much about the personality of the wearer. . . . I love paradox. If I were a tall, statuesque woman, I would probably have worn tiny, delicate jewels. Liking simple, often severe clothes, I feel they need the contrast of large, colorful pieces. My hairstyle, too, is very severe, drawn back in a chignon, and this requires the added drama of necklaces and earrings. Since I am quite short, I feel that these accessories, combined with my clothes, give a definite identity. For a woman working hard in a man's world, this is important.*[78]

74 Charles Baudelaire, "On the Ideal and the Model," in *Art in Paris 1845–1862: Reviews of Salons and Other Exhibitions*, Jonathan Mayne, trans. and ed. (London: Phaidon Press, 1965), 81.

75 Charles Baudelaire, "XI. In Praise of Cosmetics," from "The Painter of Modern Life," in *The Painter of Modern Life and Other Essays*, 33.

76 Rubinstein, *My Life for Beauty*, 126.

77 Advertisement, *Vogue* 71, no. 2 (January 15, 1928): 99.

78 Helena Rubinstein, "Why I Love Jewels," undated manuscript, Helena Rubinstein archive, L'Oréal Luxe, Paris.

Rubinstein produced myriad pamphlets, brochures, and even hardcover books. They offered beauty and health tips, exercise instructions, guides to good posture and hygiene, and secrets to finding one's own style. Many were available by mail order or at the salons. These three are from 1931, 1938, and c. 1950.

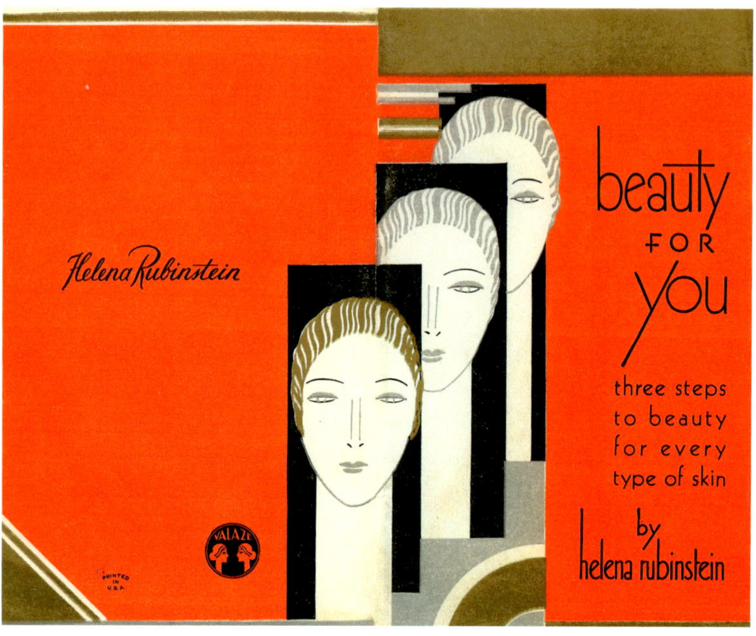

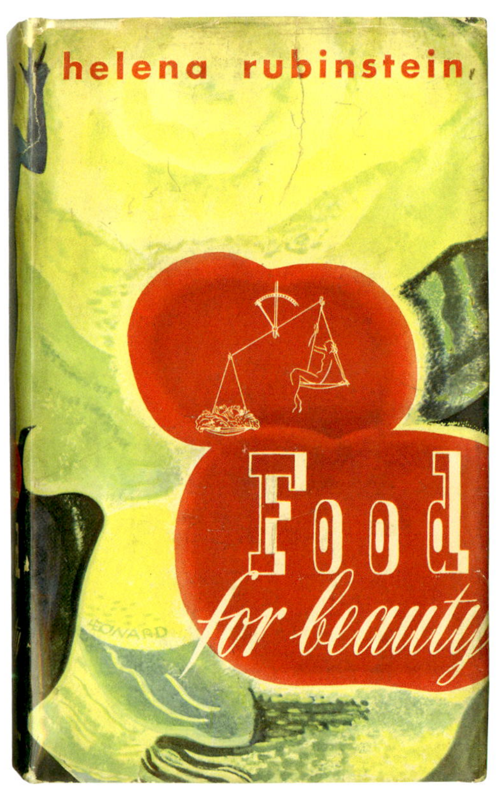

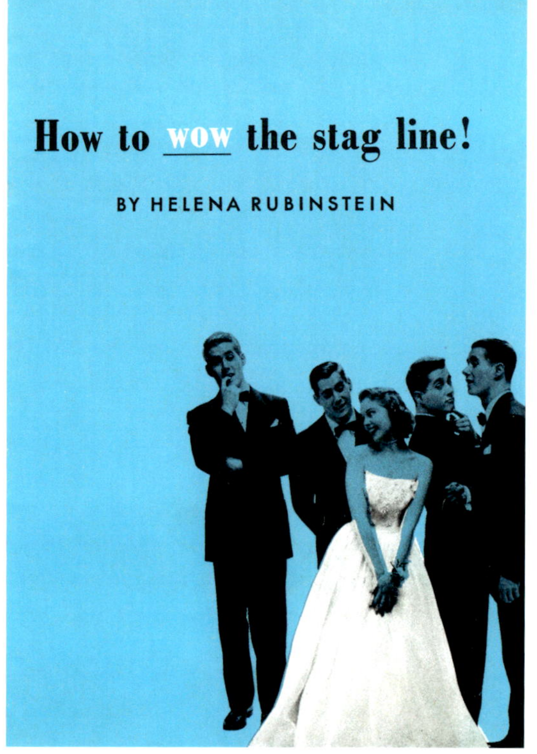

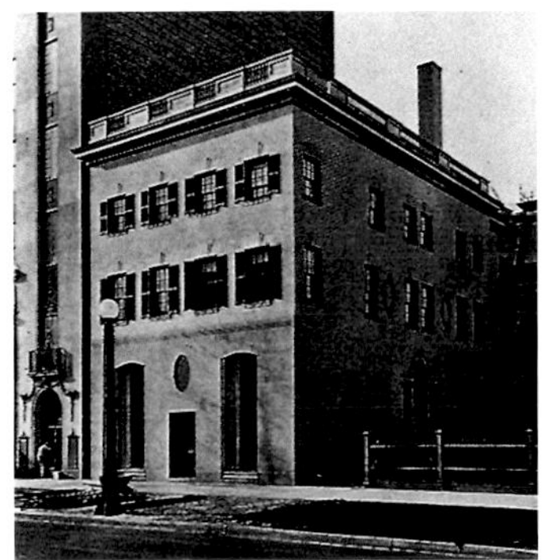

Facade of the Helena Rubinstein salon in Chicago, from *Good Furniture*, May 1928.

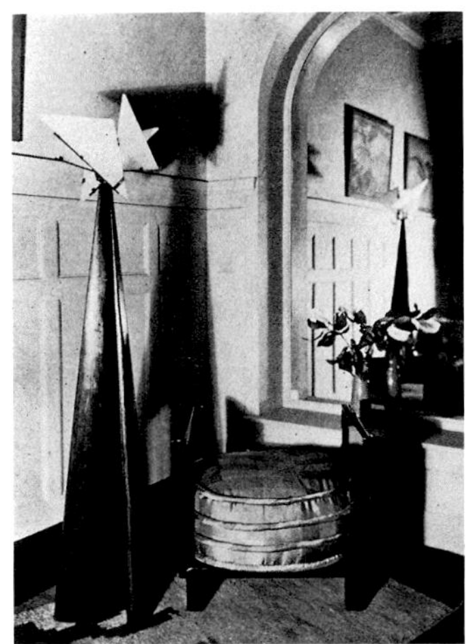

Interior of the Chicago salon, with a Pierre Chareau lamp called *La Religieuse*, from *Good Furniture*, May 1928.

Art Moderne

If Paris and London in the 1920s were the source of Rubinstein's modernist style and unidealized notions of beauty, as well as much of her art collection, the United States was a clean slate, an opportunity to try out her business methods on a large and eager population. Following her experience in London with Ernö Goldfinger, in 1928 Madame opened two new salons in New York and Chicago. Here too she used architecture to convey the idea of both taste and modernity. *Good Furniture* magazine called the latter "A Beauty Salon in Art Moderne," and described it as "the most extensive example in Chicago of modern art interior decoration adapted to a commercial establishment."[79] Likening the shop to Madame's famous Parisian and New York counterparts, the article praised the salon's conversion of an old Georgian Revival building, mentioning its new, flat facade and tall, deeply inset windows, an echo of what Madame had learned from Goldfinger. The building achieved just the right balance of classical ornamentation and pristine modernism. The interior decor, the article noted, quoting the director of the Chicago Academy of Fine Arts, was "the first comprehensive example in the United States of the application of modern art to the interior decoration of a commercial building."[80] In this context "modern art" and "art moderne" are names for what today we usually call Art Deco.

The author praised Rubinstein's early patronage of modern art:

> *One of Madame Rubinstein's chief reasons for planning her three beauty shops in the modern manner is to acquaint her patrons with distinguished examples of modern art. Because women of wealth so seldom take the time to visit museums and galleries of art, Madame Rubinstein believes that many of them do not learn to appreciate the beauty of the significant new art achievements. She wishes to influence such women to give the young modernistic artists the encouragement and patronage which they need.*

The article credited Madame with being involved in the planning of both exterior and interior architectural features. It was clearly she, for example, who had chosen the "silver leaf wallpaper" that covered the lobby ceiling, the "niches . . . lined in metallic gold leaf," and the windows "simply hung with full green velvet draperies and a metallic cloth lining next to the glass." The new salon was embellished with many of its owner's latest French Art Deco objects, such as several examples of the latest in Art Deco furniture and Pierre Chareau's famous sculptural lamp, called *La Religieuse (The Nun)*. Its tall, conical cast-iron body and crown of intersecting geometric shapes of translucent alabaster resembled a nun's habit. The lamp reminds us of the modernist question initially posed by Constantin Brancusi: where does a pedestal end and a sculpture begin?

In addition to Elie Nadelman, Madame introduced the work of the Ukrainian Chana Orloff, a School of Paris sculptor and portraitist, to Chicago, two years before Orloff had her first exhibition in the United States, as well as sculptures by Boris Lovet-Lorski and paintings by Louis Marcoussis. She displayed modernist tapestries made by Maison Myrbor in Paris, whose founder, Marie Cuttoli, had become a good friend (see page 101). Cuttoli had revived the tradition of Beauvais tapestry manufacture, employing many of her artist friends, among them Picasso, Matisse, Léger, and Georges Braque, to provide cartoons that were executed in the low-warp weave for which the Beauvais workshops were famous. Even Madame's friend, the couturier Paul Poiret, was represented with

79 "A Beauty Salon in Art Moderne: Modern Art in Commerce," *Good Furniture* (May 1928): 242–44; Slesin, *Over the Top*, 46.

80 "A Beauty Salon in Art Moderne," 242. The article goes on to say that "Professor Carl N. Werntz took fifty of his students on a tour of study of Madame Rubinstein's remarkable new shop."

rugs distinguished by elaborate floral designs and dark dramatic borders. Poiret's clothing designs had begun to lose their novel vitality by the end of the 1910s, and he had turned to the decorative arts, founding Atelier Martine in 1912.

Rubinstein's new modernist salon in New York, at 8 East 57th Street, similarly showcased contemporary interior design and decorative arts. According to *The New Yorker*, Madame had chosen the brownstone for its extraordinary staircase. It was the only interior feature she retained; everything else was gutted.[81]

With her new salon, Madame began to exercise more confidently her passion for decor. She continued to import European designers who could imagine Art Deco in a new, American mode. She worked again with Paul Frankl, who had by now become a leading figure in the field of decorative arts. Aided by an American, Donald Deskey, whom he had hired to design screens, Frankl had created a stylistic idiom for American design. The 57th Street salon featured his "Skyscraper" furniture, made in varied styles and kinds of wood and lacquer, and often employing synthetic materials like Bakelite and linoleum. This was a stripped-down version of European Deco, eschewing ornamentation in favor of a cleaner, more industrial line. Frankl's non-American perspective allowed him to put into practice what he had learned from the French Art Deco designers, as well as the Bauhaus and De Stijl schools—a fact not lost on Madame, who consistently employed immigrant artists and designers. The 1930s were to prove her a conjurer of a new breed of hybrid salon—part museum, part fashion house, part department store. Rubinstein knew how to blur boundaries.[82]

At this juncture in her career Rubinstein began to pay greater attention to the fashion industry, acquiring signature clothes for herself. She also began to focus more on the burgeoning world of magazine publishing—the nexus for beauty, art, fashion, and design. A vehicle for this cross-pollination was the modish window display. While shops and department stores had been using window displays for at least a century, by the 1920s the window space in stylish shops had become a site for elaborately staged presentations and scenes, often with a modernist inflection. Some even showed art along with their goods: Bonwit Teller, the most experimental, began to display mannequins along with African art in 1927.

The celebrated industrial designer Raymond Loewy noted the common roots of modernism and fashion. Writing for Bonwit Teller in 1928, he declared that "true modernism is good taste! Bonwit Teller are modernists in that they interpret in dress that which the age expresses in art."[83] The entwinement of modernism and *la mode* within popular, chic department-store displays was further amplified in the fashion magazines. During the next decade Madame, attentive as always to the interaction of the cultural and the commercial, developed friendships with key publishers and editors, for example, inviting *House & Garden* to publicize her new home in Paris, and *Vogue* to cover all her New York events.

Life magazine devoted eight pages to Rubinstein in 1941, featuring her home and life with her glamorous second husband, the affable Prince Artchil Gourielli-Tchkonia, a gentleman of possibly spurious Georgian nobility, more than twenty years her junior. She had married him in 1938 and now possessed a title beyond that of Madame: the press was happy to refer to her as Princess Gourielli.

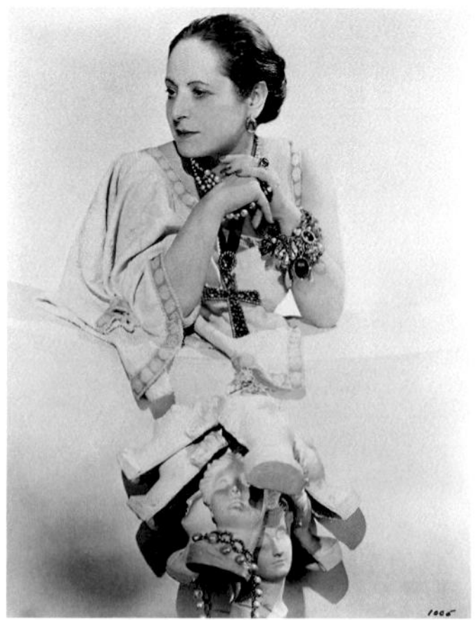

Cecil Beaton's 1938 photograph of Rubinstein in a Schiaparelli sari dress emphasizes her love of heavy jewelry, seen not only in the extraordinary collection she wears but also in the cascading busts beneath her.

81 Jo Swerling, "Profiles," *New Yorker* 4, no. 19 (June 30, 1928): 20–22. While the article is a substantive profile of Rubinstein, it is full of inaccuracies that Rubinstein herself blithely introduced regarding her early life and the start of her business. About her family years, she seems to have revealed only that she was "undistinguished in childhood and early girlhood, except her complexion, about which her boy friends wrote poetry."

82 See Clifford, "Helena Rubinstein's Beauty Salons," 91.

83 Loewy, quoted in Terry Smith, *Making the Modern* (Chicago: University of Chicago Press, 1993), 361, cited in Clifford, "Helena Rubinstein's Beauty Salons," 91.

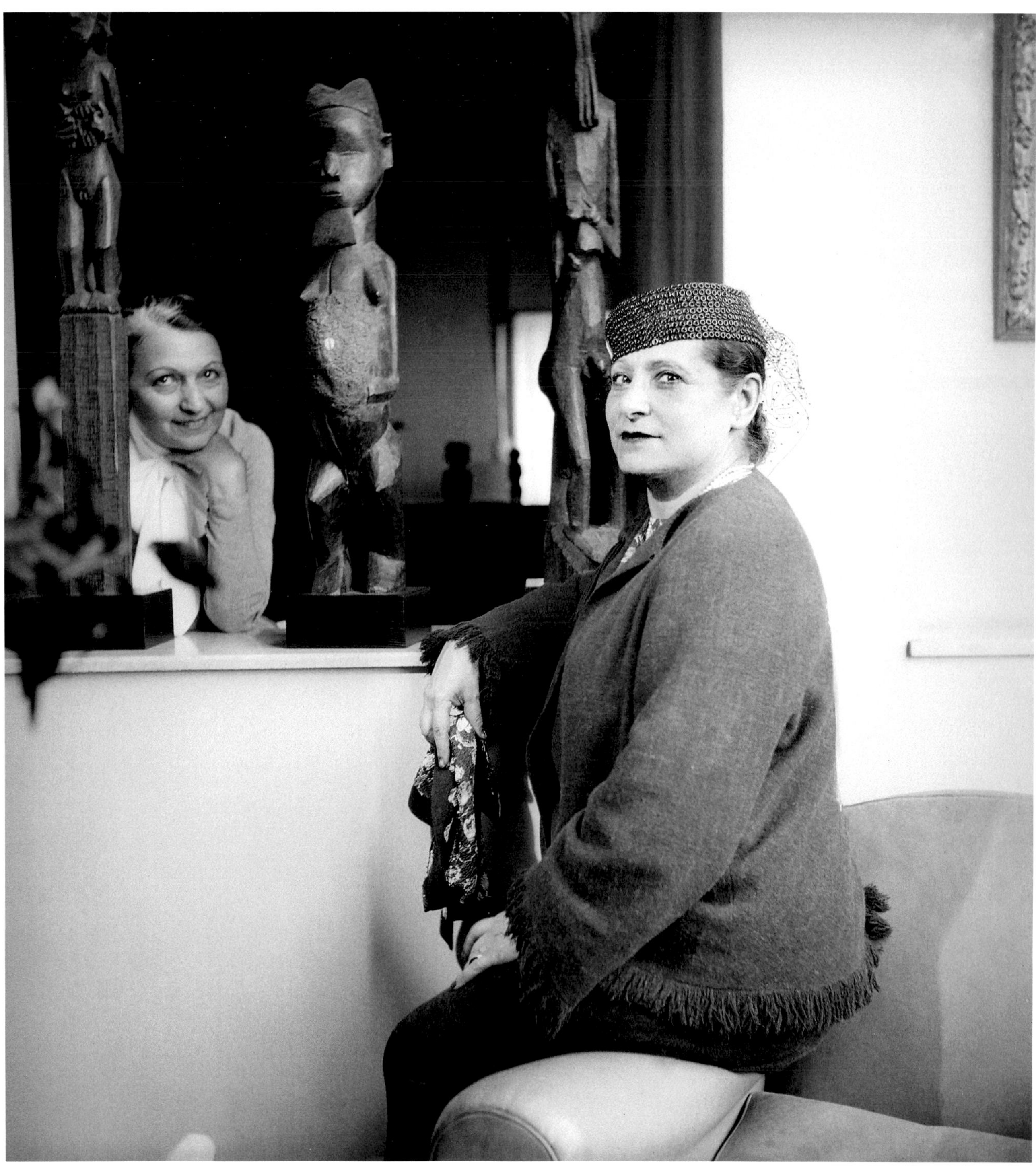

Marie Cuttoli and Helena Rubinstein, 1934.

Boris Lovet-Lorski
God Unknown, 1926
Marble, 10½ in. (26.7 cm) high
Berry-Hill Galleries, New York

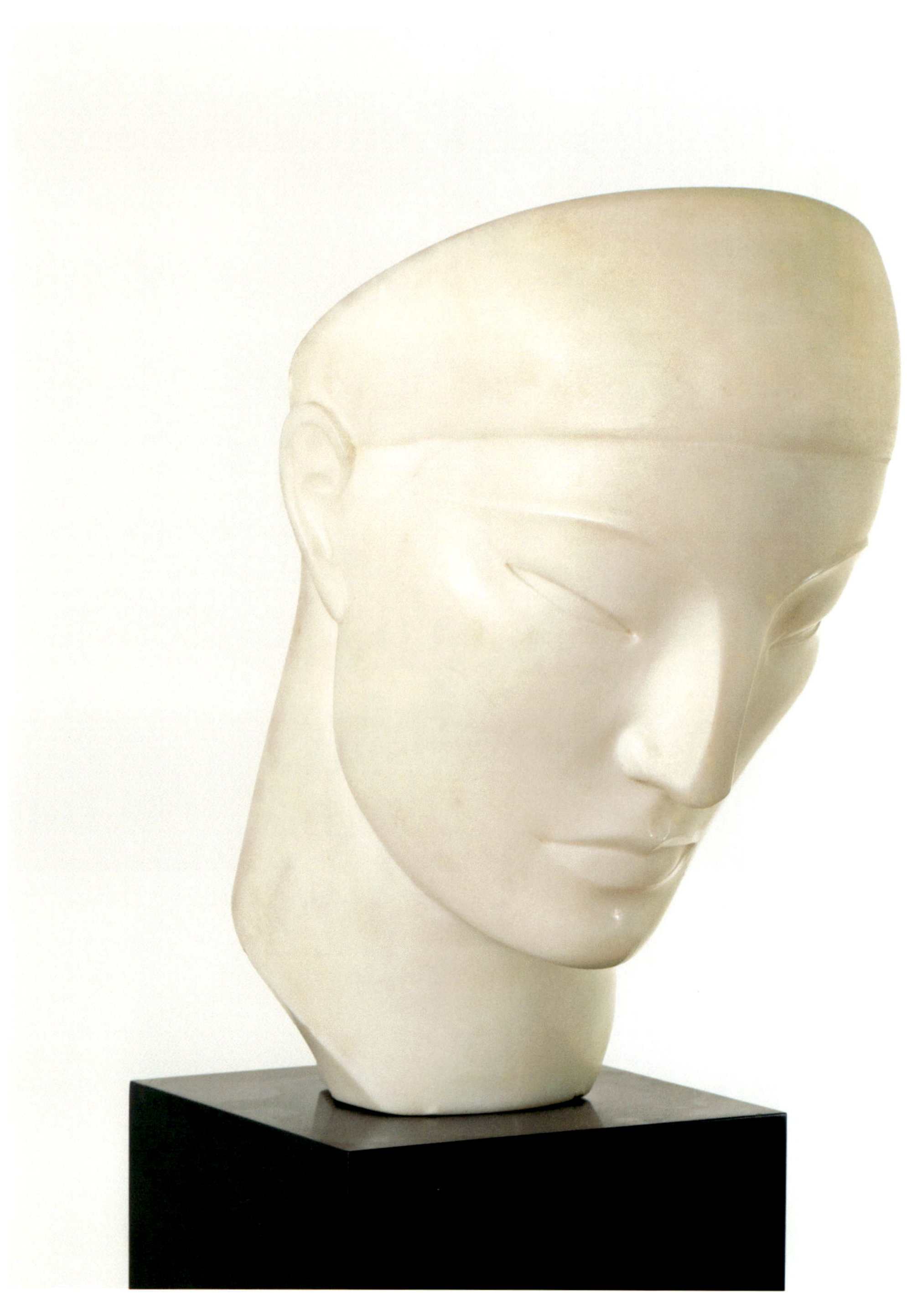

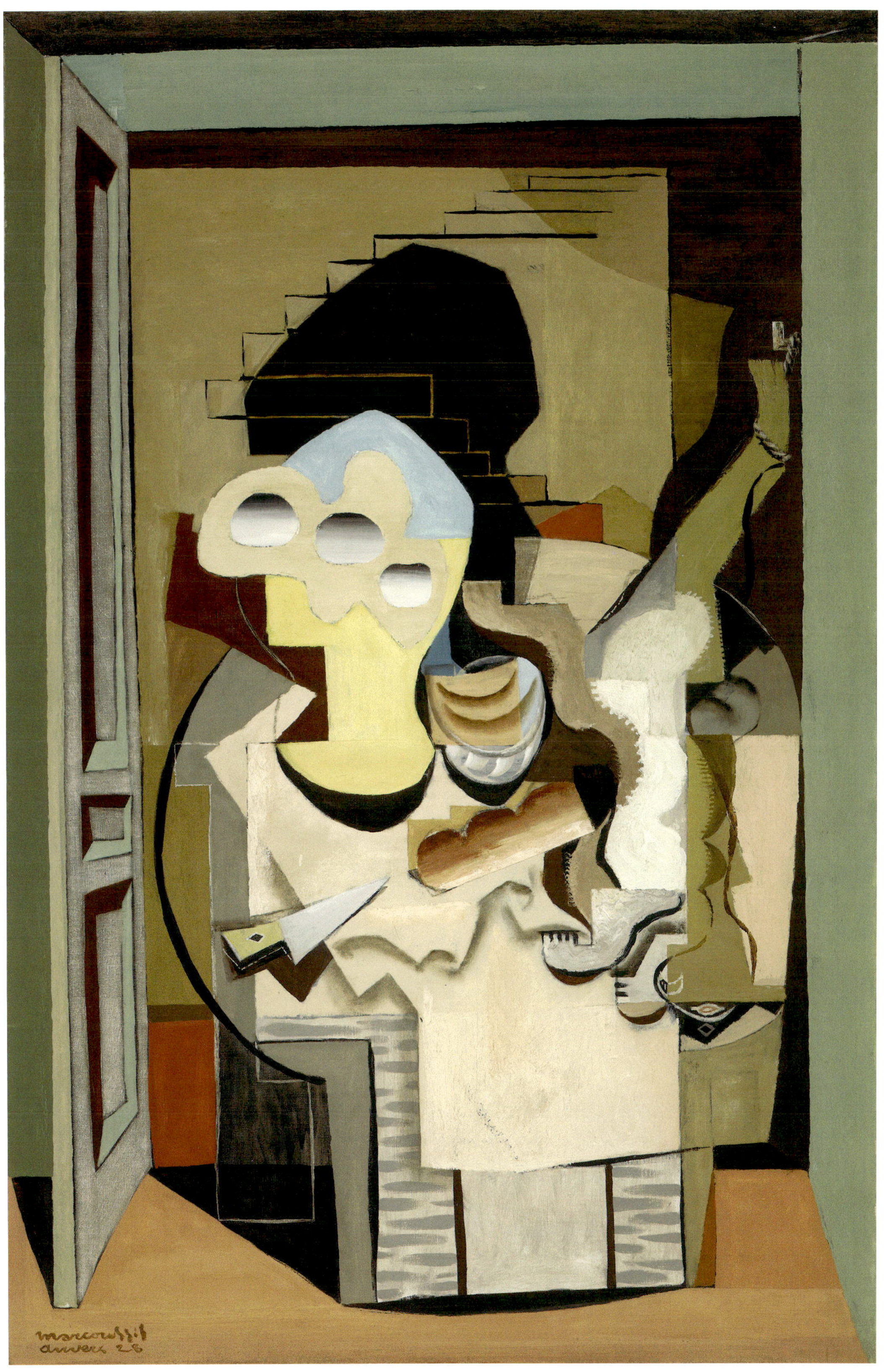

Louis Casimir Marcoussis
Anvers, 1928
Oil on canvas, 56¾ × 37 in. (144.2 × 94 cm)
Yale University Art Gallery, New Haven, Connecticut,
Charles B. Benenson, B.A. 1933, Collection

With his brand of wry Cubism, Marcoussis alludes to the love and toil of domesticity. A table bears an assembly of culinary tools and victuals, including a menacing knife and the hanging carcass of an animal. Rubinstein was ambivalent about her domestic role; Marcoussis, a good friend, was clearly sympathetic. A French artist of Polish Jewish origin, he knew a thing or two about conflict.

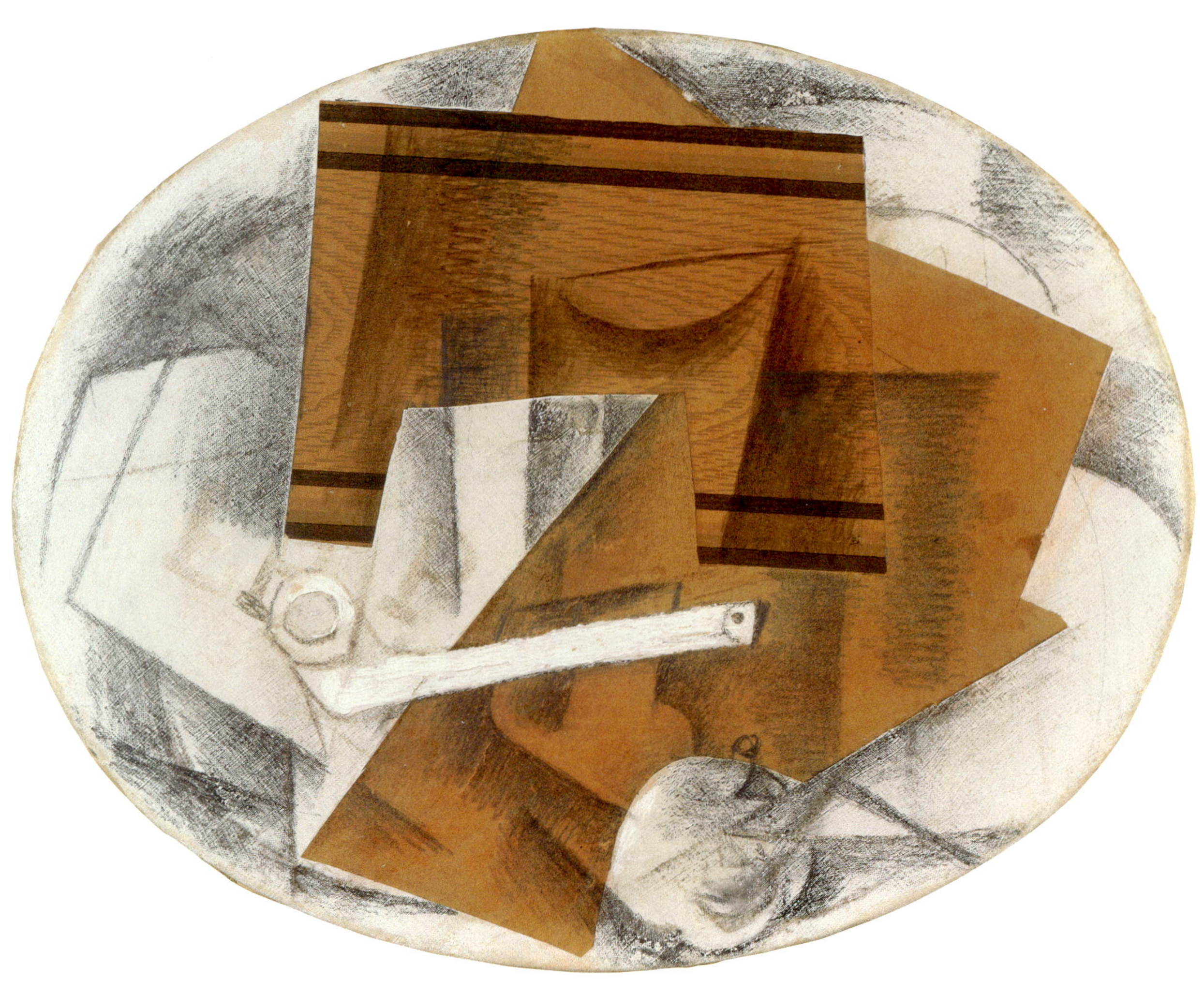

Georges Braque
Still Life with Pipe and Glass, c. 1913
Charcoal, paint, and pasted paper on canvas
10¼ × 13¼ in. (26 × 33.7 cm)
Private collection, Greenwich, Connecticut

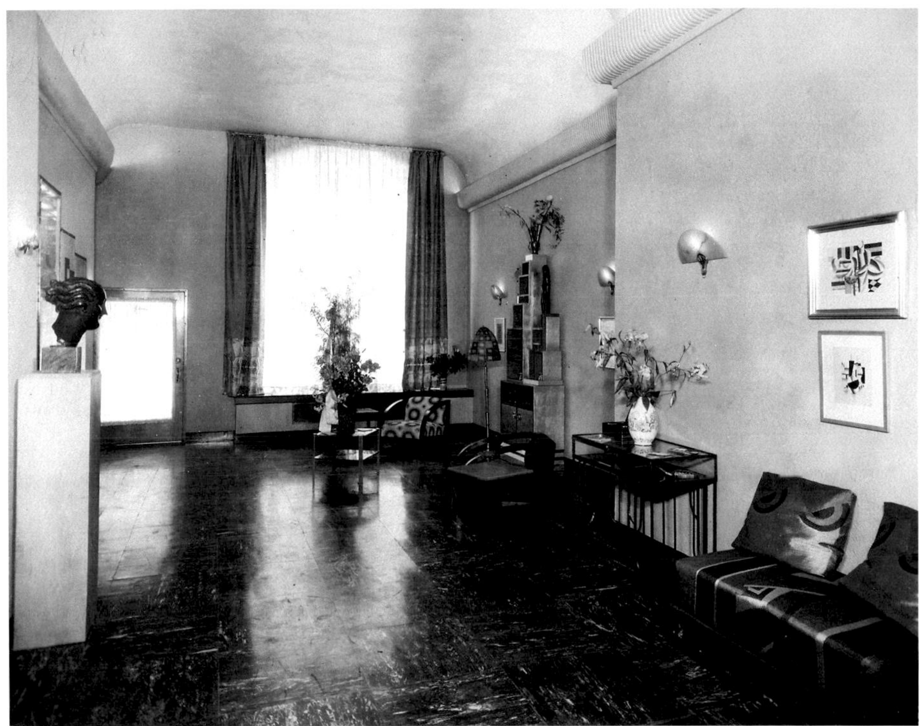

Helena Rubinstein salon, 8 East 57th Street, New York, 1928, interior design by Paul T. Frankl, assisted by Donald Deskey. The use of new materials and the absence of traditional ornament can be seen in the salon's balancing of bare walls with spare, modernist works. The clean lines of Léger's drawings on the right are echoed in the plain pedestals upon which Nadelman's busts are placed, or the austere lines of the settee and its neighboring wrought-iron table. The linoleum floor, applied in easily installed, prefabricated modular units, was also a modernist import. Linoleum had been widely used by European architects and designers such as Josef Hoffmann and Bruno Paul since the turn of the century.

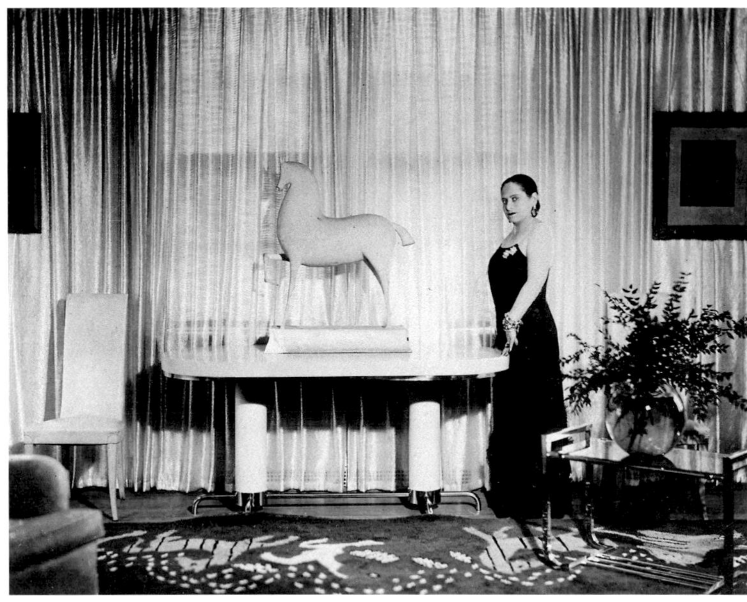

Deskey also designed Rubinstein's home at 895 Park Avenue. Elie Nadelman's plaster horse and a Jean Lurçat carpet are seen here in 1934.

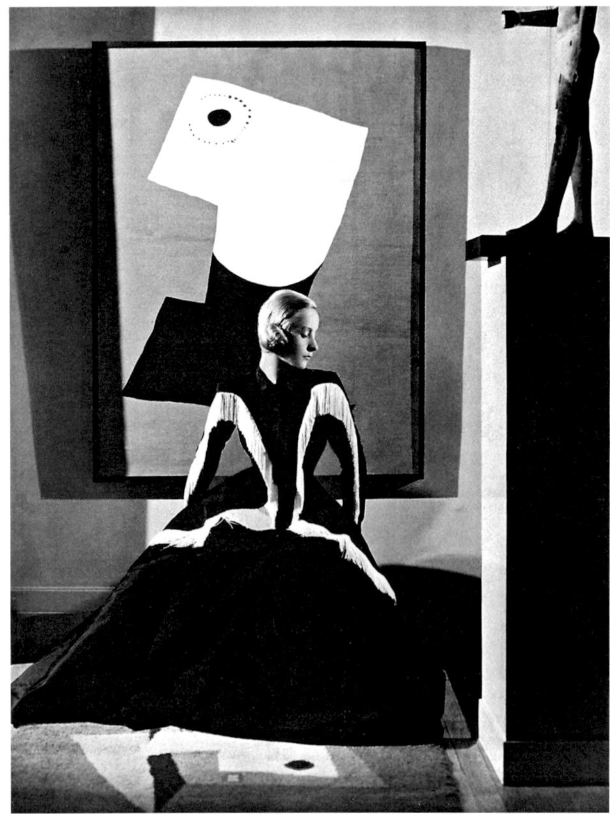

A model in Balenciaga with Joan Miró's 1927 *Portrait*, photographed in Rubinstein's Paris home, 1939.

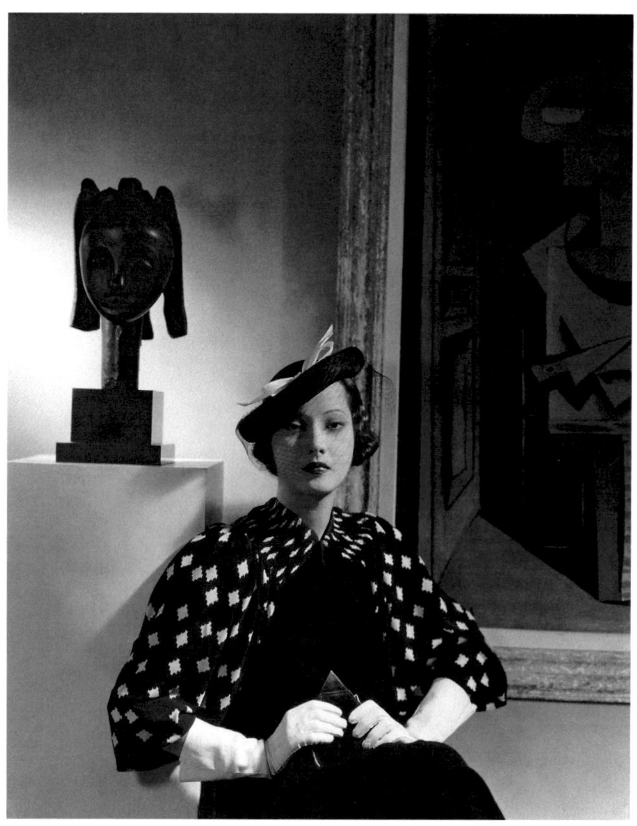

The actress Merle Oberon photographed by Edward Steichen in New York in 1935 for *Vogue*, with a Fang reliquary head and Louis Marcoussis's 1928 painting *Anvers*.

Rubinstein used her own spectacular homes for fashion shoots and publicity photographs for her business. At the time this was unprecedented, though over the next three decades the use of noted photographers and grand private homes became a signature of fashion magazines. Her art collections were often featured as prominently as the models.

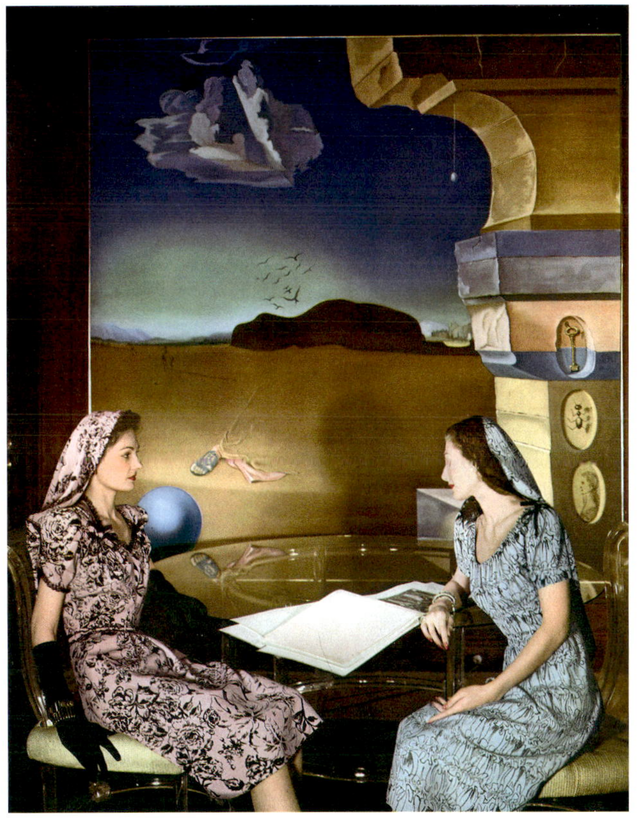

Models wearing Adele Simpson fashions, photographed for *Vogue* at 625 Park Avenue, New York; a Dalí mural is in the background.

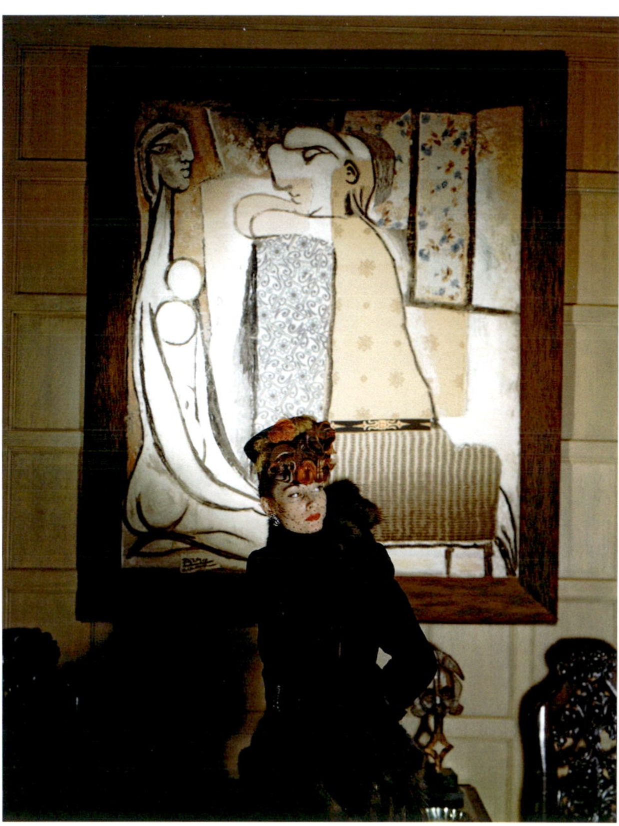

A *Vogue* model in 1944, with Picasso's 1934 tapestry *Confidence*, at 625 Park Avenue.

Overleaf: Rubinstein's art collections serve as a backdrop to a fashion shoot for *Life* magazine in her Paris apartment, 1963.

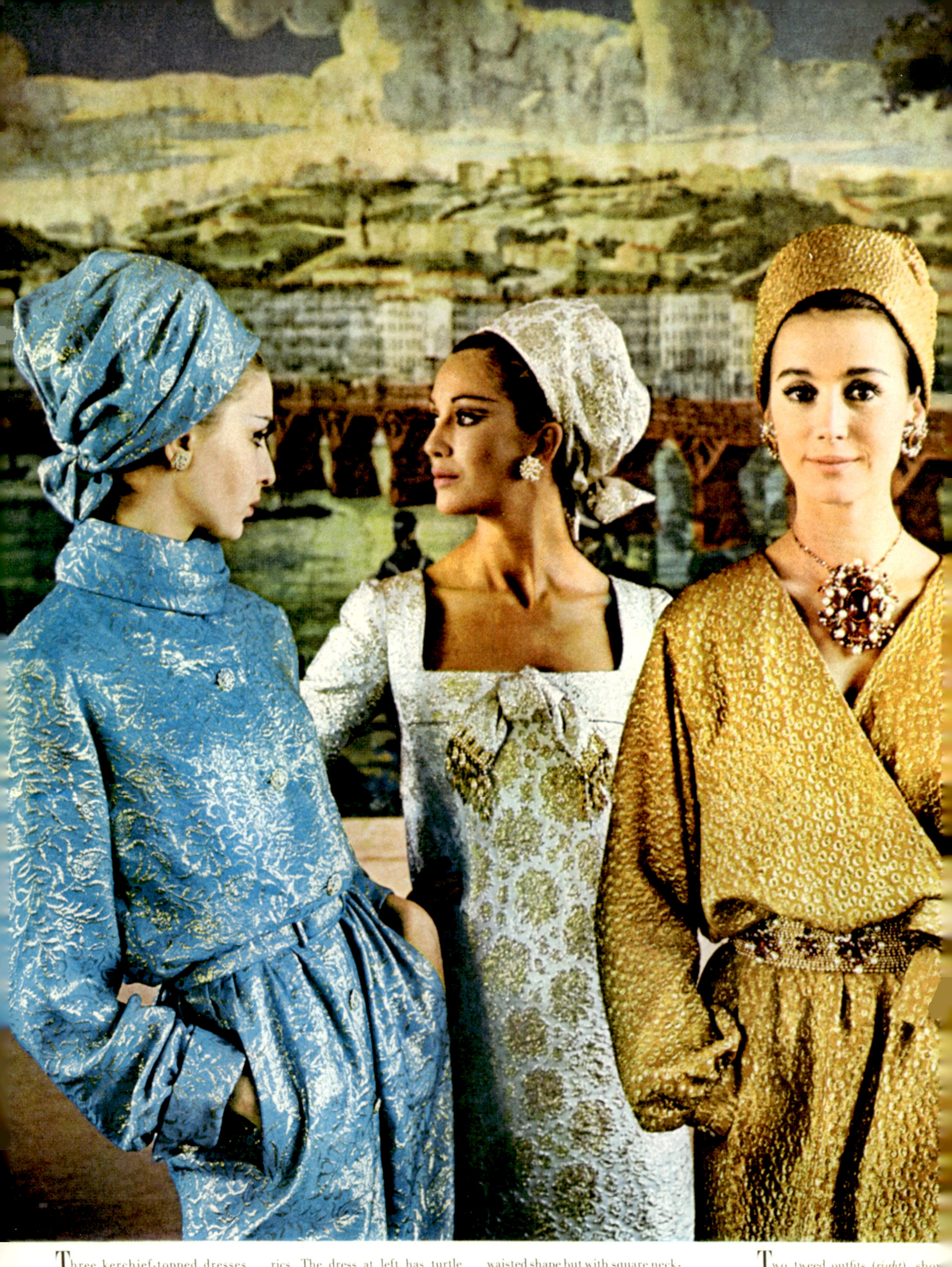

Three kerchief-topped dresses from Dior are the epitome of casual shapes done in sumptuous fabrics. The dress at left has turtle neck and buttons up front. The center dress has the popular unwaisted shape but with square neckline. Dress at right has wrapped top, is worn with huge fake jewel.

Two tweed outfits (*right*), show in Madame Rubinstein's conserv tory, are trimmed with fur. Suit

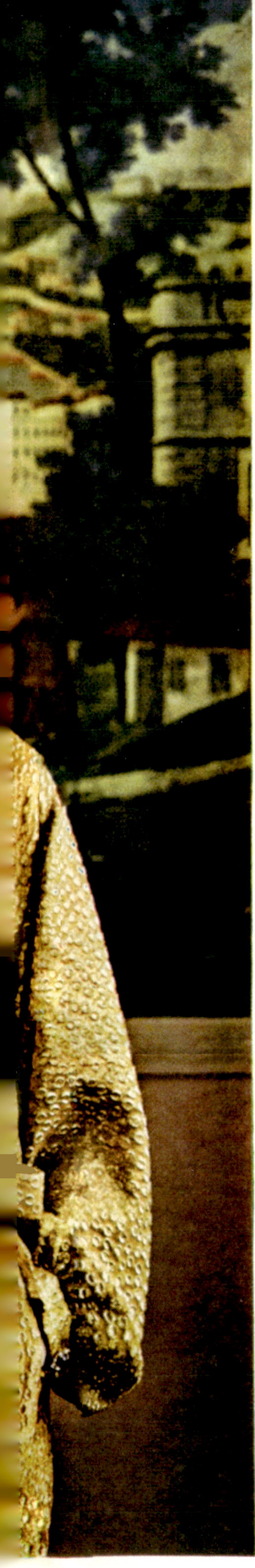

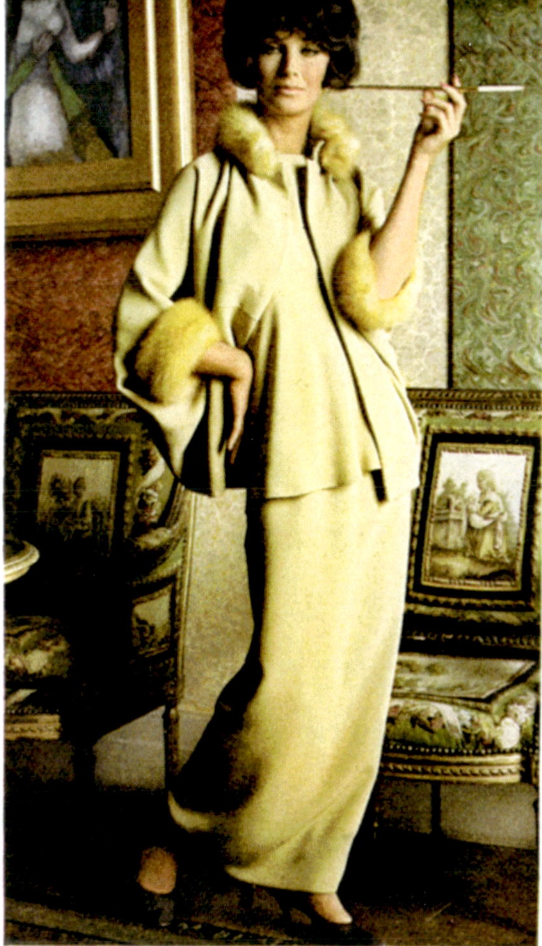

Crepe dinner outfit with '30s droop and matching fox fur trim is from Cardin. Chairs are Louis XVI.

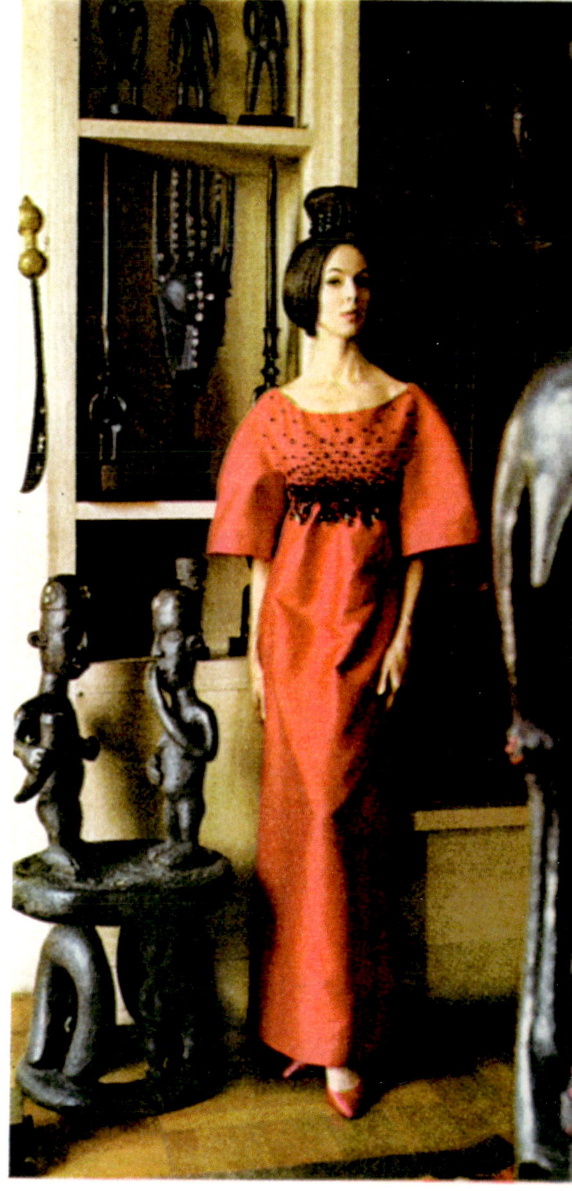

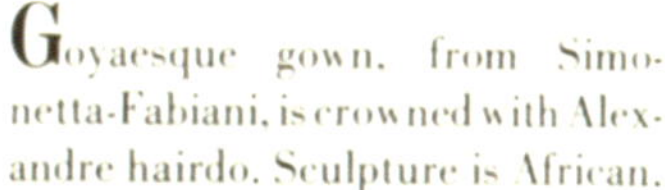

Goyaesque gown, from Simonetta-Fabiani, is crowned with Alexandre hairdo. Sculpture is African.

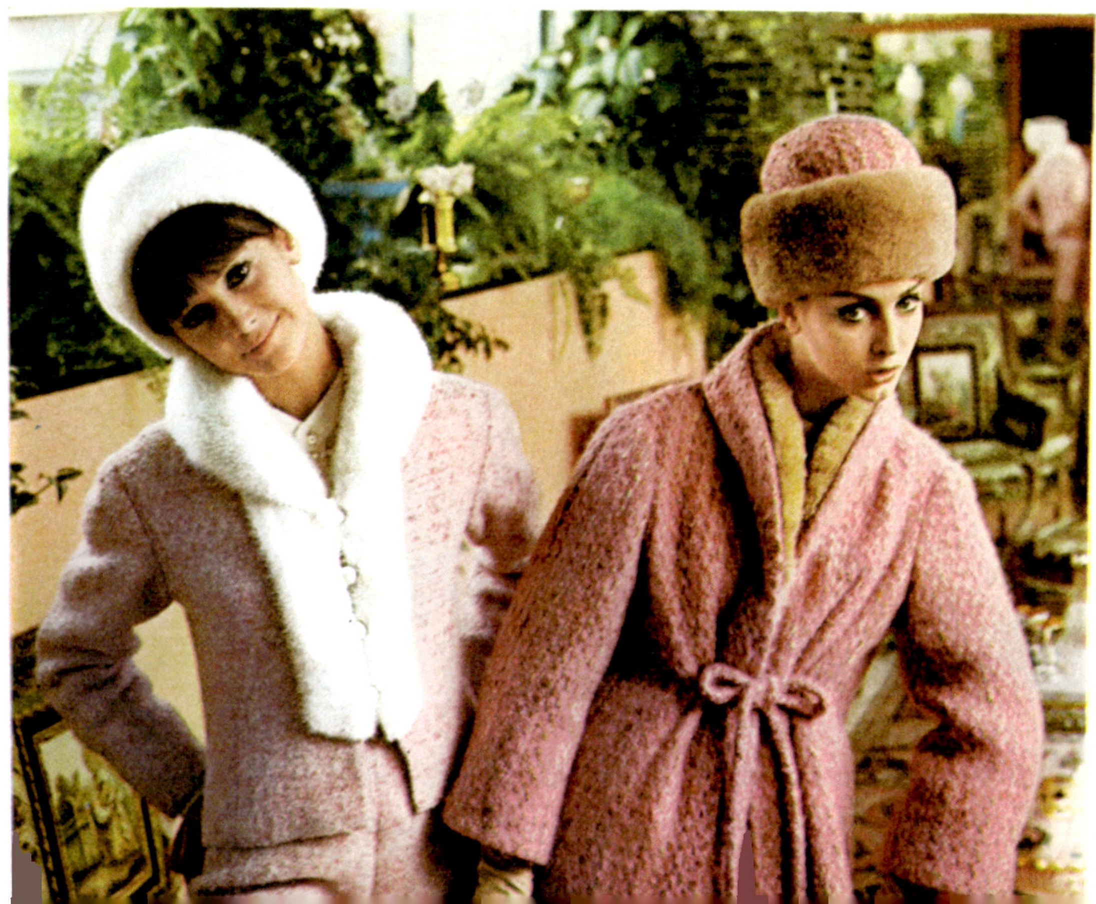

leftith white mink is from Nina Ric. Coat faced with guanaco and maning hat come from Laroche.

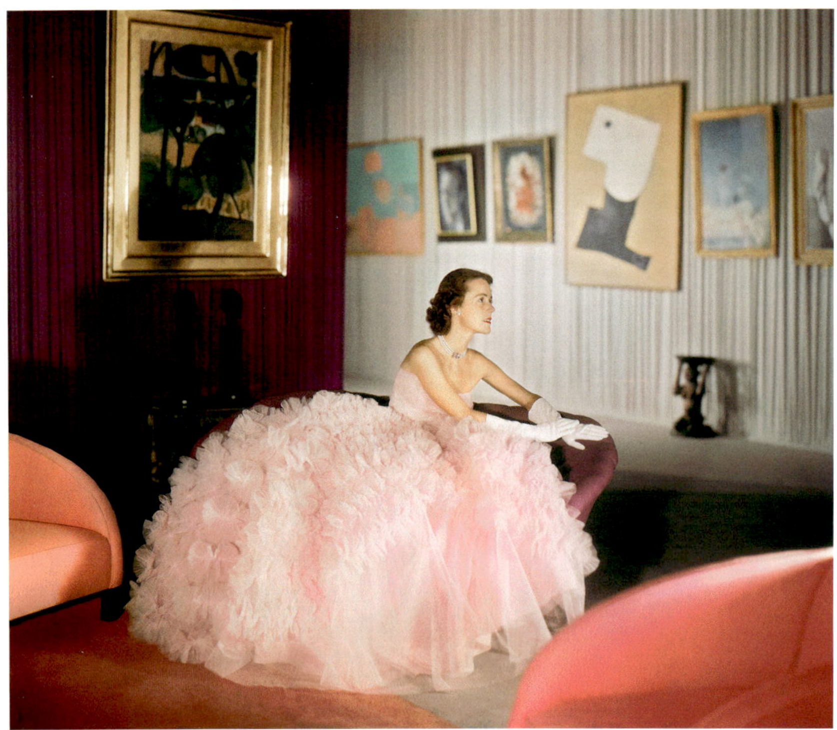

The socialite Mrs. R. Fulton Cutting II poses in the art gallery of Rubinstein's home at 625 Park Avenue in 1950. On the pleated fabric walls are works by Matisse, de Kooning, Tchelitchew, Brauner, Miró, and others. Baule and Luba sculptures stand to either side.

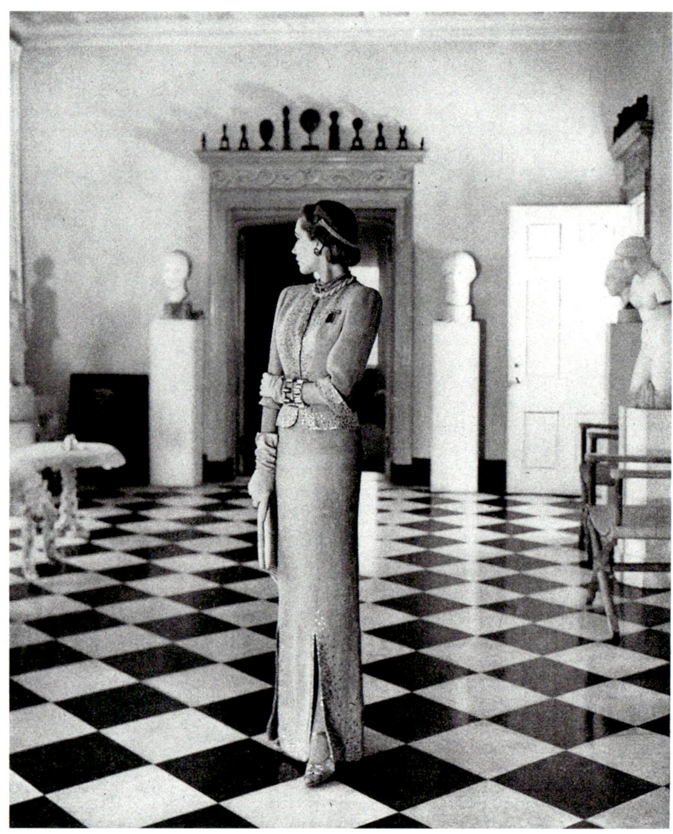

In a 1944 photo shoot for *Vogue*, a model stands in the foyer of the apartment at 625 Park Avenue, surrounded by Nadelman and African sculptures.

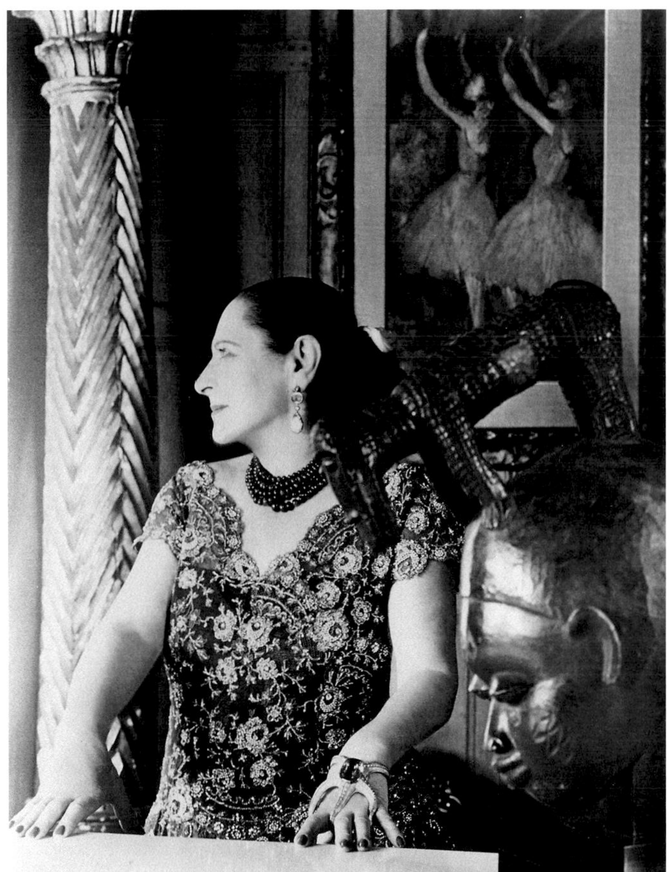

Rubinstein in a 1957 publicity shot, dressed in a Christian Dior gown of Chantilly lace, intricately embroidered with sequins and beads. She wears her famous starfish hand ornament, said to have been worn originally by Sarah Bernhardt. Madame stands in dramatic profile between a Degas pastel, *Two Dancers, Arms Raised*, and a Yoruba helmet mask from her legendary African art collection.

High Fashion, High Art

The introduction of fashion into the Rubinstein salon began with her own personal connections to figures in the fashion world. Madame cultivated alliances on both sides of the Atlantic—from Carmel Snow, American fashion editor of *Vogue* and later editor of the American edition of *Harper's Bazaar*, to Poiret, Coco Chanel, and Elsa Schiaparelli in Paris. Rubinstein had been one of Schiaparelli's first clients, and they shared a particular artistic sensibility. She responded to the designer's playful and varied artistic approaches to the female form, and to Schiaparelli's liberal use of historical references in her clothes and accessories. There were nods to classical Greece, the Orient, and Africa in her fabrics; the flashier materials—lamé and silk jacquard shot through with metallic thread—thoroughly appealed to Madame, as did the designer's interest in the circus, a theme she loved.

Madame, like Schiaparelli, mixed sources and influences without constraint.[84] With one foot planted in New York, the capital of magazine art direction, and one in Paris, the capital of fashion, she easily maintained her role as an exemplar of foreign chic and influence in the United States. In the course of the 1930s this cachet began to ebb as the luxury salon business gave way to mass marketing and retail; nevertheless, her exoticism, her collections of modern and African art, her jewels and eccentricities continued to fascinate, providing much fodder for publicity.

When the Museum of Modern Art asked Rubinstein to lend to its groundbreaking exhibition *African Negro Art* in 1935, she happily contributed seventeen works, including an exquisite large Bakota *Mbulu Ngulu* reliquary figure from Gabon; a Fang reliquary head composed of varied geometries—oval head, circular face, cylindrical neck, lozenge-shaped eye; and a rare Fang four-faced helmet mask, each face a different size (see pages 114 and 115). The exhibition, organized by James Johnson Sweeney and comprising more than six hundred sculptures and textiles, was the first major museum effort to foreground such work as fine art rather than ethnographic objects.[85]

Around the time the show opened, Rubinstein released a publicity shot she had commissioned from George Maillard Kesslere, who had painted her portrait almost a decade before (see pages 49 and 116). It portrays Madame as a connoisseur, proudly exhibiting one of her masks from the Ivory Coast. Although her gloves were meant to suggest the accouterments of a conservator, they were designed by Chanel in black velvet with enormous straw cuffs, a juxtaposition of materials that subtly speaks to her equation of Western and African cultures.[86] She wears a close cap with a thick braid that frames her face in the style of classical Greek and Roman portrait busts—or Nadelman's modernist versions of them (see page 74).

The photograph draws an explicit connection between her face and that of the sculpture she holds. The accompanying press release underscored this mixed appeal: "Today, Negro sculptures . . . are recognized

84 See Clifford, "Helena Rubinstein's Beauty Salons," 91.

85 It is striking that within a year of opening, the new museum was mounting a show of non-Western art—spurred by the interest in it of Picasso and the Cubists, but also by a progressive, globalized sensibility.

86 See Clifford, "Helena Rubinstein's Beauty Salons," 103.

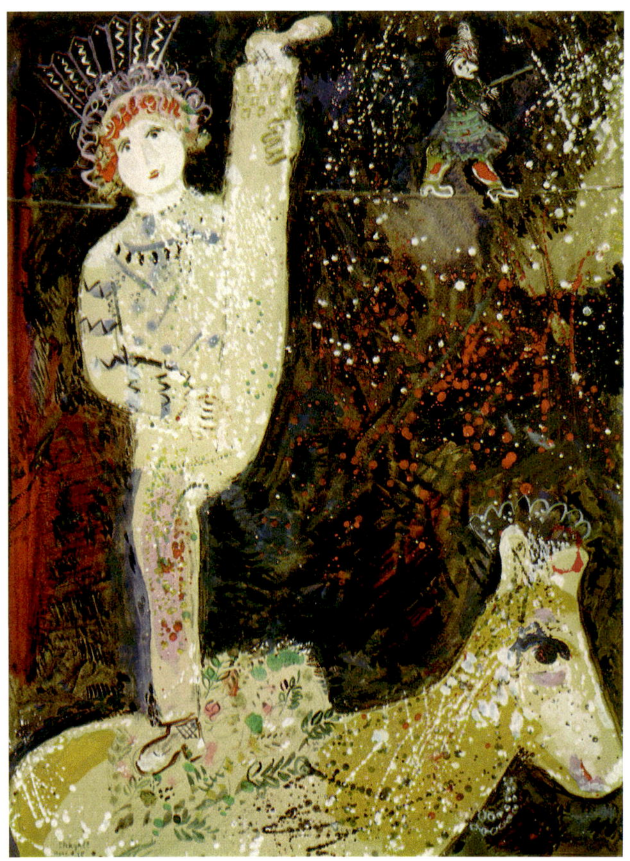

Marc Chagall
Circus Scene, 1926
Gouache, 24 × 18½ in. (61 × 47 cm)
Location unknown

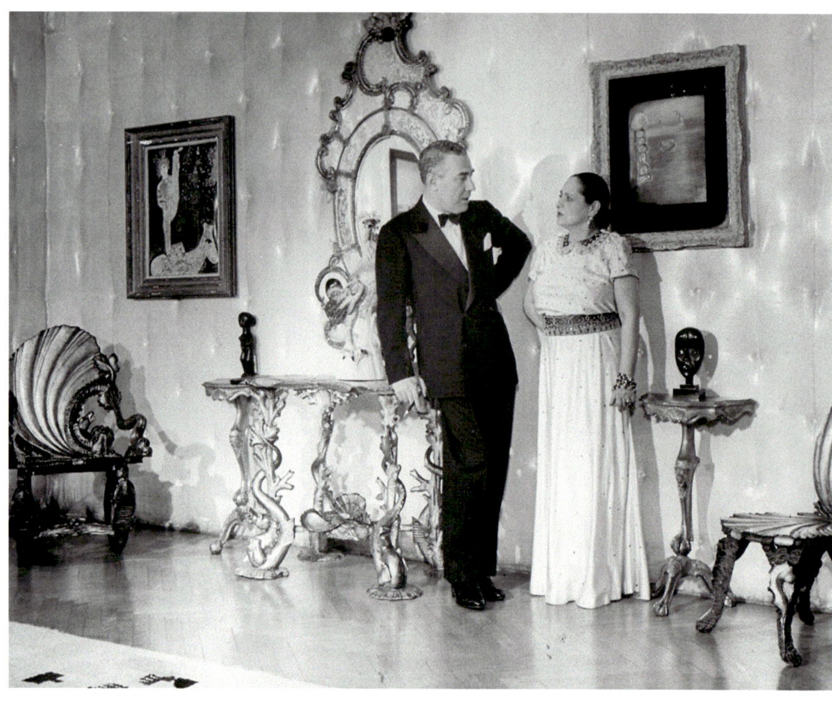

Princess Gourielli, in Schiaparelli, and Prince Artchil Gourielli at home, photographed by Alfred Eisenstaedt, c. 1941. Chagall's *Circus Scene* is visible on the wall behind them.

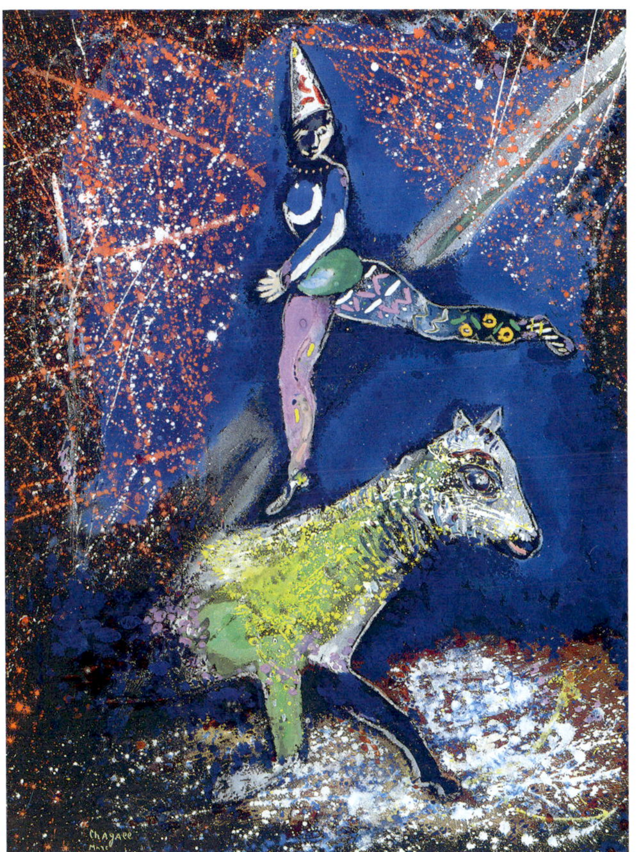

Marc Chagall
The Acrobat on Horseback, 1927–28
Gouache and ink, 24 × 18 in. (61 × 45.7 cm)
Collection of Julian Robertson

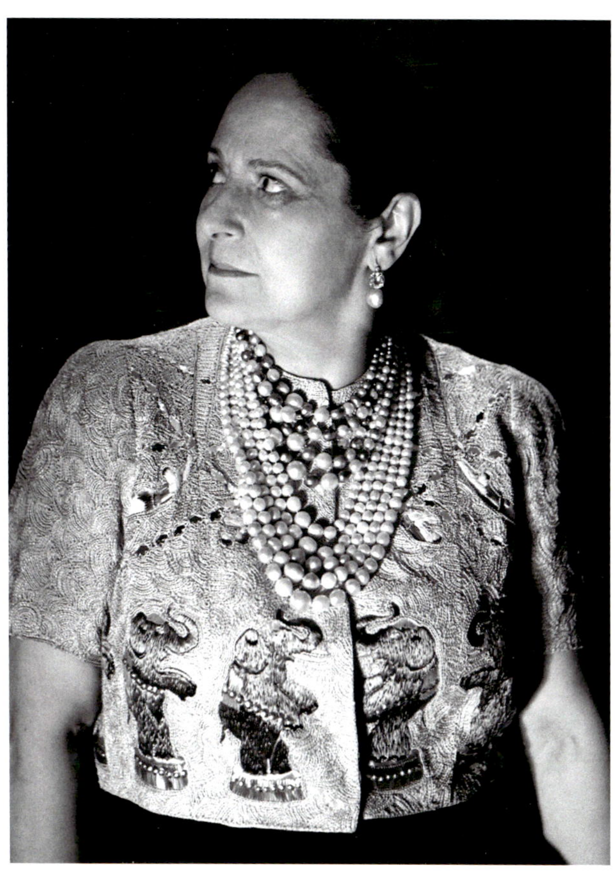

Rubinstein's celebrated Schiaparelli bolero jacket, thickly embroidered with elephants, from the designer's 1938 Circus collection.

Fang reliquary head
Gabon, nineteenth century
Wood, 13¾ in. (34.9 cm) high
Private collection

Fang mask
Gabon, nineteenth century
Wood, kaolin, 14¼ in. (35.6 cm) high
Detroit Institute of Arts, Founders Society Purchase, New Endowment Fund, General Endowment Fund, Benson and Edith Ford Fund, Henry Ford II Fund, Conrad H. Smith Fund

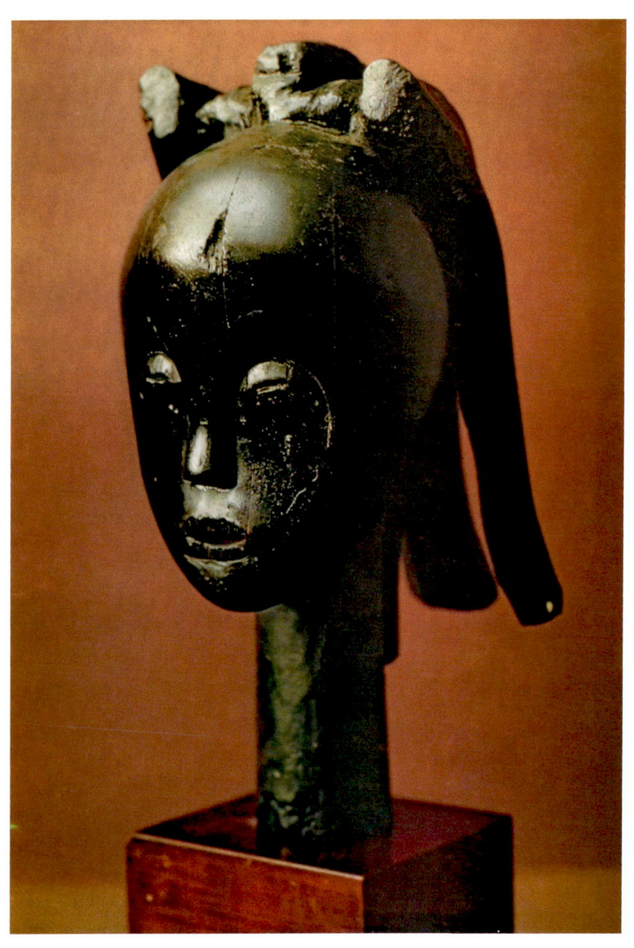

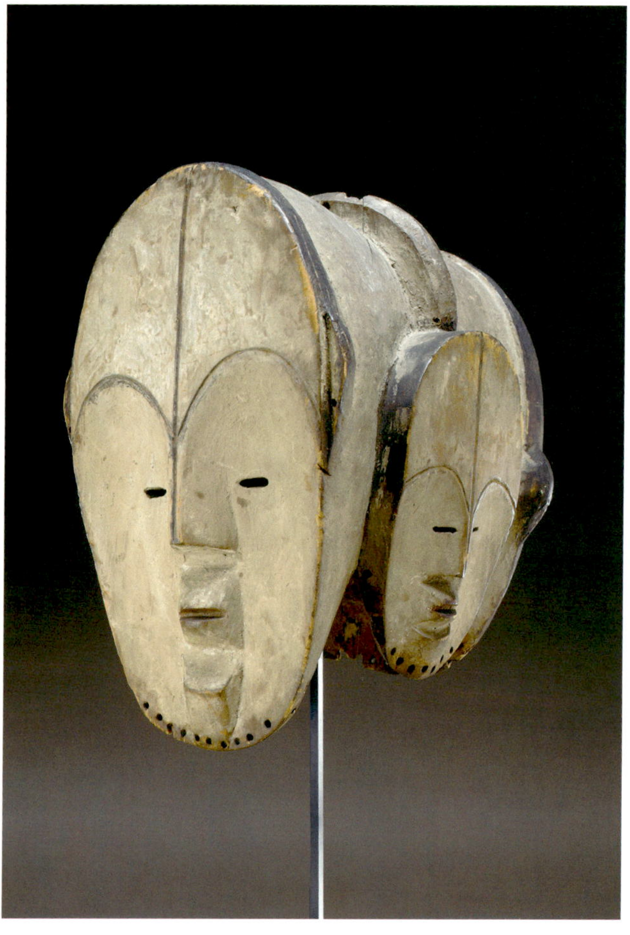

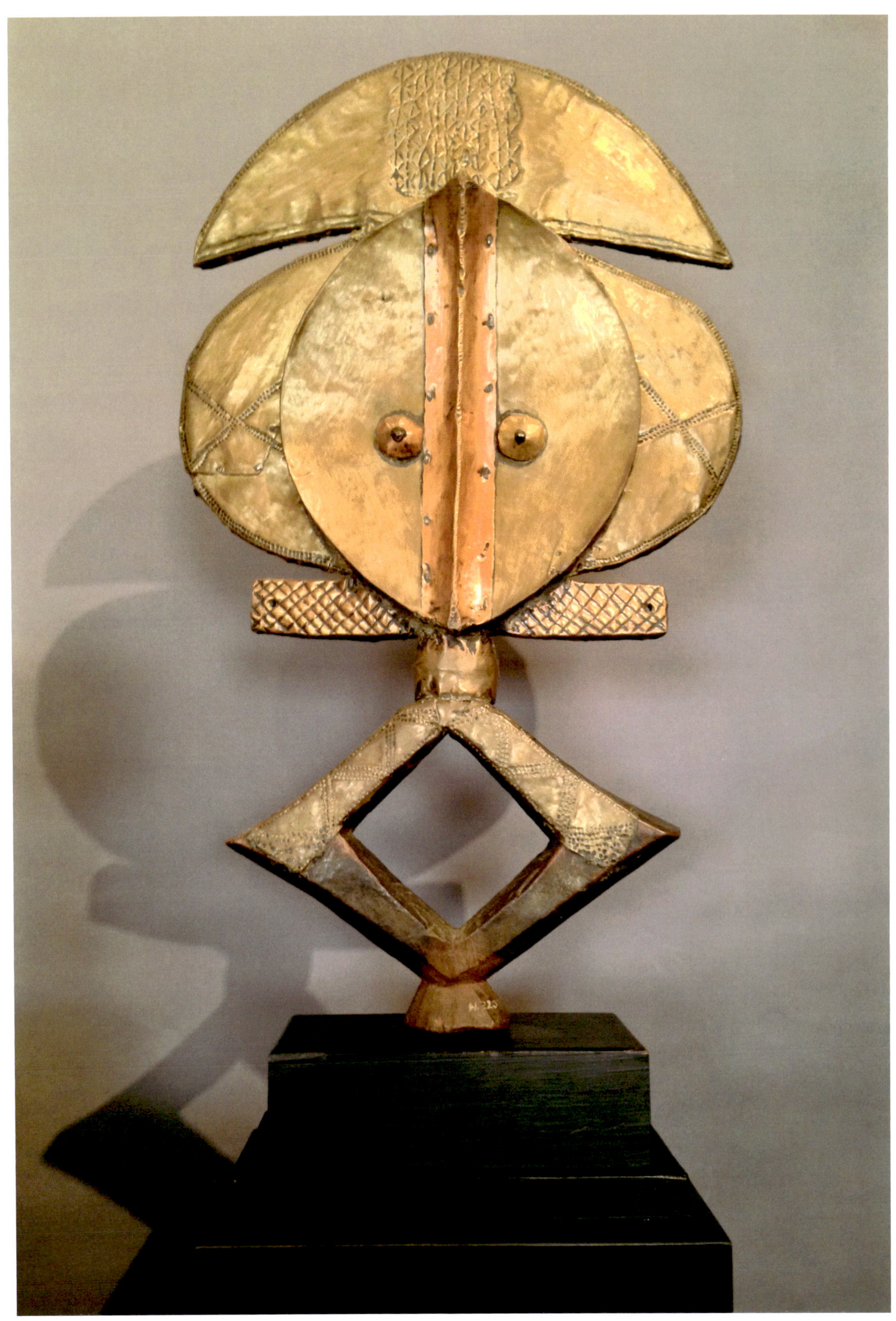

Bakota reliquary guardian figure
Gabon, date unknown
Wood, brass, and copper, 25½ in. (64.8 cm) high
Private collection

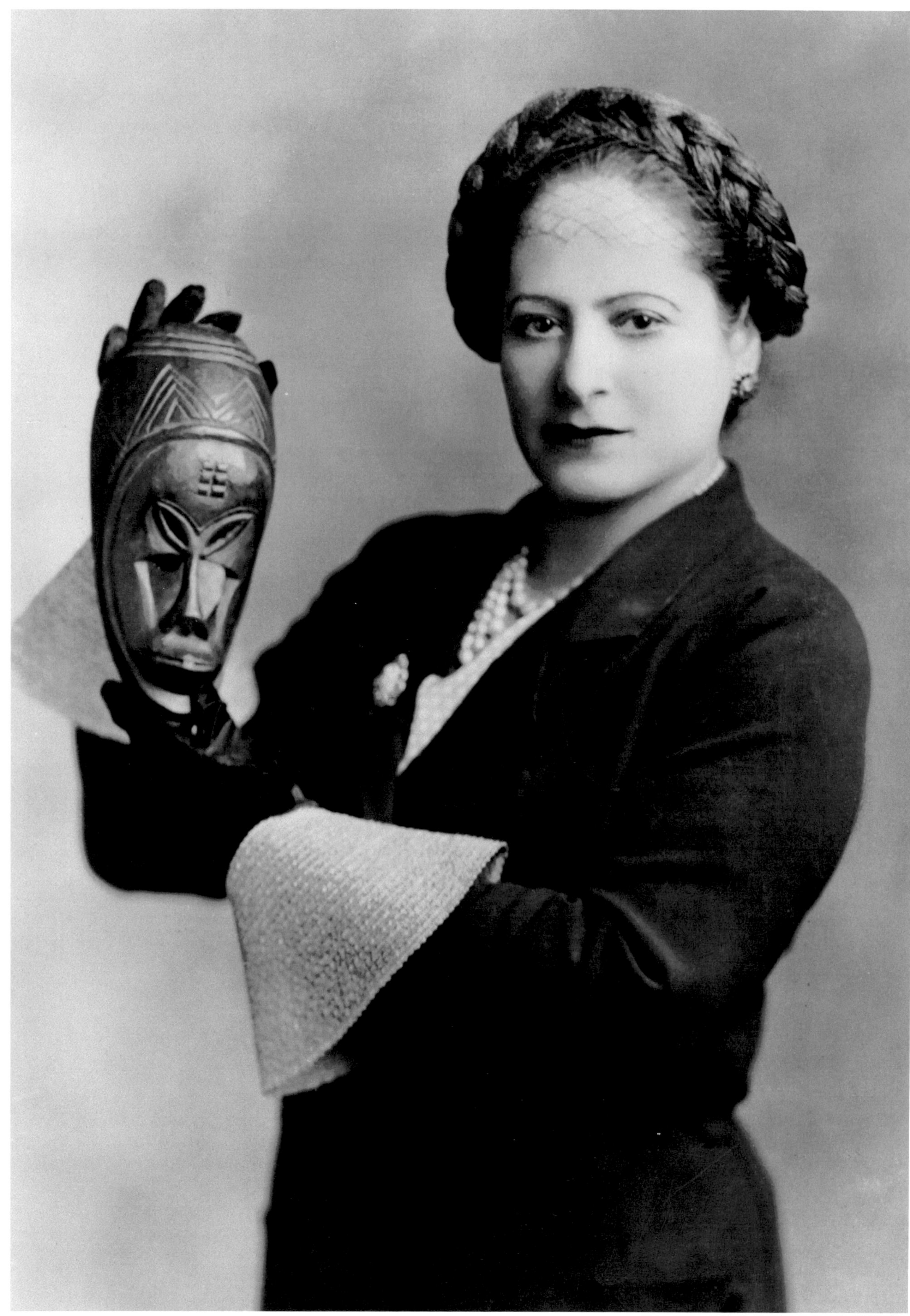

Helena Rubinstein with an African mask, 1934.

as having a true aesthetic value and a peculiar beauty all of their own, entirely different, but no less interesting than the more conventional, long-accepted standards of Greek sculptural beauty."[87] Madame's calculated positioning of herself in two worlds—the artistic vanguard and high fashion—served to distinguish and distance her from Arden. It also helped solidify her exoticism at a moment when the flourishing world of fashion magazines and upscale retail stores had begun to embrace the avant-garde.

In 1936, Rubinstein was finally able to acquire a building on Fifth Avenue, between 55th and 56th streets, and opened a flagship store, down the block from her competitor with the fancy red door. Its unadorned ultramodernist limestone facade was designed by Harold Sterner and famously displayed her name in widely spaced sans-serif, lowercase letters—h e l e n a r u b i n s t e i n.[88] Lewis Mumford, the architecture critic for *The New Yorker*, called it "the best recent shop front" on Fifth Avenue.[89] *Harper's Bazaar* was equally enthusiastic. "From across the street her salon is a luxurious façade. Once inside the door it is a gigantic and splendid boudoir."[90]

The opening of the salon was timed to coordinate with the Museum of Modern Art's popular exhibition *Fantastic Art, Dada, Surrealism*. As one entered the doors, one was met with a spectacle, a surreal decor comprising a mélange of period styles—from Rococo to Victorian to contemporary—intended to jolt the senses. The interior, designed by Ladislas Medgyes and Martine Kane, presented the boldest panoply yet of Madame's eclecticism. There were theatrically daring color contrasts and imposing royal-blue silk draperies held back dramatically by passementerie tassels to reveal floor-to-ceiling mirrored walls that staged an endless repetition of the space. The round reception area was fitted out with Victorian Belter sofas upholstered in white silk, placed against freestanding walls papered in metallic blue, save only for Nadelman's suite of large terracotta statuettes, *The Four Seasons*, each on its own wall. In the center of the room a plaster urn, poised above a commanding tufted seating unit, provided a source of light (see page 119). Along the hallway beyond, one passed Giorgio De Chirico's mythological mural of gods and white horses among classical ruins, which Madame had commissioned, in front of Jean-Michel Frank's oak-and-leather chairs, which faced a pair of colossal carved marble urns on pedestals. The seven-floor salon included a library, decorated with works from Madame's collection: Nadelman's *Two Nudes*, Modigliani drawings, a carpet designed by Léger, Frank lamps, and several portraits of Madame (see page 33).[91]

The grandness of the establishment finally allowed her to create displays that echoed those of a museum. She installed her collection of miniature rooms—dollhouse-size dioramas showing rooms decorated in various period styles. They ranged from a mid-eighteenth-century French Rococo room with Louis XV furniture and an early eighteenth-century Queen Anne dining room through the mid-Victorian English style of the 1860s, and even included an Austrian country kitchen of the same period. It was as if Rubinstein were representing her lifelong, encyclopedic experimentation with playful decorative fantasies in her many homes. The display seemed at once to define her past and justify its unceasing contemporary transformation.

On the street facade, she turned her display windows into performance spaces. Shortly after the salon opened, she enacted a set of quasi-Surrealist *tableaux vivants* of well-known paintings, such as Edouard Manet's *The Balcony* and Picasso's *Woman in a Blouse*, with live models placed behind a gilded frame (see page 125). The event caused such a stir

87 Helena Rubinstein Foundation archives, Special Collections, Fashion Institute of Technology Library, New York.

88 This was a nod toward the influence of her first husband, Edward Titus, and his many modernist literary friends, among them e. e. cummings; Woodhead, *War Paint*, 237. But her use of such lowercase lettering dated to at least the 1920s and had appeared on product labels (see page 82) as well as in the fluorescent sign on her Grafton Street salon (see page 88).

89 "The Sky Line," *New Yorker* 12, no. 47 (January 9, 1937): 48, 50–51. Mumford praises the considered integration of the old building and its new facade, describing it as "a design that makes a more conscious use of modern materials and constructional devices. . . . the shop's facade fits into the old-fashioned building above without submitting to it." *Life* acclaimed the salon as Madame's "toniest"; see "The Business of Beauty Is the Business of Rubinstein," *Life* 2, no. 9 (March 1, 1937): 39.

90 Carola De Peyster Kip, "Worn Out and Repaired," *Harper's Bazaar* 71 (February 1937): 102.

91 The establishment also included rooms for classes, private massages, and other services, as well as an auditorium for lectures and public programs.

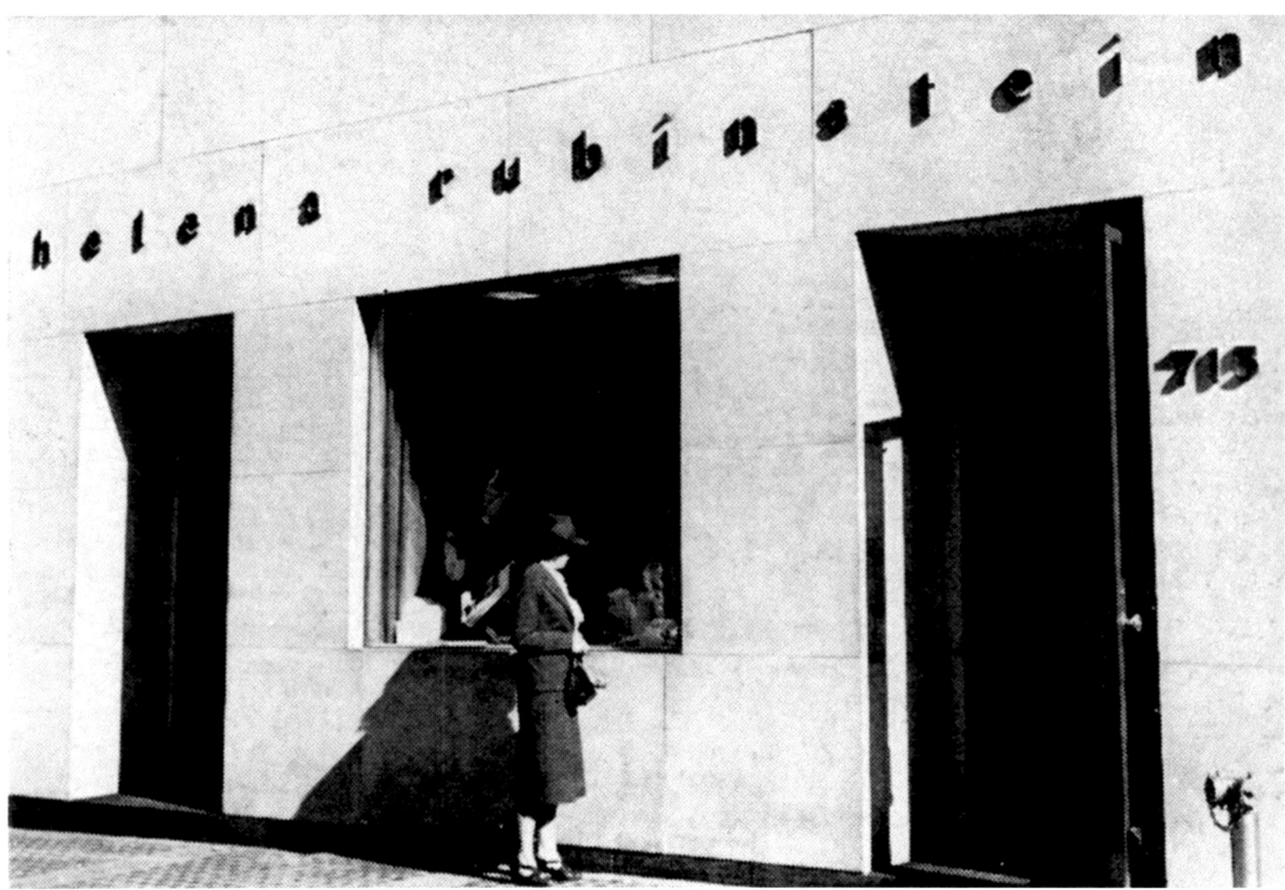

Helena Rubinstein salon, 715 Fifth Avenue, New York, 1941.

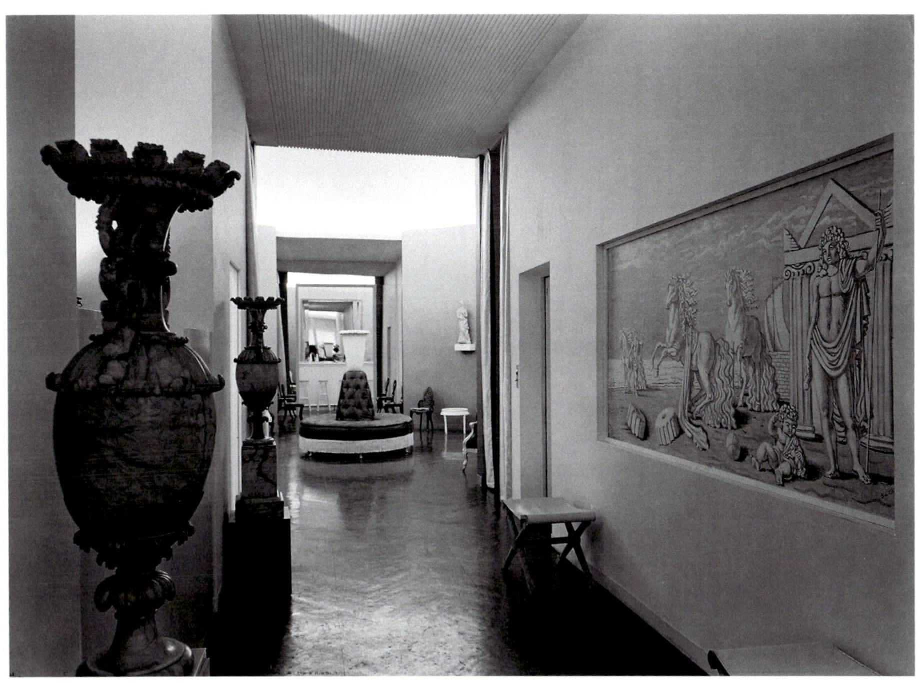

Hallway off the waiting room of the Helena Rubinstein Salon at 715 Fifth Avenue, with Giorgio De Chirico's mythological mural at right, flanked by Jean-Michel Frank's oak-and-leather stools; interior designed by Ladislas Medgyes and Martine Kane.

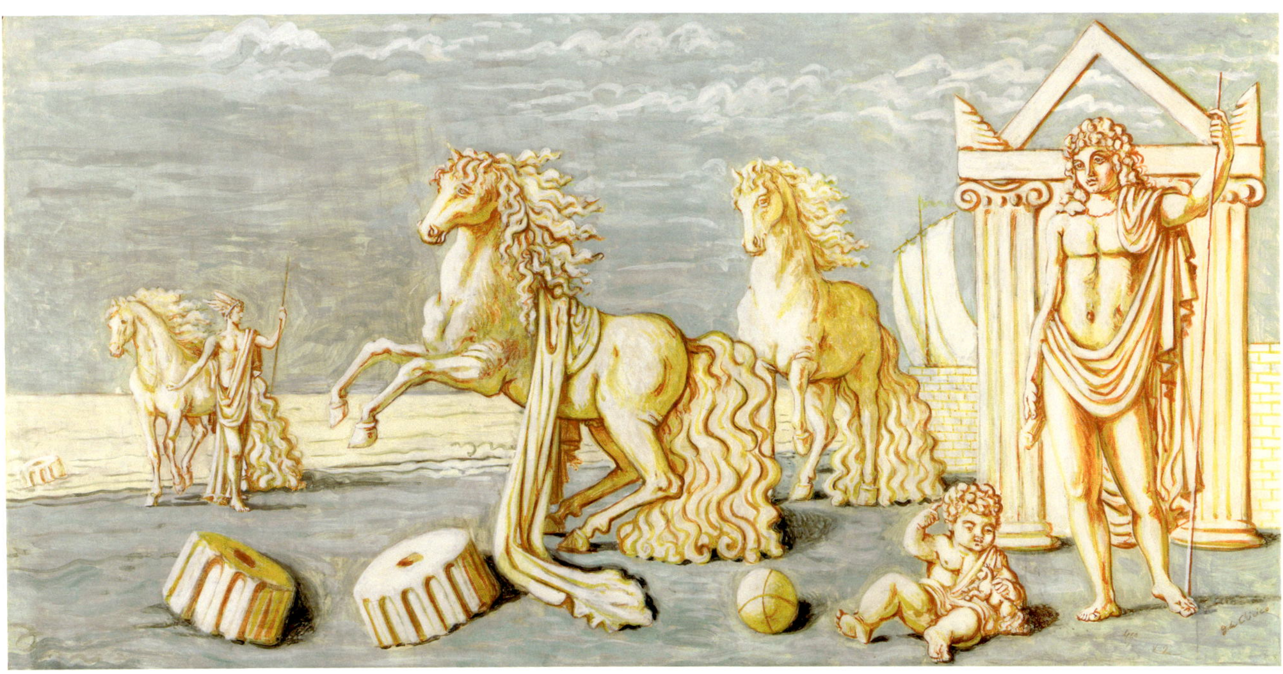

Giorgio De Chirico
Deities by the Seashore, 1936
Oil on Masonite, 48 × 96 in. (121.9 × 243.8 cm)
Galerie Andrea Caratsch, Zurich

Slightly Surrealist photographs by Martin Munkácsi in *Harper's Bazaar*, February 1937, juxtapose workers fixing the roof of the Metropolitan Museum of Art with women having their beauty "repaired" at the Rubinstein salon.

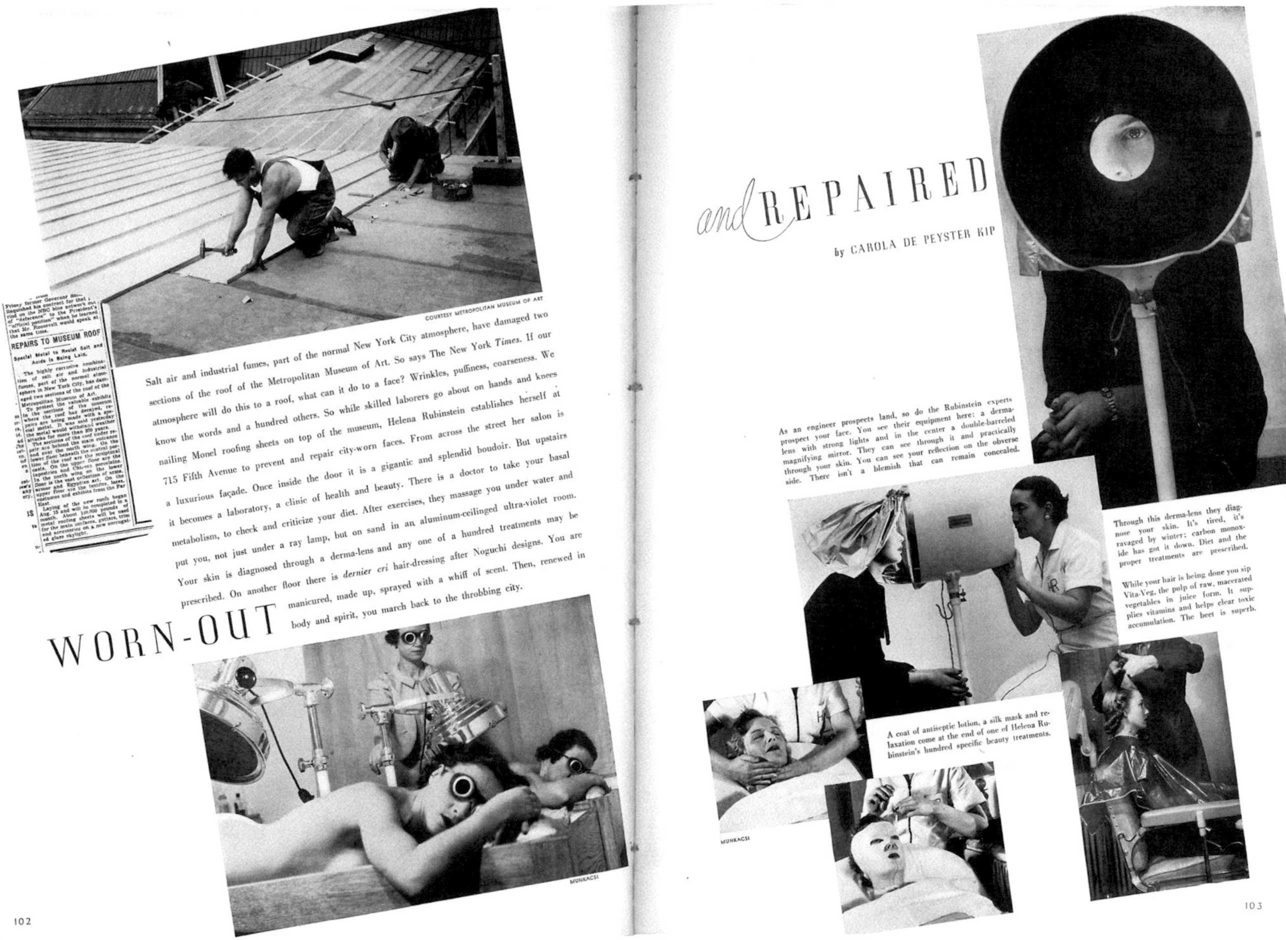

Friday former Governor Smith relinquished his contract for that period on the NBC blue network out of "deference" to the President's "official position" when he learned that Mr. Roosevelt would speak at the same time.

REPAIRS TO MUSEUM ROOF

Special Metal to Resist Salt and Acids Is Being Laid.

The highly corrosive combination of salt air and industrial fumes, part of the normal atmosphere in New York City, has damaged two sections of the roof of the Metropolitan Museum of Art.

To protect the valuable exhibits in the sections of the museum where the roof has decayed, repairs are being made with a special metal. It was said yesterday the metal would withstand weather attacks for more than 300 years.

The sections of the roof under repair are behind the main entrance and over the north wing. On the lower floor beneath the central portion of the roof are the sculptural casts. On the upper floor are the tapestries and Chinese porcelains. In the north wing on the lower floor is the vast collection of arms, armor and Egyptian art. On the upper floor are the textiles, laces, costumes and exhibits from the Far East.

Laying of the new roofs began Aug. 15 and will be completed in a month. About 110,000 pounds of metal roofing sheets will be used for the main surfaces, gutters, trim and accessories on a new corrugated glass skylight.

COURTESY METROPOLITAN MUSEUM OF ART

WORN-OUT

Salt air and industrial fumes, part of the normal New York City atmosphere, have damaged two sections of the roof of the Metropolitan Museum of Art. So says The New York *Times*. If our atmosphere will do this to a roof, what can it do to a face? Wrinkles, puffiness, coarseness. We know the words and a hundred others. So while skilled laborers go about on hands and knees nailing Monel roofing sheets on top of the museum, Helena Rubinstein establishes herself at 715 Fifth Avenue to prevent and repair city-worn faces. From across the street her salon is a luxurious façade. Once inside the door it is a gigantic and splendid boudoir. But upstairs it becomes a laboratory, a clinic of health and beauty. There is a doctor to take your basal metabolism, to check and criticize your diet. After exercises, they massage you under water and put you, not just under a ray lamp, but on sand in an aluminum-ceilinged ultra-violet room. Your skin is diagnosed through a derma-lens and any one of a hundred treatments may be prescribed. On another floor there is *dernier cri* hair-dressing after Noguchi designs. You are manicured, made up, sprayed with a whiff of scent. Then, renewed in body and spirit, you march back to the throbbing city.

MUNKACSI

102

and REPAIRED

by CAROLA DE PEYSTER KIP

As an engineer prospects land, so do the Rubinstein experts prospect your face. You see their equipment here: a derma-lens with strong lights and in the center a double-barreled magnifying mirror. They can see through it and practically through your skin. You can see your reflection on the obverse side. There isn't a blemish that can remain concealed.

Through this derma-lens they diagnose your skin. It's tired, it's ravaged by winter; carbon monoxide has got it down. Diet and the proper treatments are prescribed.

While your hair is being done you sip Vita-Veg, the pulp of raw, macerated vegetables in juice form. It supplies vitamins and helps clear toxic accumulation. The beet is superb.

A coat of antiseptic lotion, a silk mask and relaxation come at the end of one of Helena Rubinstein's hundred specific beauty treatments.

MUNKACSI

103

that the governing board charged with monitoring Fifth Avenue's business practices ordered Rubinstein to dismantle the window immediately. *Life* magazine reported on "Rembrandt and Manet and Picasso à la Rubinstein," successfully publicizing Madame's art-world cachet and alluding to her collection.[92]

In the avant-garde of the late 1920s, Surrealist art had begun to compete with more abstract forms of modernism, and to appear in literary forms as well, in tandem with a popular interest in fantasy imagery and the psychology of dreams. Savvy marketers were quick to recognize the value of Surrealist design and art for commercial purposes. In particular, Paris couturières like Schiaparelli merged fashion and art, collaborating with artists such as Jean Cocteau, Salvador Dalí, and Man Ray. By the mid-1930s the movement had gone mainstream. The June 1937 edition of *Vogue* published Cecil Beaton's photograph of Wallis Simpson, shortly before her marriage to Edward VIII, wearing a Schiaparelli evening dress with a scarlet waistband bearing a lobster painted by Dalí. Madame soon realized—along with Schiaparelli, Man Ray, and Dalí—that the commercial viability of the Surrealist movement was greater in the United States than in Europe.[93]

Although there is little documentation of Rubinstein's various salon window displays, her activity partook of the period's extensive appropriation of Surrealist spectacle, intended for a vanguard audience. Popular reception reached its commercial epiphany in 1939, when Salvador Dalí decorated Bonwit Teller windows with a bathtub awash with disembodied arms, a taxidermic buffalo head and stuffed pigeons, and female mannequins with blood streaming from their eyes. When he discovered that the store's management had decided independently to clothe the mannequins, the artist became enraged; in the ensuing histrionics he and the bathtub accidently went flying through the store's window.[94]

Two years prior, during the Museum of Modern Art's Surrealism show, Rubinstein sent a cable to Man Ray in Paris, expressing interest in his painting *Observatory Time—The Lovers*, a disembodied pair of lips floating in the sky, whose allusion to a couple making love had roused its share of notoriety at the museum. The painting had already been featured in a fashion spread in *Harper's Bazaar*, in which a model reclining on a couch echoed the erotic silhouette in the sky above her (see page 126). Madame wished to borrow the work to exhibit in the window of her new salon.[95]

Surrealist style also influenced the packaging design of Rubinstein's expanding line of beauty products—not only for skin care, but also makeup and perfume—that were part of her growing commercial empire. She employed her interior designer, Martine Kane, among others, to develop boxes and cases, always with an eye to what was up-to-the-minute and distinctive. Madame was equally concerned with look and functionality. As early as 1926 she had created a lipstick shaped like a pair of lips and a lipstick container in a supposedly Cubist style (see pages 80 and 83).

In her own several homes and salons she was surrounded by imaginative constellations of objects and new design ideas. As fashion and home decor magazines proliferated, she used them in innovative ways. She knew that her homes were essential to the prosperity of her company, and that they had to cater to a new world of retail, governed by an expanding cultural concept of fashion. In the early thirties she acquired one of the most historic *hôtels particuliers*, or private mansions, in Paris, at 24, quai de Béthune on the Ile St.-Louis. She knew that the restoration of this seventeenth-century building, with its panoramic views, would make it an incomparable asset, anchoring her social status in Paris.

92 "Mme. Rubinstein's Living Art Blocks Fifth Avenue Traffic," and "The Business of Beauty Is the Business of Helena Rubinstein," *Life* 2, no. 9 (March 1, 1937): 39–40.

93 America, particularly New York, was receptive to the new, willing to accept a mixture of high art and commercialism that Paris disdained. In her biography, Schiaparelli acknowledged her debt to the American market, largely crediting it for her success: "America had always been more hospitable and friendly to me. She had made it possible for me to obtain a unique place in the world. France gave me the inspiration, America the sympathetic approval and the result." *Shocking Life: The Autobiography of Elsa Schiaparelli* (London: V & A Publications, 2007), 112.

94 Such publicity contributed to the artist's disrepute and loss of art-world credibility. His already politically strained relationship with the European Surrealists also collapsed; they excommunicated him from the Surrealist movement for his pranks. For a range of critical takes on fashion's use of Surrealism, see Dickran Tashjian, *A Boatload of Madmen: Surrealism and the American Avant-Garde, 1920–1950* (New York: Thames and Hudson, 1995); Richard Martin, *Fashion and Surrealism* (New York: Rizzoli, 1987); Lewis Kachur, *Displaying the Marvelous: Marcel Duchamp, Salvador Dali, and Surrealist Exhibition Installations* (Cambridge, MA: MIT Press, 2001).

95 The picture of the model appeared in *Harper's Bazaar* (November 1936): 63. Man Ray had taken a similar picture in Paris with a nude woman on the couch in his studio at 8 rue du Val-de-Grace. He says in his memoir that the loan was intended for Rubinstein's new "beauty emporium" on Fifth Avenue; see *Self Portrait* (London: André Deutsch, 1963), 257–58.

Three miniature rooms: a French Rococo salon, an early twentieth-century Montmartre artist's studio, and a mid-Victorian English parlor. Tel Aviv Museum of Art.

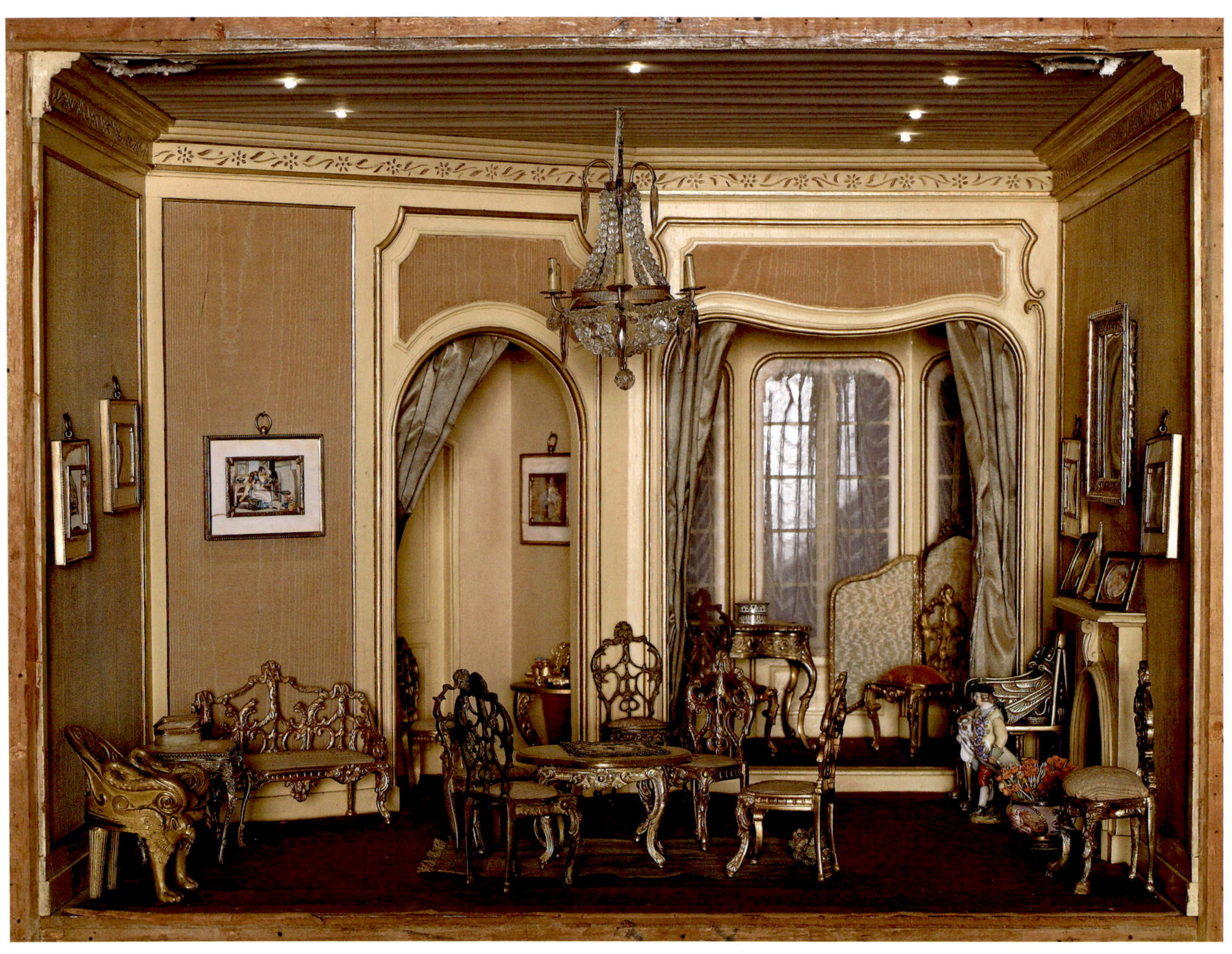

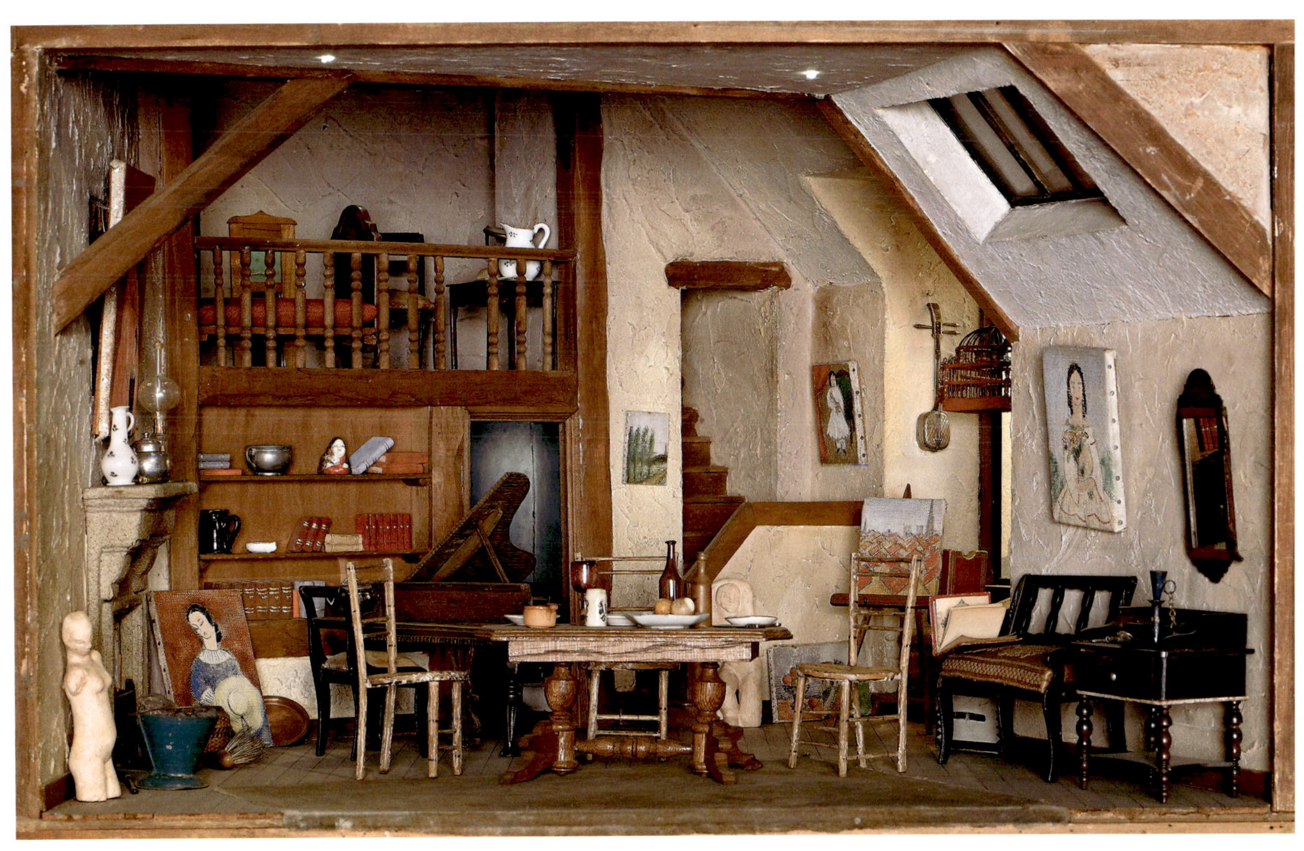

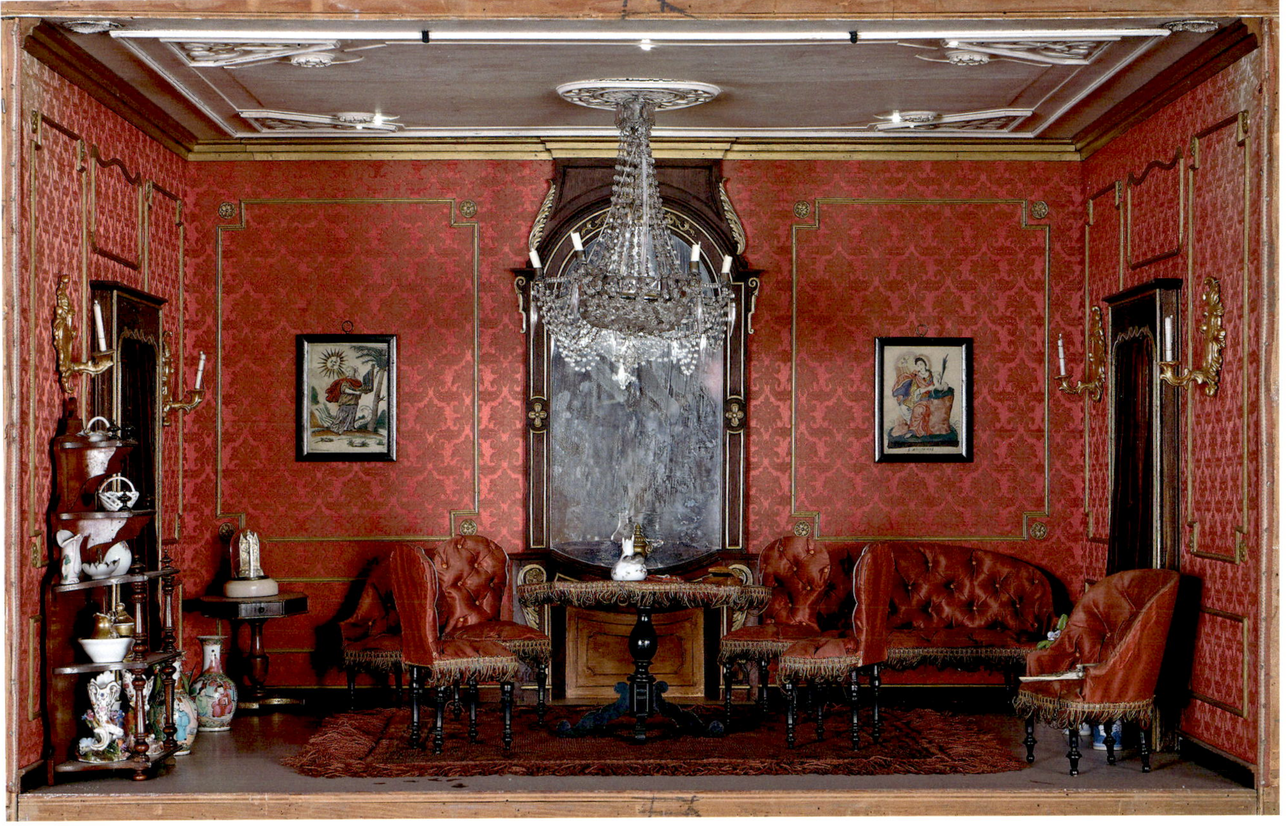

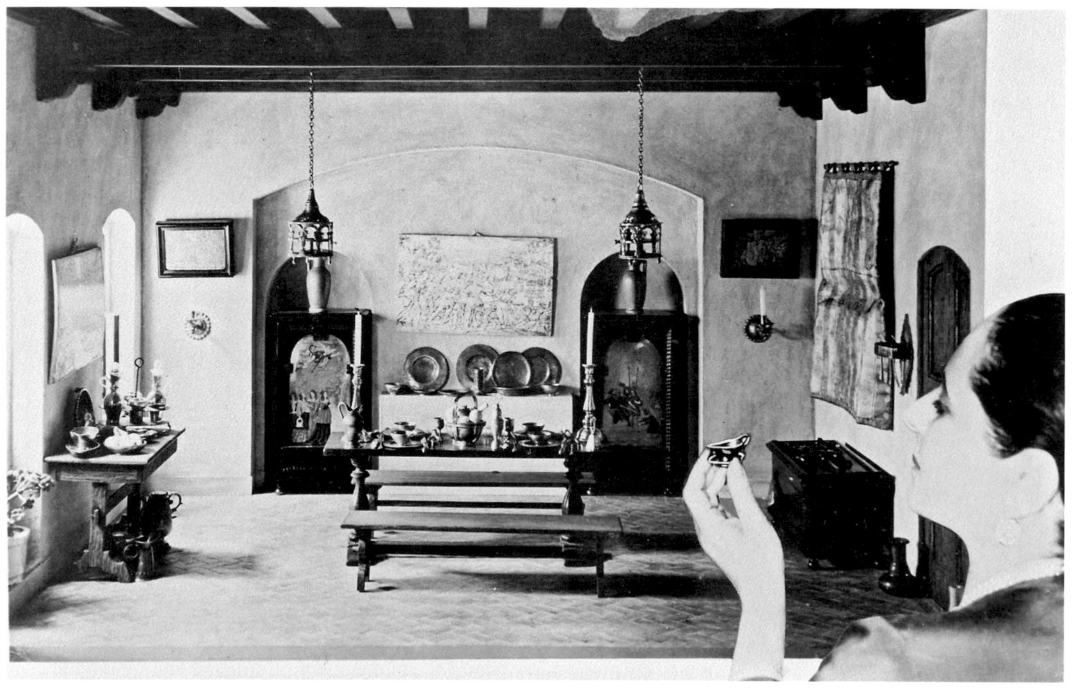

Helena Rubinstein with her Spanish Baroque miniature dining room.

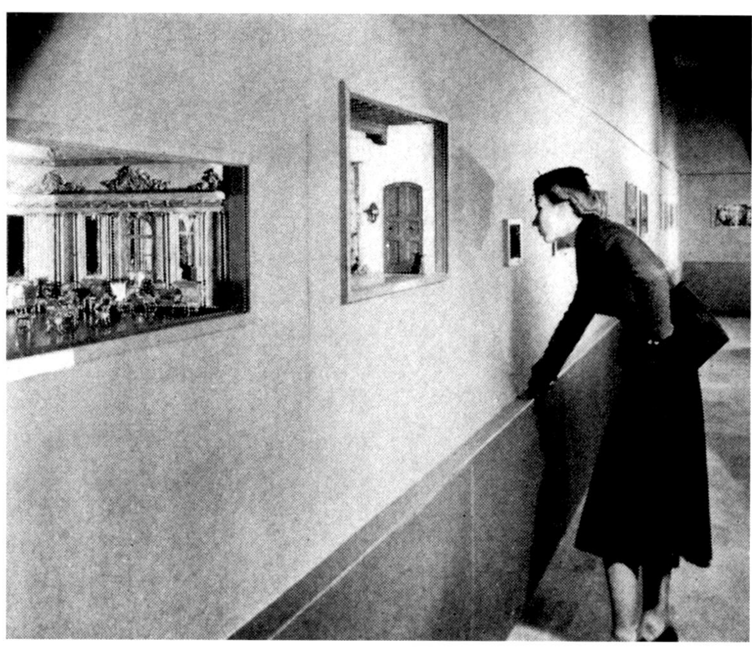

Helena Rubinstein's miniature rooms installed in her salon at 715 Fifth Avenue, New York, 1937.

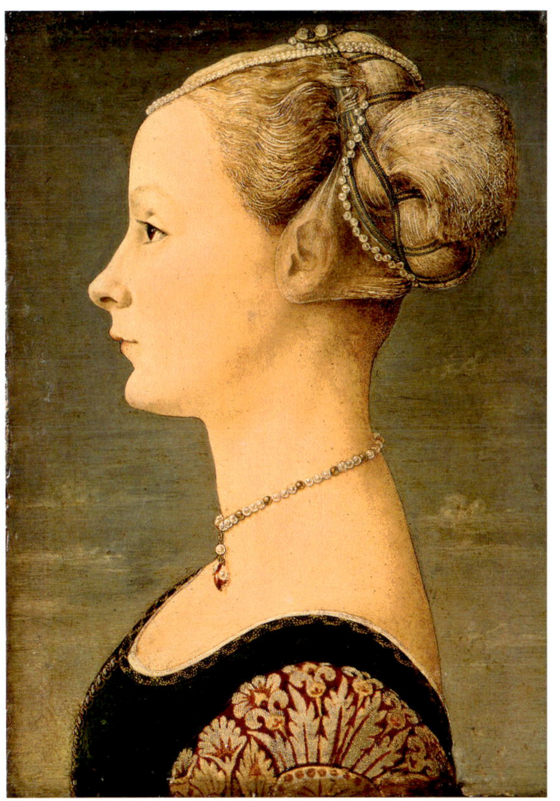

Piero del Pollaiuolo
Portrait of an Unknown Woman, c. 1470–72
Tempera and oil on panel, 18 × 12⅞ in. (45.5 × 32.7 cm).
Museo Poldi Pezzoli, Milan

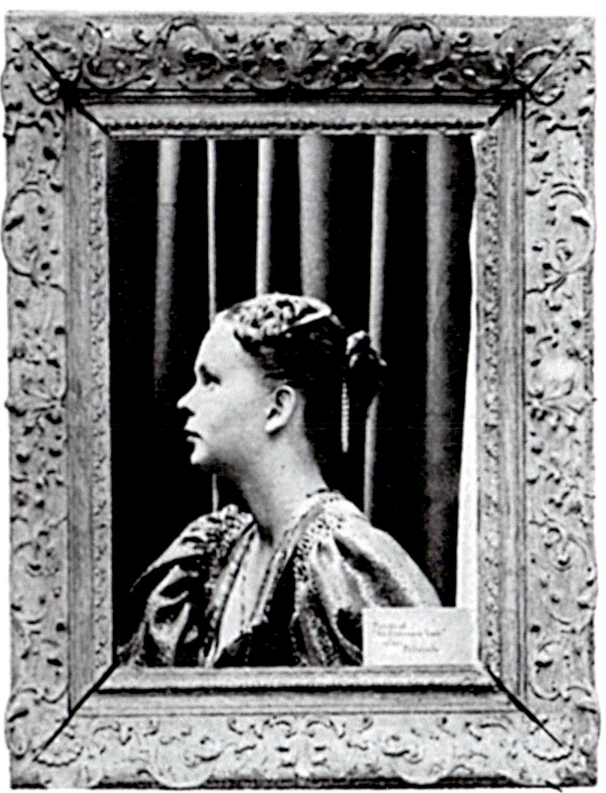

A "living model" in the salon window at 715 Fifth Avenue, 1937, enacts a Renaissance painting.

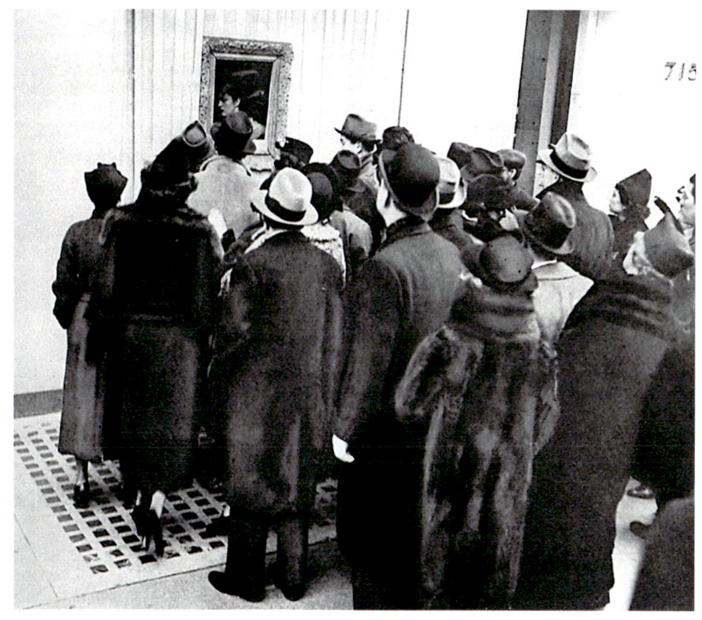

"Living models," posing behind frames, staged famous paintings such as Picasso's *Woman in a Blouse* in the window of Helena Rubinstein's newly opened salon at 715 Fifth Avenue, drawing crowds and publicity.

Man Ray's 1934 painting *Observatory Time–The Lovers* was featured in a 1936 fashion shoot with a supine model. Rubinstein loved the painting and borrowed the dramatic lips for her packaging.

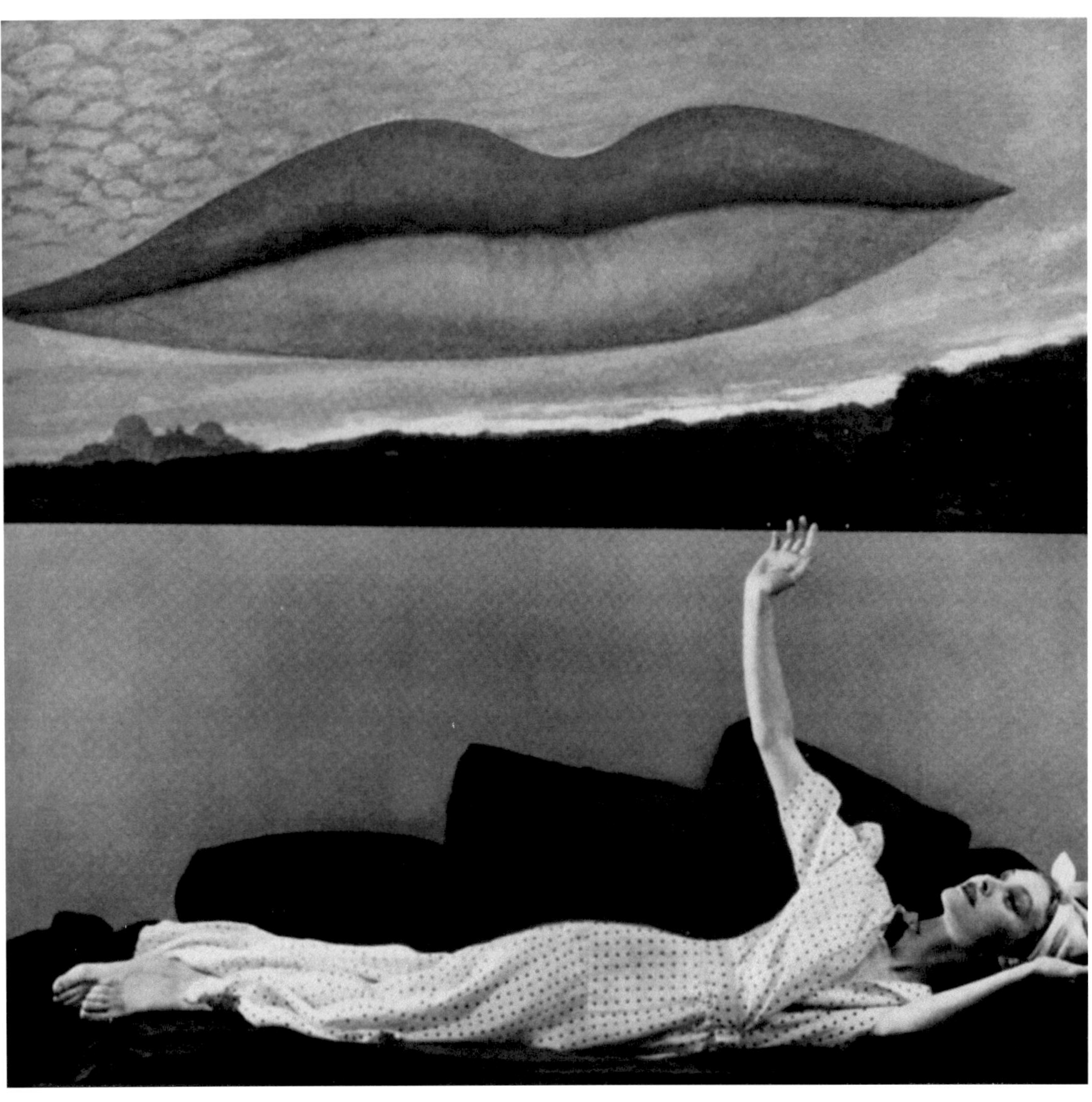

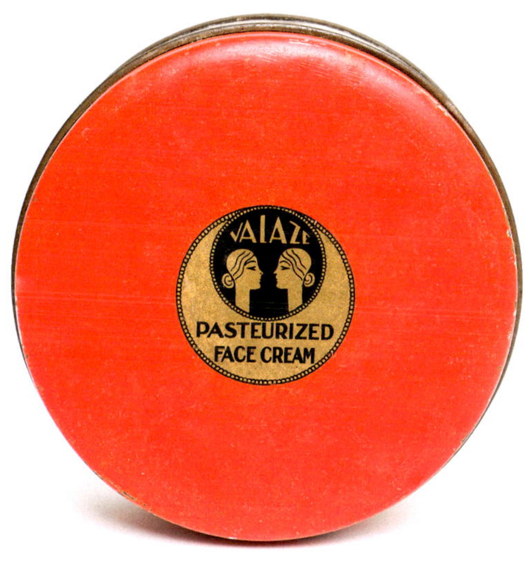

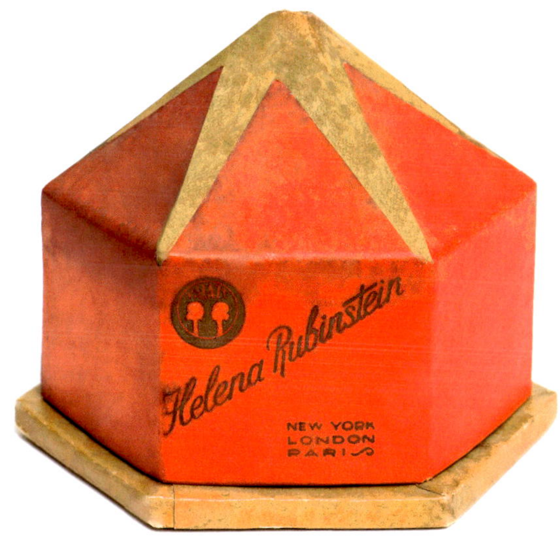

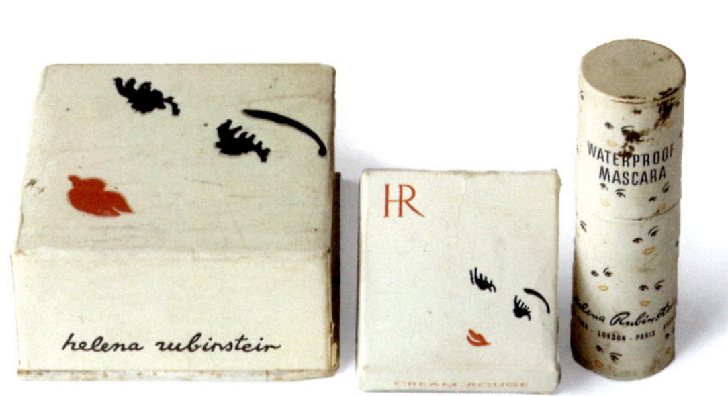

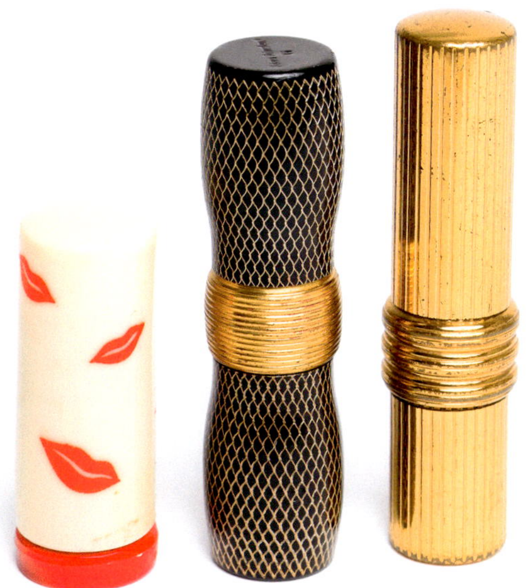

Among Rubinstein's distinctive packaging designs are (*clockwise from top*) a Valaze Pasteurized Face Cream tin, c. 1930, with an Art Deco version of the original logo of two women in profile; a 1927 "modern-istic" box (in the words of *Vogue*) for a water-lily powder, inspired by Orientalist and Art Deco design; an hourglass Convertible lipstick case, c. 1958; the 1942 Red Lips lipstick container inspired by Man Ray; and a suite of waterproof makeup products with floating eyes and lips from the 1940s.

The decor of the Rubinstein rooms (in both the salons and her homes) was always wildly eclectic—a mix of historical periods, offbeat new materials, and idiosyncratic color schemes. In the 1930s she added the madcap imagery of Surrealism to the stew. She began to use her apartments in Paris and New York more and more for fashion and publicity shoots, both to promote her own products and as settings for magazine features on couture (see pages 106–10). This gave her an excuse to redecorate frequently and extravagantly. (A country home in Connecticut was somewhat calmer and more private.) Her New York apartment, in particular, became a social and public stage. In its staid, classical dining room she hung her collection of Mexican naive portraits of women and children. Decorative paintings of whimsically baroque female personae were also featured on the walls of the hair salon in the Fifth Avenue emporium.[96] Such creative and cultural pluralism fostered a progressive sense of beauty—not unrelated to her notion that beauty needed to be maintained and, above all, endlessly reconceived.

Competition was increasing and Rubinstein dared not rest on her laurels or relax into complacency. She sang the praises of self-invention to the women who were her clients, and reinvented her settings with each new campaign of decoration. At the same time, she presented herself as perpetually, unchangingly young in most reproductions. She was in her sixties, no longer the delicate, pale-skinned young beauty of the Edwardian era. Rubinstein had achieved enormous success by her early thirties, in part by using her own image as a constant, ubiquitous advertisement for her products, the experience of her salons, and her philosophy of beauty and self-invention—all of which she marketed relentlessly. The fresh face of her formative years was gradually eclipsed by the image that prevailed after World War I: that of a middle-aged, elegantly tailored, yet matronly businesswoman. She did not hesitate to show herself this way in publicity photographs (see page 132). Even so, most of the numerous painted portraits she commissioned of herself, many done when she was well past middle age, depict her as young (see page 133). It is only the last portraits that show her true appearance: "Despite her expensive clothes and jewelry and lavish surroundings, she has the face of a Jewish grandmother, hard and frail at the same time. And that is what she was despite appearances, that is who she had never stopped being: the 'little lady from Kraków.'"[97]

Possibly the most famous of these later realistic renderings is the English painter Graham Sutherland's imposing conception of her, seen from below, poised in a royal red Balenciaga gown, hawk-eyed, with crossed hands adorned with flamboyantly jeweled rings and sharp red fingernails (see page 135). Her initial response to the canvas was not sanguine: "Look at me . . . so old . . . so savage . . . like a witch!" She was shocked, as she recorded in her memoir, to "see herself in such a harsh light"; she hated the "incredibly bold, domineering interpretation of what I had never imagined I looked like."[98] But after the work was publicly displayed and decreed a masterpiece, her sentiments evidently changed. As she later confessed, "the picture grew on me."[99] The woman depicted by Sutherland had been running a global business with the singular command of a queen for more than six decades. He later recalled:

> *In many ways she was to me a real mystery woman. . . . But I have an acute "sense" of her presence—even now of the contained energy burning away behind the stillness. . . . My impression was strong in thinking that neither pictures, furniture nor objects meant more to her than a foil for her electric, contained and strong vitality . . . I was able to observe her*

96 These may have been painted by the decorative artist Federico Pallavicini, who had made similar work for her apartment.

97 Fitoussi, *Helena Rubinstein: The Woman Who Invented Beauty*, x. For the reference to "the little lady from Kraków" see Elaine Brown Kieffer, "Madame Rubinstein: The Little Lady from Krakow Has Made a Fabulous Success of Selling Beauty," *Life* 11, no. 6 (July 21, 1941): 36–40, 43–45.

98 O'Higgins, *Madame*, 235.

99 Slesin, *Over the Top*, 207.

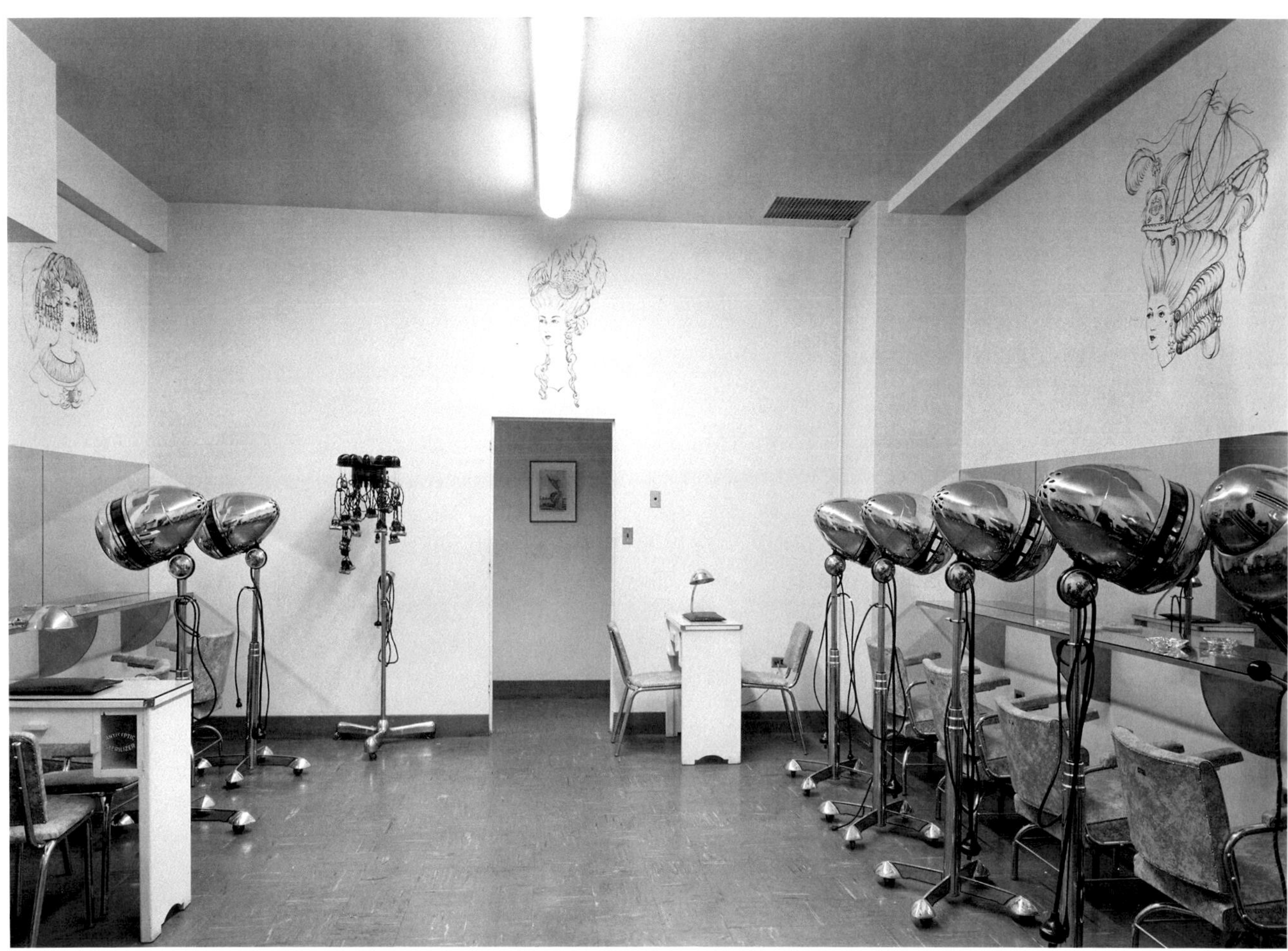

Hair-styling room, Helena Rubinstein salon, 655 Fifth Avenue, New York, 1948, with pictures of fantasy hairstyles, possibly by Federico Pallavicini, decorating the walls, borrowed from seventeenth- and eighteenth-century paintings. At left is a coiffure from Diego Velázquez's portrait of the Infanta Maria Theresa of Spain; at right is Marie Antoinette's hairstyle, featuring a sailing ship perched on top of an elaborate wig.

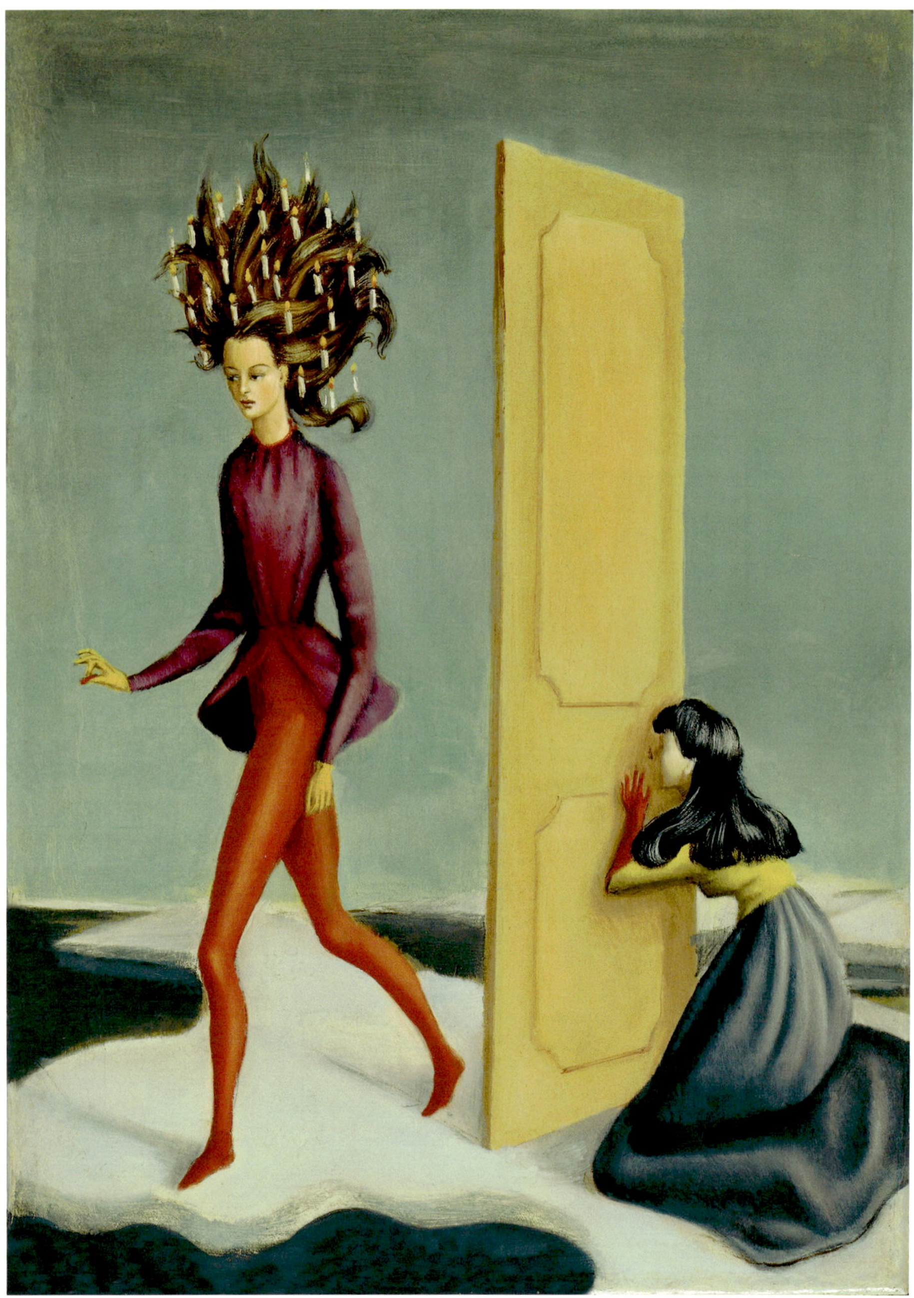

Leonor Fini
Two Women, 1939
Oil on canvas, 13⅜ × 9⅝ in. (34 × 24.5 cm)
The Ulla and Heiner Pietzsch Collection, Berlin

This painting, by one of the Surrealist movement's most prominent women, suggests that changes in fashion had made possible a novel and complex code of looking, quite independent of the masculine gaze. It represents a new phenomenon—the woman as voyeur.

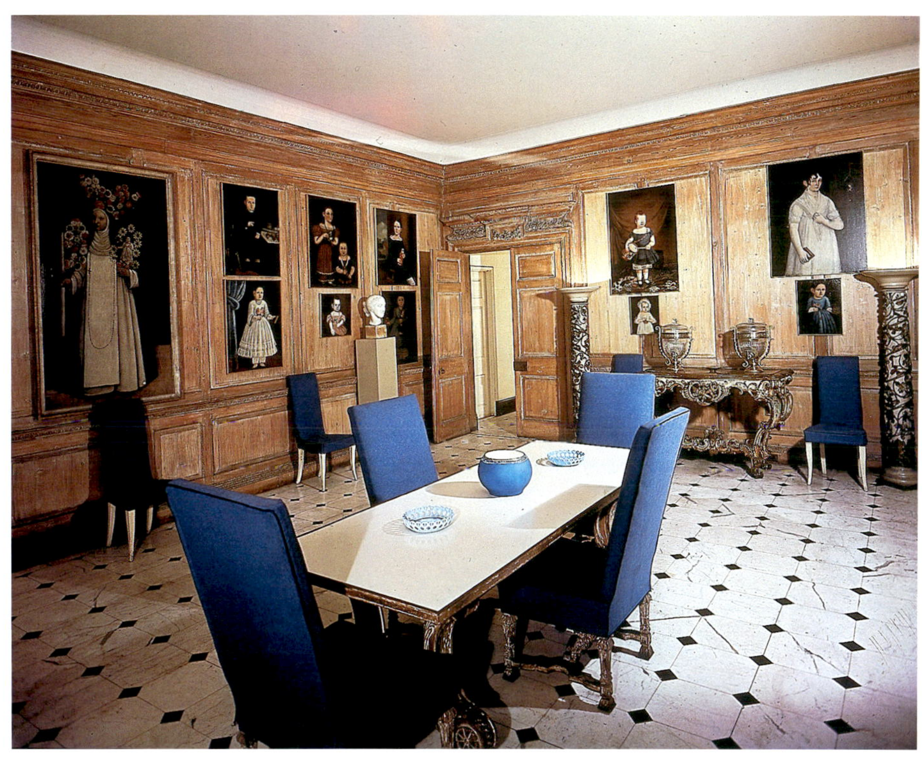

Helena Rubinstein's dining room at 625 Park Avenue, date unknown. On the paneled wall hang numerous folk paintings, most of which Madame collected in Mexico. The sculpture is by Elie Nadelman.

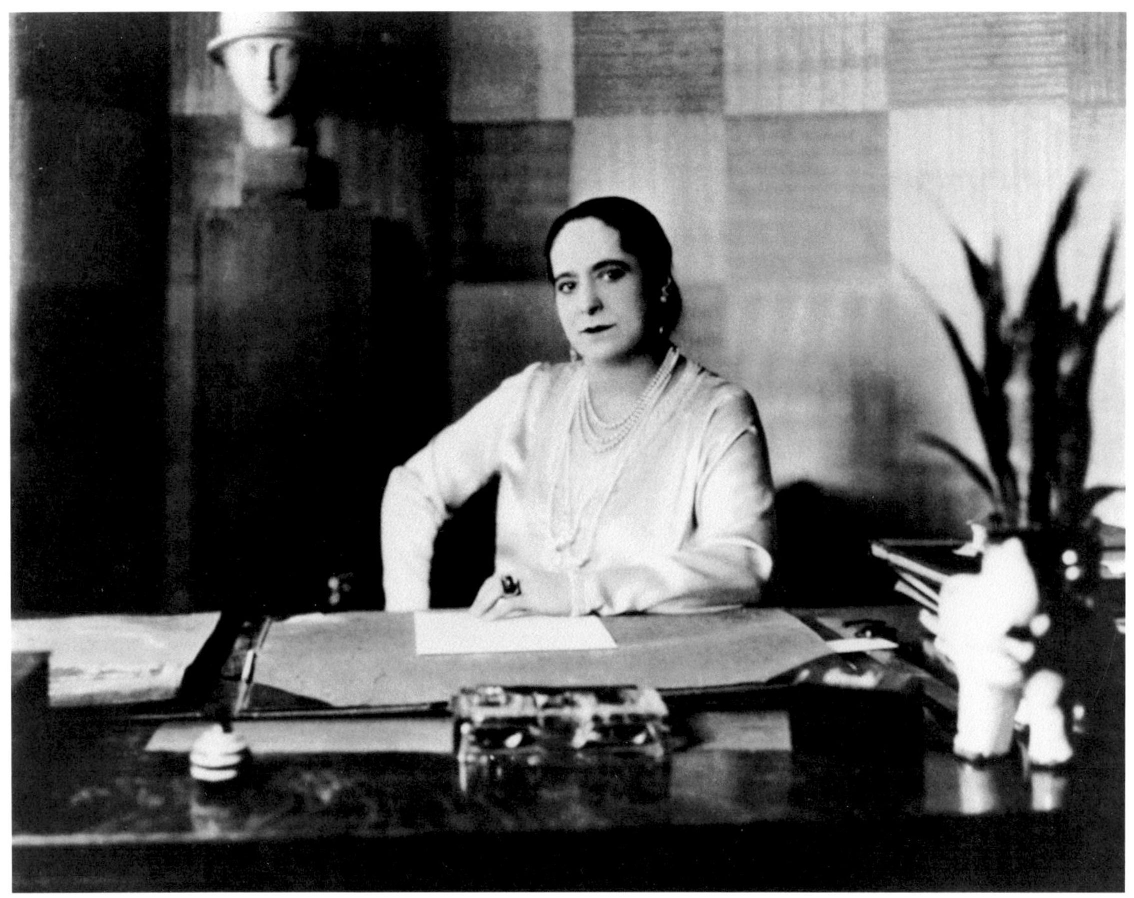

Helena Rubinstein in her New York office, c. 1928. She was a famous workaholic for whom business was all-consuming, impinging drastically on domestic life, a fact that she eventually acknowledged in her memoirs.

Marie Laurencin
Portrait of Helena Rubinstein, 1934
Oil on canvas, 33 × 27 in. (83.8 × 68.6 cm)
Private collection, Stowe, Vermont

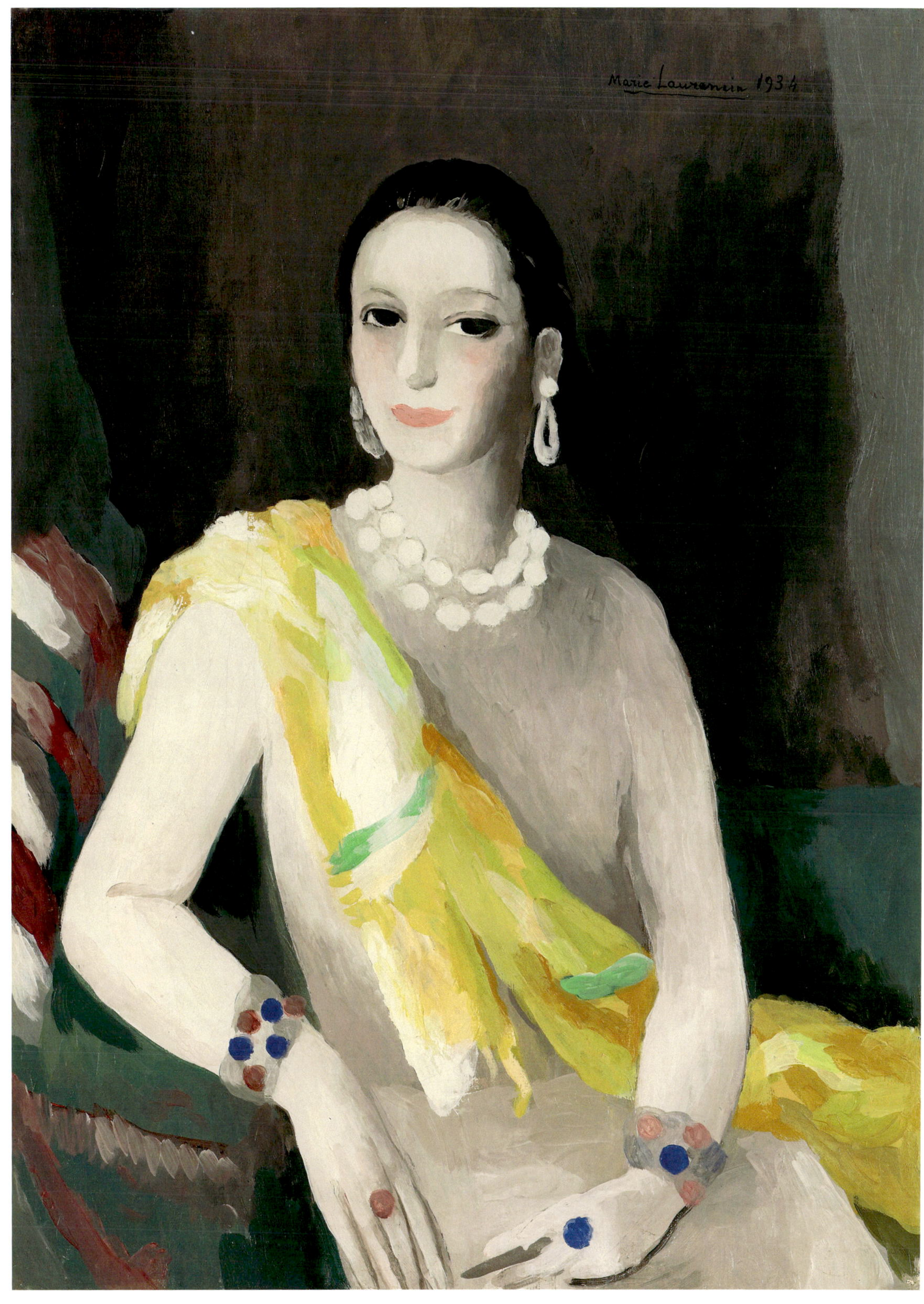

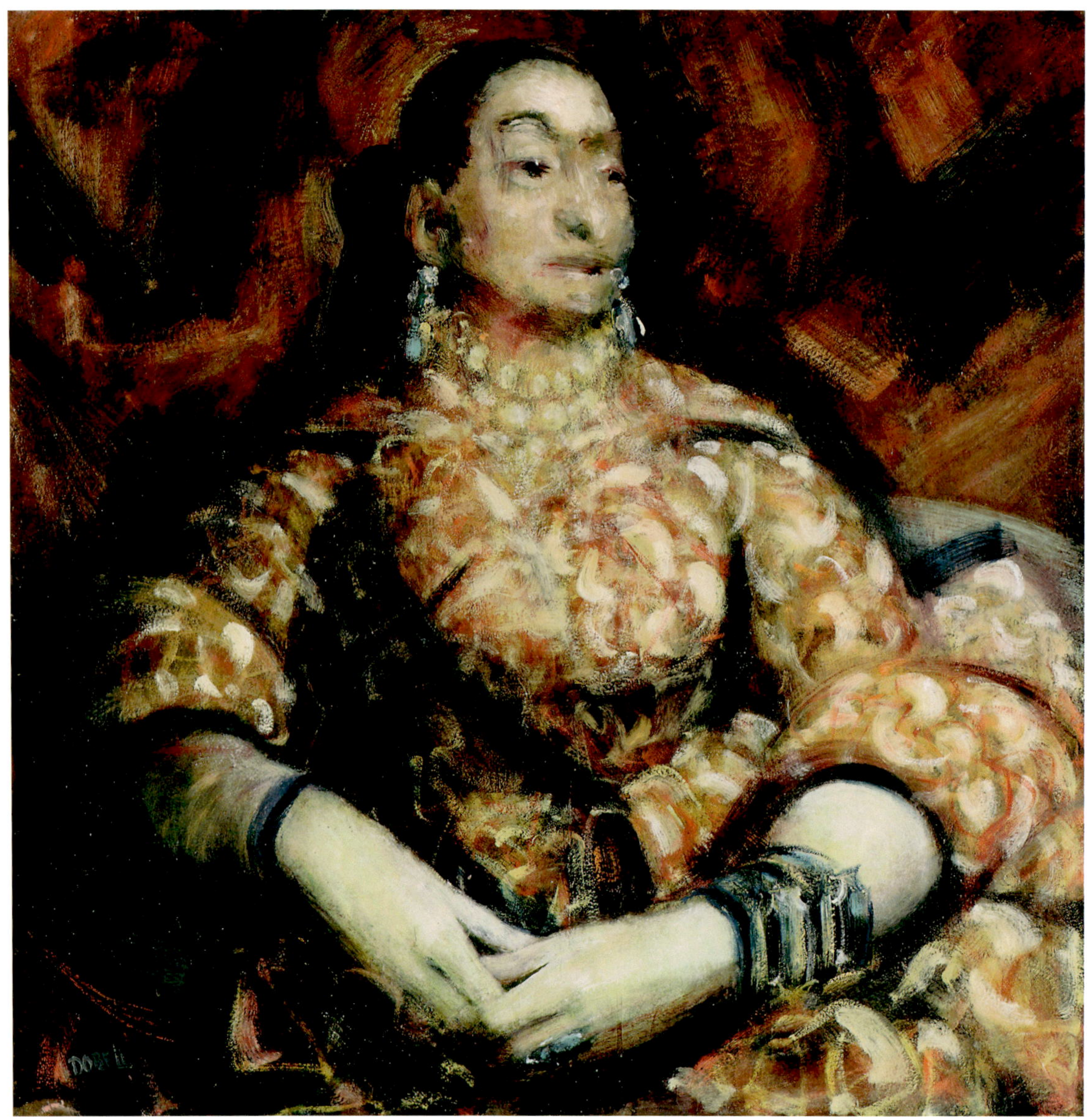

William Dobell
Helena Rubinstein, 1957
Oil on composition board, 37⅝ × 37⅝ in.
(95.6 × 95.6 cm)
National Gallery of Victoria, Melbourne,
Felton Bequest, 1964

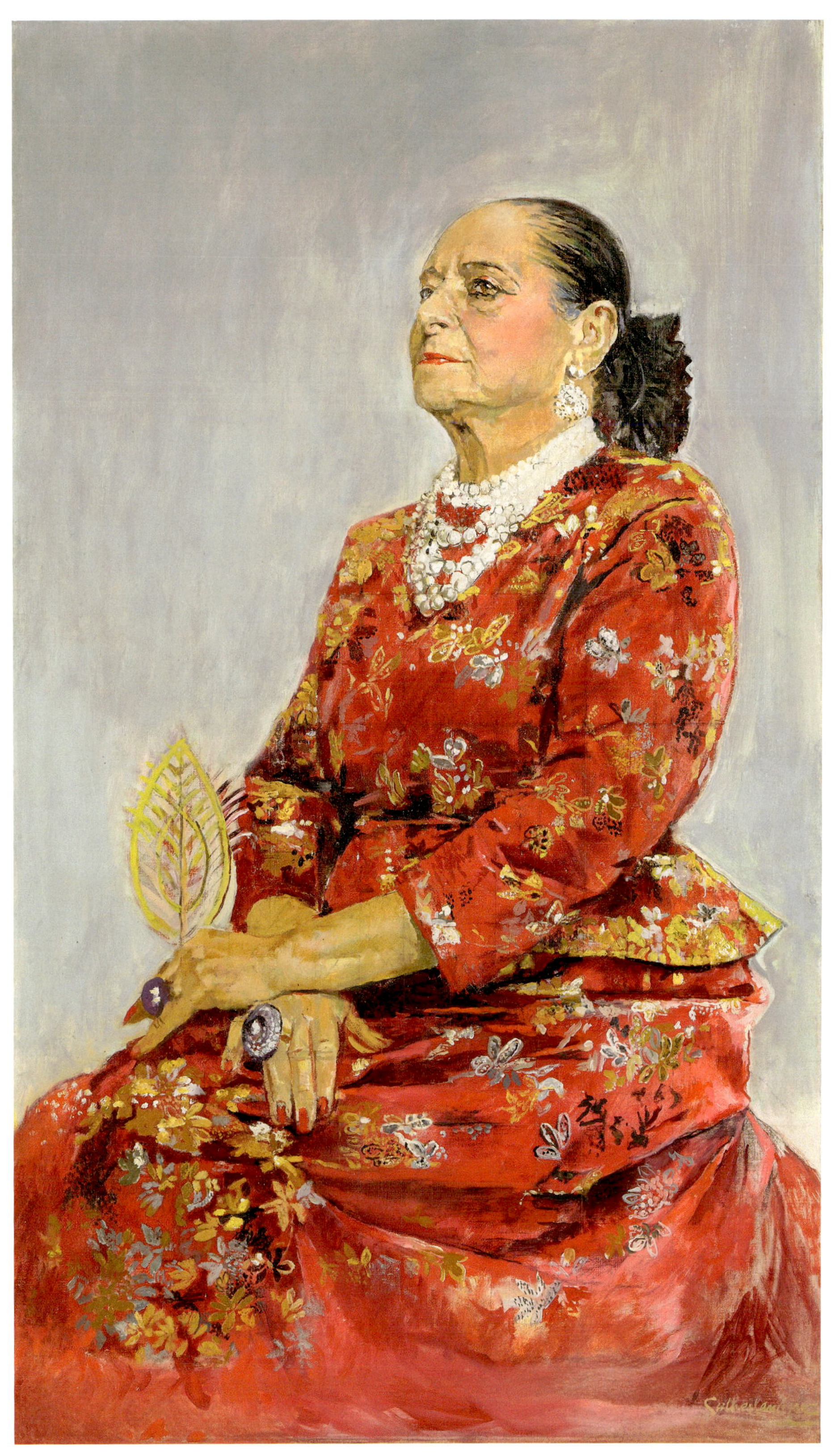

Graham Sutherland
Helena Rubinstein in a Red Brocade Balenciaga Gown, 1957
Oil on canvas, 61¾ × 36½ in. (156.9 × 92.7 cm)
Daniel Katz Gallery, London

buying—and bargaining—over a table-full of costume jewelry by the gross and I drew her, unaware of my presence, in her Balenciaga dress, looking like an empress . . . showing that rare, almost deprecating, but enchanting smile; it gave me the material in which I was able to work. She was, in a word—magnificent—minute and monosyllabic, with the force of an Egyptian ruler.[100]

Painted the same year as the Sutherland work, the Australian artist Sir William Dobell's portrait (of which he did eight variations) was doubtless based on photographs as well as on the Sutherland portrait.[101] Dobell depicts Madame as an aging warrior, a stout, ruthless Genghis Khan in repose, seated regally before a heavily brocaded wall. He orientalizes her by exaggerating her ethnicity and dramatizing the Balenciaga garment, using loose swirls of paint to convey its intricate pattern and the weight of its thickly woven fabric. The artist replaces Sutherland's comparatively demure diamond and pearl jewelry with a pair of long, exotic dangling turquoise earrings, whose shades of blue echo in a massive bracelet and ring, reflecting in a ghostly manner on her milk-white arms. She is, in Dobell's likeness, a melancholic figure whose eyes seem fixed on the past. Nevertheless, he has presented her as colossal, mythic, theatrical. Together these two striking portraits convey a complex femininity, the image of a woman who has seen her share of battle. Rubinstein, who loved large, chunky jewelry, once likened it to armor; "although I no longer need the added courage the handsome jewelry once gave me," she wrote in her memoirs, "it was not easy being a hard-working woman in a man's world many years ago."[102]

By 1934 the Depression had badly affected her business in America; unresolved family issues—principally the decision to finalize her divorce from Edward—and nonstop travel added to her fatigue and low spirits. That summer she retreated to a clinic in Germany for a time, but by autumn she had rallied. She hired the much-admired architect Louis Süe to work on a new, glorious home in Paris on the Ile St.-Louis. This was to be both a grand residence in the *ancien régime* manner and a public display of her business's prosperity. And at the age of sixty-two, with self-esteem untarnished, she commissioned two more portraits.

The first was by Marie Laurencin, a member of the Parisian avant-garde and the circle of Picasso (see page 133). She painted Madame in her characteristic delicate palette, the so-called *forme féminine*.[103] Rubinstein is depicted as an Indian princess, seated in a relaxed but stately pose, a subtly yellow-greenish shawl draped over one shoulder. She is heavily bejeweled, with elongated looped earrings, a double strand of huge pearls, and matching jeweled cuffs and rings. Typical of many of Laurencin's portraits, any resemblance to the sitter was entirely subjective.[104] At a minimum, the resemblance is to a Helena Rubinstein of forty years earlier.

The second work, *Head of Helena Rubinstein Encrusted with Sequins*, by the Russian Pavel Tchelitchew, has an almost grotesque quality, but captures his subject's complexity as a figure of femininity and power. Here too she is presented as a young woman. Tchelitchew had begun his career working as a stage designer in Berlin, before moving to Paris in the early 1920s, and retained a sense of atmospheric theatricality in his work. As if to make her face glow, Tchelitchew coats Madame's features with real gold sequins; more sequins glitter in her hair like a halo. Beneath this coruscating surface, she is enveloped in her own luminous sheen, while the gravitas of her darkened, heavy eyelids seems to allude to a beauty queen's endless fight with time. The painting typifies Tchelitchew's effort to depict what

100 Woodhead, *War Paint*, 368.

101 Known for his subjective manner of portraiture, Dobell was once sued by two unsuccessful entrants for the well-respected Archibald Prize for failing to observe certain "rules" of portraiture in favor of producing what was described in court as caricature.

102 Rubinstein, *My Life for Beauty*, 101.

103 In the 1920s the French critic Louis Vauxcelles characterized Laurencin's portraits as a model of femininity, even referring to such an ideal as "un Laurencin." See his contribution on the artist in *L'Histoire générale de l'art français, de la Révolution à nos jours* (Paris: Librairie de France, 1922–25), vol. 2, 321; quoted in Gill Perry, *Women Artists and the Parisian Avant-Garde: Modernism and "Feminine" Art, 1900 to the Late 1920s* (Manchester, UK: Manchester University Press, 1996), 107.

104 In 1923 Coco Chanel invited Laurencin to paint her portrait; she obligingly produced a sleek Chanel wearing a slinky, bare-shouldered gown. Chanel rejected the painting on the grounds that it did not look like her.

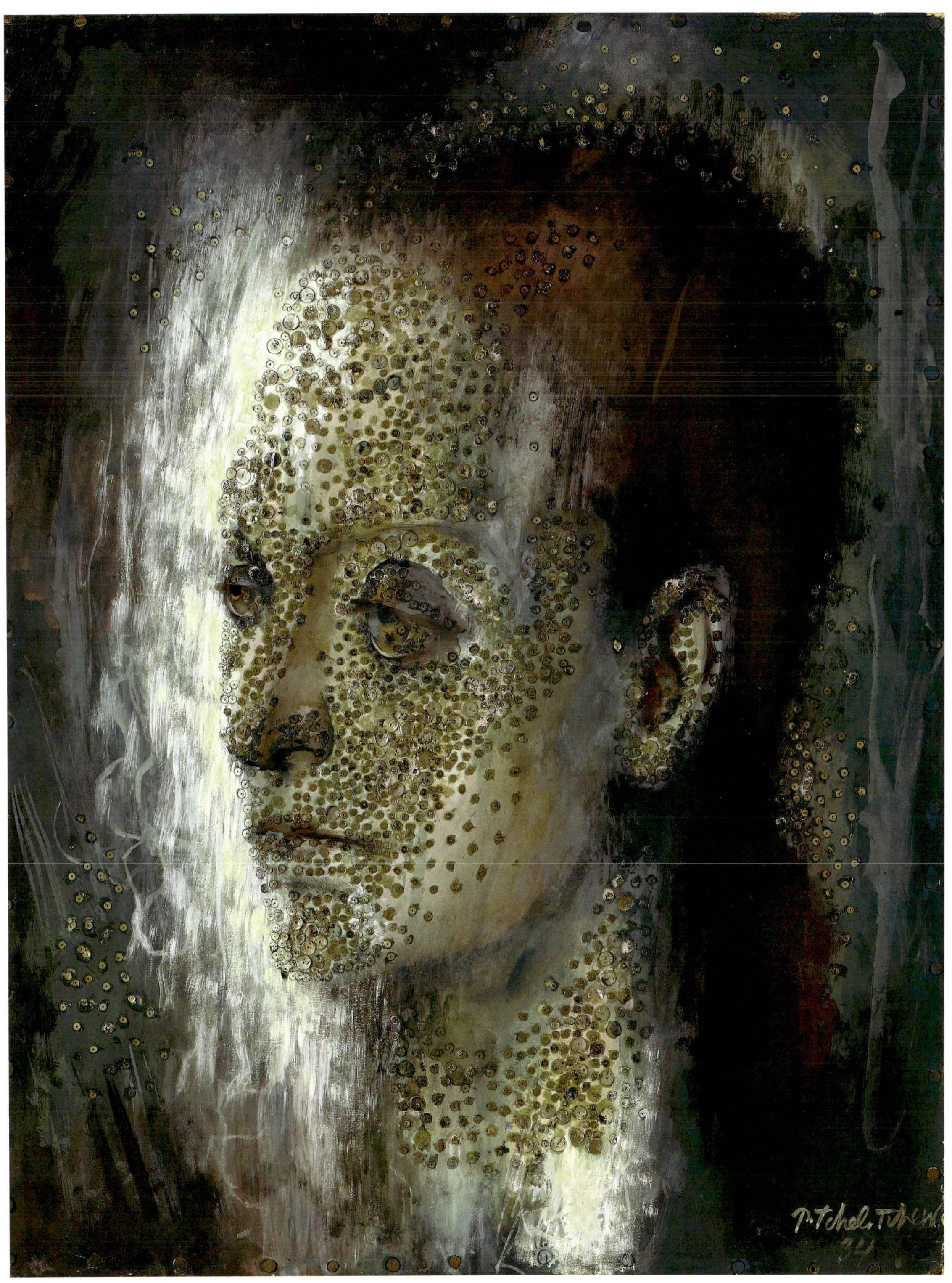

Pavel Tchelitchew
Portrait of Helena Rubinstein Encrusted with Sequins, 1934
Gouache, oil, ink, and sequins on board, 26 × 19¾ in. (66 × 50.2 cm)
Private collection

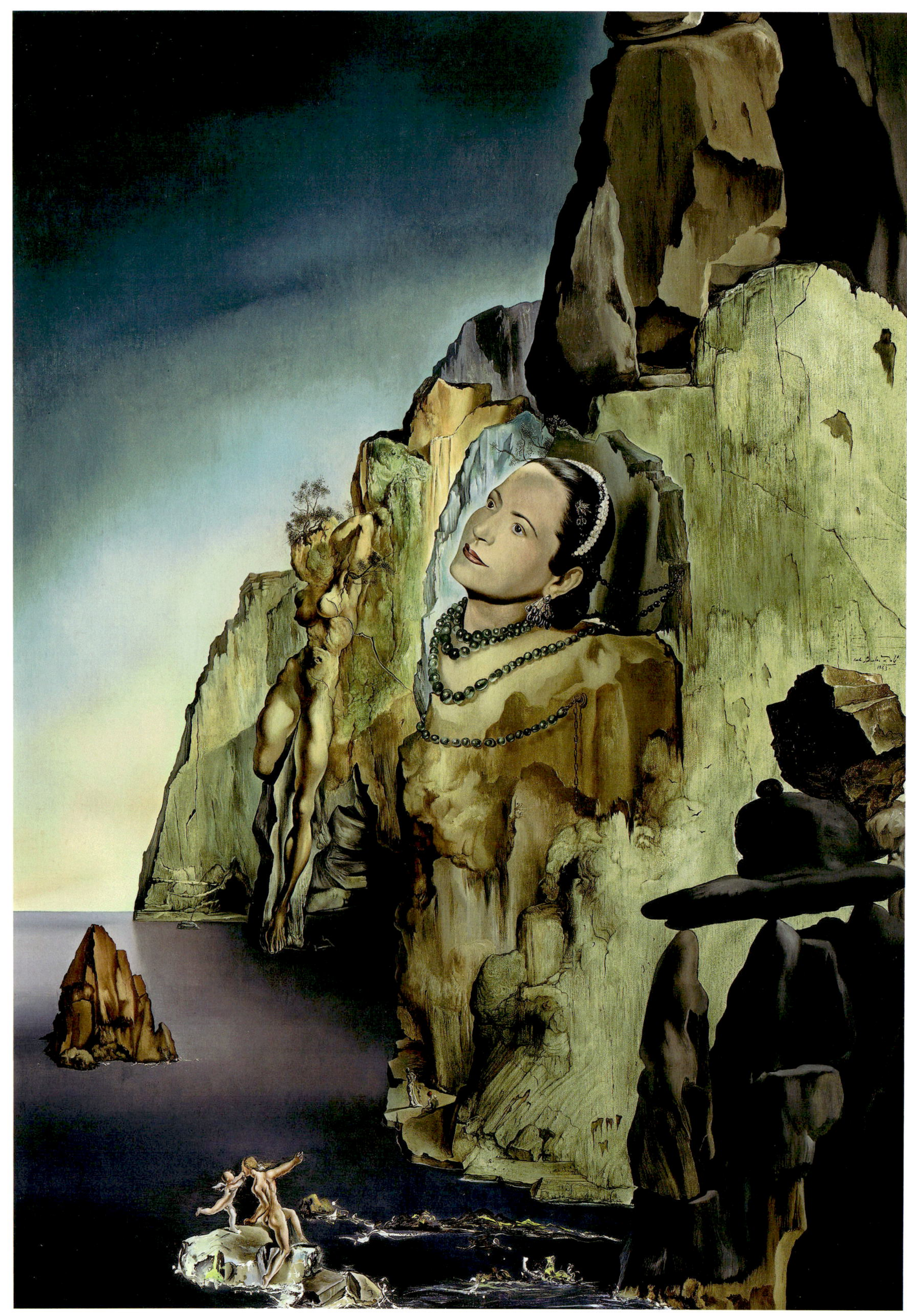

Salvador Dalí
Princess Artchil Gourielli–Helena Rubinstein, 1943
Oil on canvas, 35 × 25¼ in. (88.9 × 64 cm)
Private collection

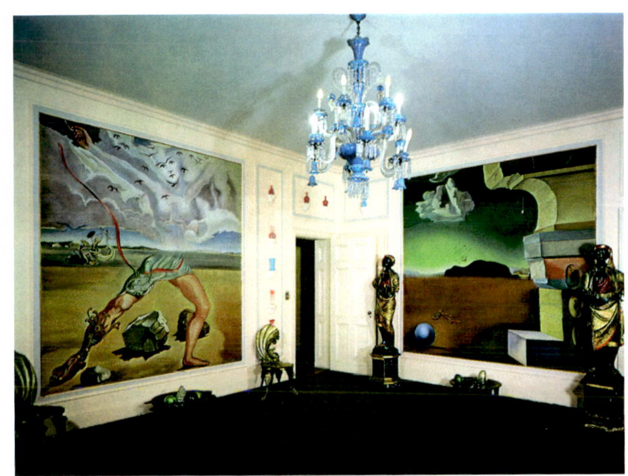

Salvador Dalí, *Heroic Noon* (*left*) and *Evening* (*right*), murals in situ in Rubinstein's apartment at 625 Park Avenue.

has been referred to as an "inner landscape," a kind of transcendent, protopsychedelic imagery that dissolves the body's opacity.[105]

Of the dozens of portraits of Madame, perhaps the best known is that done a decade later by Salvador Dalí, whom she helped to welcome to New York in 1940 after the outbreak of World War II. They had probably known one another in Paris in the thirties, but how well acquainted they had been is uncertain.[106] He had been a serious member of the Surrealists, but abandoned both the group and his ideological flirtations with Communism when the war came. In New York, Dalí indulged his fondness for publicity and his interest, shared with Madame, in popularizing Surrealism among consumers. For his commercial shenanigans in these years he was excommunicated from the movement by André Breton.

In 1942 Rubinstein commissioned Dalí to paint three large murals, *Fantastic Landscape: Dawn, Heroic Noon, and Evening*, to decorate a card room in her triplex apartment at 625 Park Avenue. Her aim seems to have been to distract competitors during her well-known bridge games. The following year, when she was seventy, he painted her portrait as well. The title of the work, *Princess Artchil Gourielli–Helena Rubinstein*, stresses her dual persona as self-made magnate and noble lady of leisure.

Dalí depicts an implausibly youthful Madame chained by her pearl and emerald necklaces to a stone cliff, like a latter-day Andromeda. The tilt of her head and the skyward focus of her frozen, expressionless gaze are emblematic of countless fashion photographs. Though monumentally conceived, the portrait occupies a relatively small part of the painting. As in many Dalí confections, the carefully rendered details are worthy of a Renaissance painting, despite their eccentricity—from the sheer, stony cliffs to a configuration of vertical rocks at right that precariously balance a huge oyster shell, opened to a breastlike form whose nipple is a pearl. To her left is a full-length nude, erotically straddling a phallic stone; her head, turned in the manner of a classical nude, merges with the cliff face, and her hair is a tuft of sparse green growth on the barren coastline. The woman's upper body, fissured like the cliff behind her, is slowly coming apart. Below, unnoticed, Venus and Cupid cavort on a reef; a solitary outcropping behind them, with a craggy, aged stone face, stands in the sea like a hopeless guardian. In the Greek myth, Andromeda is rescued by Perseus; for Madame, though, there will be no escape from time.

A similar theme of mortality informs the artist's series of murals, *Fantastic Landscape*, with its three individual titles indicating the day's progression from dawn to dusk. The central painting, *Heroic Noon*, focuses on the protagonist, a heroic female figure so formidable she can barely be contained within the mural's frame. A hallucinatory creature, she is perfectly bifurcated at the waist by the horizon, her upper body and face a mirage of clouds and birds; her lower, terrestrial half solid flesh. In the background a goddess overpowers a male combatant—a possible allusion to sea-born Aphrodite, who rose from the water in a seashell, and is often depicted accompanied by her son, Eros. The two flanking murals are roughly symmetrical: repoussoir architectural elements frame a landscape with distant figures and slight but portentous variations: an ominously dark cloud in *Dawn* becomes a fleeting, feathery cloud by *Dusk*.

The triptych was painted for specific walls in the room, and Dalí exploited the space to achieve an illusionistic, dimensionally

105 On Tchelitchew see Alexander Kuznetsov, *Pavel Tchelitchew: Metamorphoses* (Stuttgart: Arnoldsche, 2013).

106 Edward Titus, as editor of *This Quarter*, published an important issue on Surrealism, including a piece by Dali, in 1932, its last year of existence.

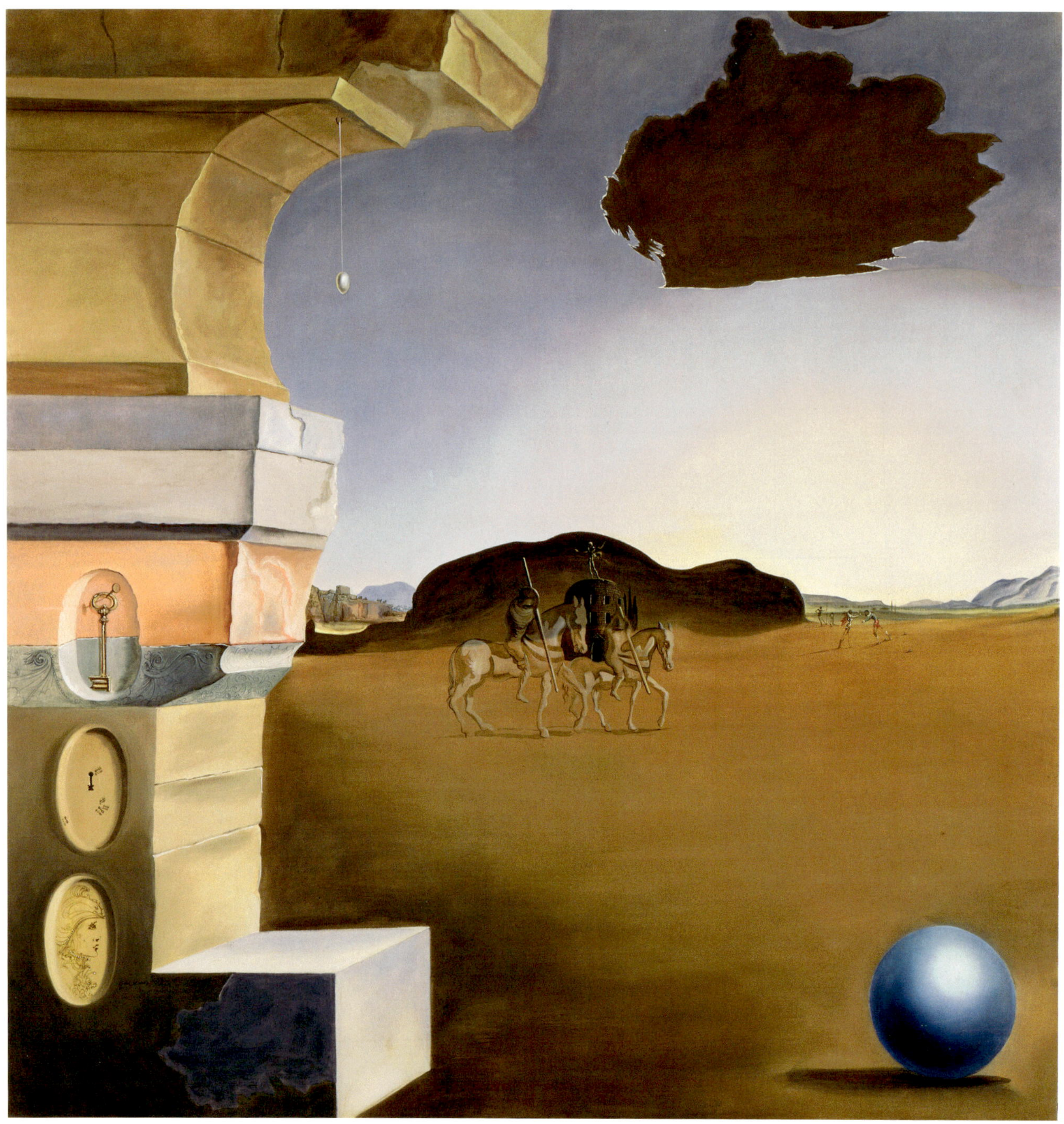

Salvador Dalí
Fantastic Landscape I (Dawn), 1942
Oil on canvas, 97⅜ × 97¼ in. (247.3 × 247 cm)
Yokohama Museum of Art, Japan

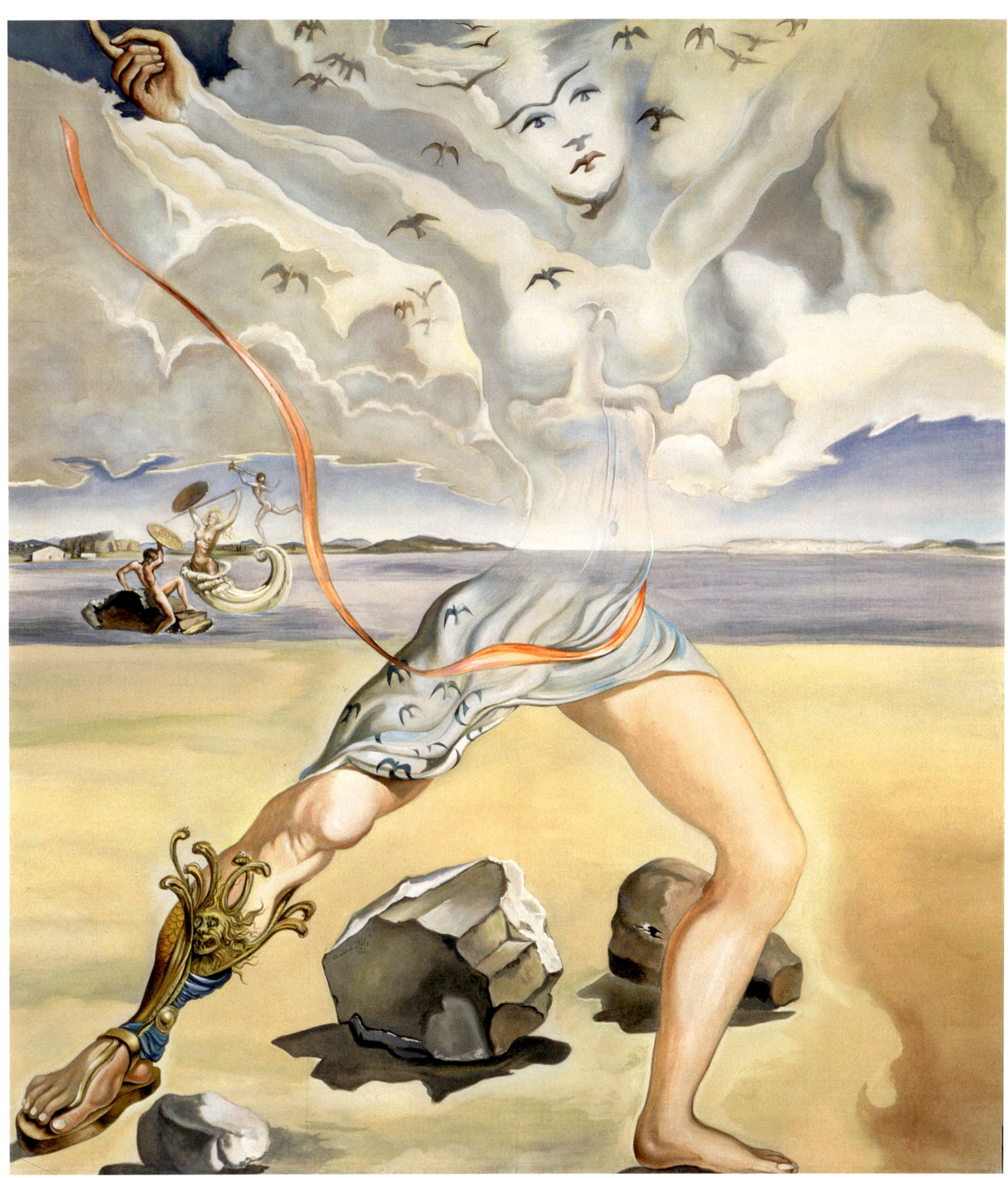

Salvador Dalí
Fantastic Landscape II (Heroic Noon), 1942
Oil on canvas, 98¾ × 88¼ in. (250.8 × 224.2 cm)
Yokohama Museum of Art, Japan

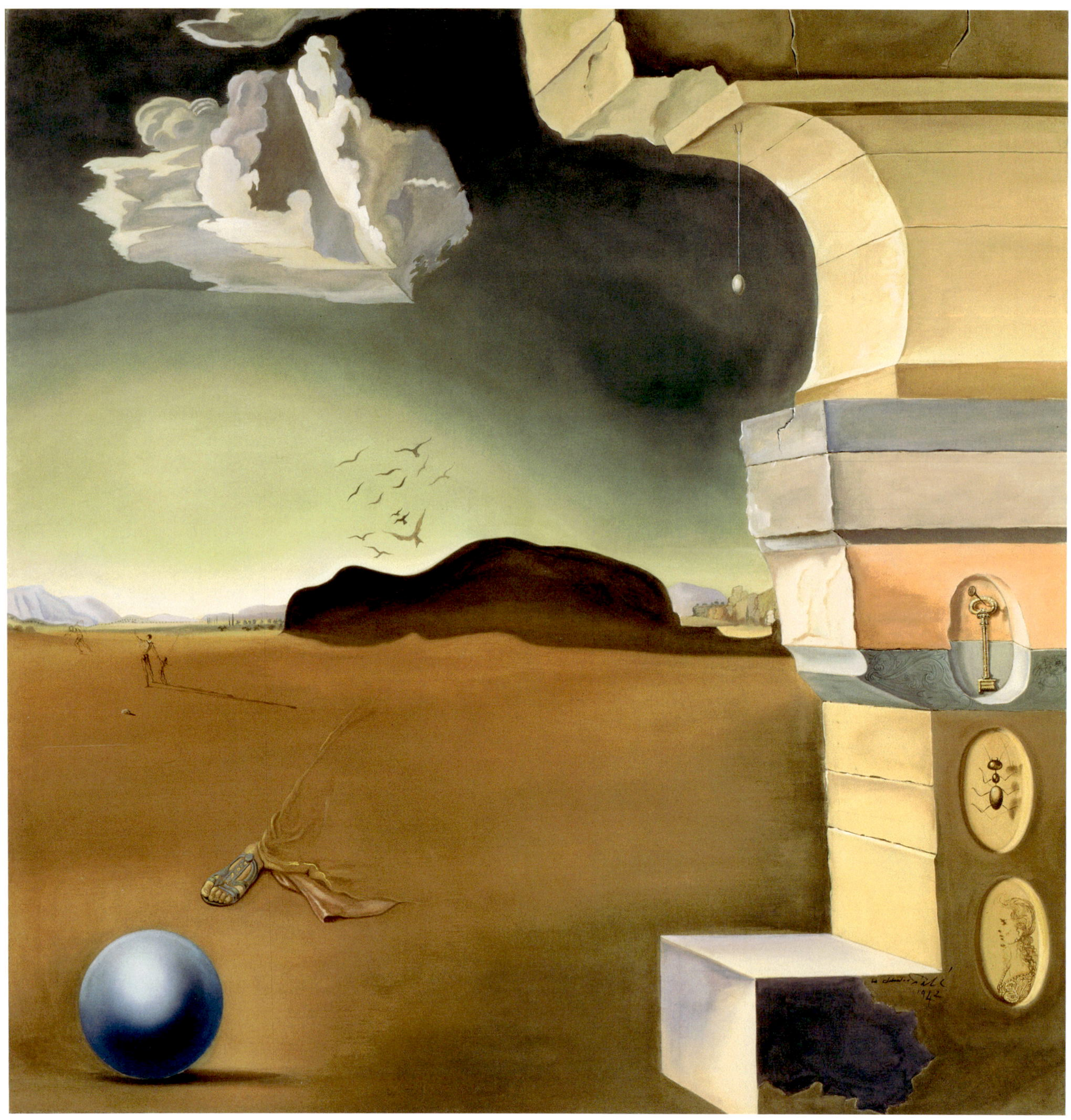

Salvador Dalí
Fantastic Landscape III (Evening), 1942
Oil on canvas, 98 × 96 in. (248.9 × 243.8 cm)
Yokohama Museum of Art, Japan

transformative, Surrealist effect. The paintings filled three walls; the fourth was an immense mirror. The viewer could only take in the whole by looking at the three paintings in their reversed reflection.[107] Madame was quite pleased with the outcome. She had been a champion of Surrealism for a decade and this spectacular commission was the crowning moment in her support. New York had become the city in which she expressed her proclivity for Surrealism, just as Art Deco had been the stylistic mainstay of her Parisian life in the 1920s.

Rubinstein remained in New York throughout World War II, watching at a distance as the old Europe of her youth and early success was systematically destroyed. As a Jew, she must have been affected, especially as she still had family in Poland and businesses throughout occupied Europe. Although she, like many wealthy women, raised money and hosted events on behalf of the Red Cross, she said little publicly about the news. After the war, she had the Paris salon redone by Louis Süe and Emilio Terry in an elevated reinterpretation of Neoclassicism, with one of Rubinstein's favorite works, Brancusi's *Bird in Space*, presiding triumphantly in the rotunda.

Postwar America

In the 1950s Rubinstein, now in her eighties, was still running her business, which remained highly lucrative. Yet the industry was changing rapidly; in particular, the newcomer Charles Revson, whom Rubinstein referred to as the "nail man," was building the Revlon company into a powerhouse. Neither he nor Rubinstein had thought much of television, the new ubiquitous medium, but Revson rapidly changed his mind after being persuaded to sponsor the runaway hit quiz show *The $64,000 Question*. The show ran for four years with Revlon's name emblazoned every week in neon lights above the contestants' dramatic sound booth.[108]

Revson took his company public in 1955. Such was Revlon's incursion into the market that Rubinstein, who had mostly relied on her company's own publicists, hired David Ogilvy, head of an up-and-coming advertising agency. But Revson's influence was overwhelming, catching both Rubinstein and Arden off guard. In particular, his ads emphasized highly sexualized depictions of young women. At the end of the decade, Madame sent an irritated memo to Ogilvy and her own creative staff: "I would be obliged if, once and for all, our packaging design did not resemble Revlon. . . . Our packaging should bear our own stamp, as should our handwriting." She signed it, as usual, "Madame Rubinstein."

As the 1960s began, the cosmetics industry exploded. Between 1955 and 1965 sales of toiletries and cosmetics quadrupled.[109] Competition within the industry intensified further; everyone seemed to be launching new perfumes, vying with every new product for the same market of increasingly prosperous American and European women. Department stores themselves reflected the latest scientific advances, presenting "charmaceuticals," aggressively hawked by hordes of trained employees in the stores' own swelling cosmetics real estate.[110]

Rubinstein's brand continued to be strong in prestige stores and the mass market of pharmacies; unlike Revson, she also still appealed to the elite with her luxury salons. In 1960 Revson also entered that niche market, although his salon was never profitable. By the mid-sixties, Revlon's advertising was growing more daring, with overt eroticism. In response, Madame decided to introduce a fragrance called L'Affaire, a name whose sexual implications were shocking at the time, and had the

107 The layout of the commission, and the way the mirror functioned to enhance the murals' visual effect, is described in T. F. James, "Princess of the Beauty Business," *Cosmopolitan* 146 (June 1959): 38. The murals are now at the Yokohama Museum of Art in Japan, hung in a traditional institutional style.

108 Revson initially did not care for television or think of it as a promotional medium, since in the 1950s transmission was solely in black and white. "We sell color," he would say. Sponsorship of the show was pitched to Rubinstein, among several other popular companies, including Chrysler, but they declined. Madame's first competitive foray into TV was to sponsor Imogene Coca and Sid Caesar's popular variety show *Your Show of Shows*. Woodhead, *War Paint*, 355–56, 373. For more on Revson see Andrew Tobias, *Fire and Ice: The Story of Charles Revson—The Man Who Built the Revlon Empire* (New York: William Morrow, 1976).

109 Nancy Koehn, "Estée Lauder: Self-Definition and the Modern Cosmetics Market," in Philip Scranton, ed., *Beauty and Business: Commerce, Gender, and Culture in Modern America* (New York: Routledge, 2001), 225.

110 Woodhead, *War Paint*, 377.

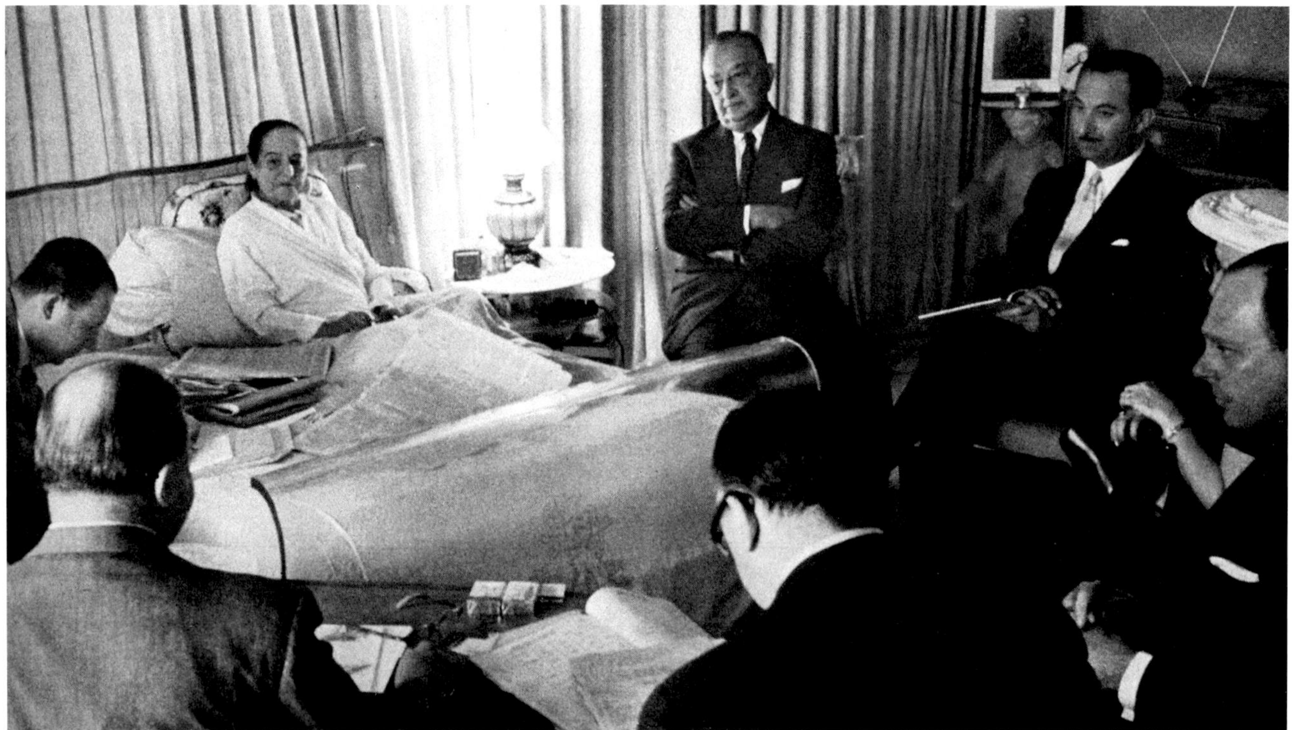

Late in life Rubinstein conducted early morning meetings from bed, where she surrounded herself with her mostly male executives. "No company moves are made without my knowing it," she declared.

company defensively debating whether or not to diffuse the sexual allusion and appear morally proper. This just before the birth control pill became widely available, an event that resounded internationally and helped usher in the sexual revolution. Indeed, the aging Rubinstein and Arden were out of sync with young female consumers.

Throughout the 1950s, and even into the 1960s, Madame appeared as active as ever, touring the world and maintaining a firm grip on her business. She visited Moscow in 1959 with her niece Mala and her assistant O'Higgins, representing the American cosmetics industry. But in truth, despite her astonishing itinerary, her continued presence at the couture runway shows, and her hands-on manner, she was slowing down. She was hospitalized on various occasions and began to conduct morning meetings at home in bed—a quirk that soon became famous.

Her avid collecting never ceased. Andy Warhol drew her portrait in the mid-1950s. Despite owning a number of works by Picasso, including early Cubist studies and a tapestry entitled *Confidence*, she wanted more (see pages 147–50). For decades she had sought to commission a portrait from him, but he had always refused. Unused to not getting her way, Madame appeared in person at his door on the French Riviera one day in 1955, and the artist, with little choice but to appease her, obliged with a series of more than thirty studies. "I'm taking down a dossier," he said, "a few police notes!" What she did not know was that he had no intention of producing anything more. Predictably, the drawings capture an impressive range of her volatile moods, from imperious to demure, and depict all of her well-known attributes—the clothes, the jewelry, the chignon, the striking manner and bearing. Unfortunately, they also reveal more than a trace of the resentment Picasso harbored toward his subject.

Sitting next to Marlene Dietrich at Yves Saint Laurent's 1958 fashion show for the House of Dior, she declared that the ordinary would never suffice for her, that she still wanted to keep up with the latest Paris creations. She was eighty-six. Madame strove never to accept the commonplace, a determination she could afford to realize. She was always, in some manner, arresting—in the way she walked "with the impulsive steps of a sandpiper," in her eccentric dress (a bowler hat crowning some idiosyncratic outfit), in the lavish jewelry she sported, in the contrasting severity of her tight, blue-black chignon swept back from the quiet intensity of her face.[111]

The Last Hurrah

Madame's collaborations with designers only increased with time, particularly toward the end of her life. In 1960, when she was eighty-eight years old, she hired the fashionable interior decorator David Hicks, a third her age, to redo her duplex apartment in London. She wanted the pied-à-terre to be as lively and inventively colorful as the recent abstract art that she had been acquiring. When the designer asked her about the color scheme, she simply cut a swatch from the purple silk Balenciaga dress she happened to be wearing. Together they produced an interior that managed to reflect both the designer's sophistication and Rubinstein's well-known exuberance, with deep violet walls and Victorian-style Belter chairs upholstered in shocking magenta.

After the rooms were done, she brought in abstract paintings by Jean-Michel Atlan and Martin Barré, recent additions to her collection. The extravagant color scheme animated the apartment into a kind of three-dimensional interpretation of the paintings. The ultimate effect,

111 O'Higgins, *Madame*, 3.

Andy Warhol
Madame Rubinstein in Kyoto, Japan, 1956
Ink with white highlights on paper, 16¾ × 22 in.
(42.5 × 55.9 cm)
Williams College Museum of Art, Williamstown, Massachusetts, Gift of Richard F. Holmes, Class of 1946

During a 1956 world tour, Rubinstein met Andy Warhol in Japan and invited him to draw her portrait.

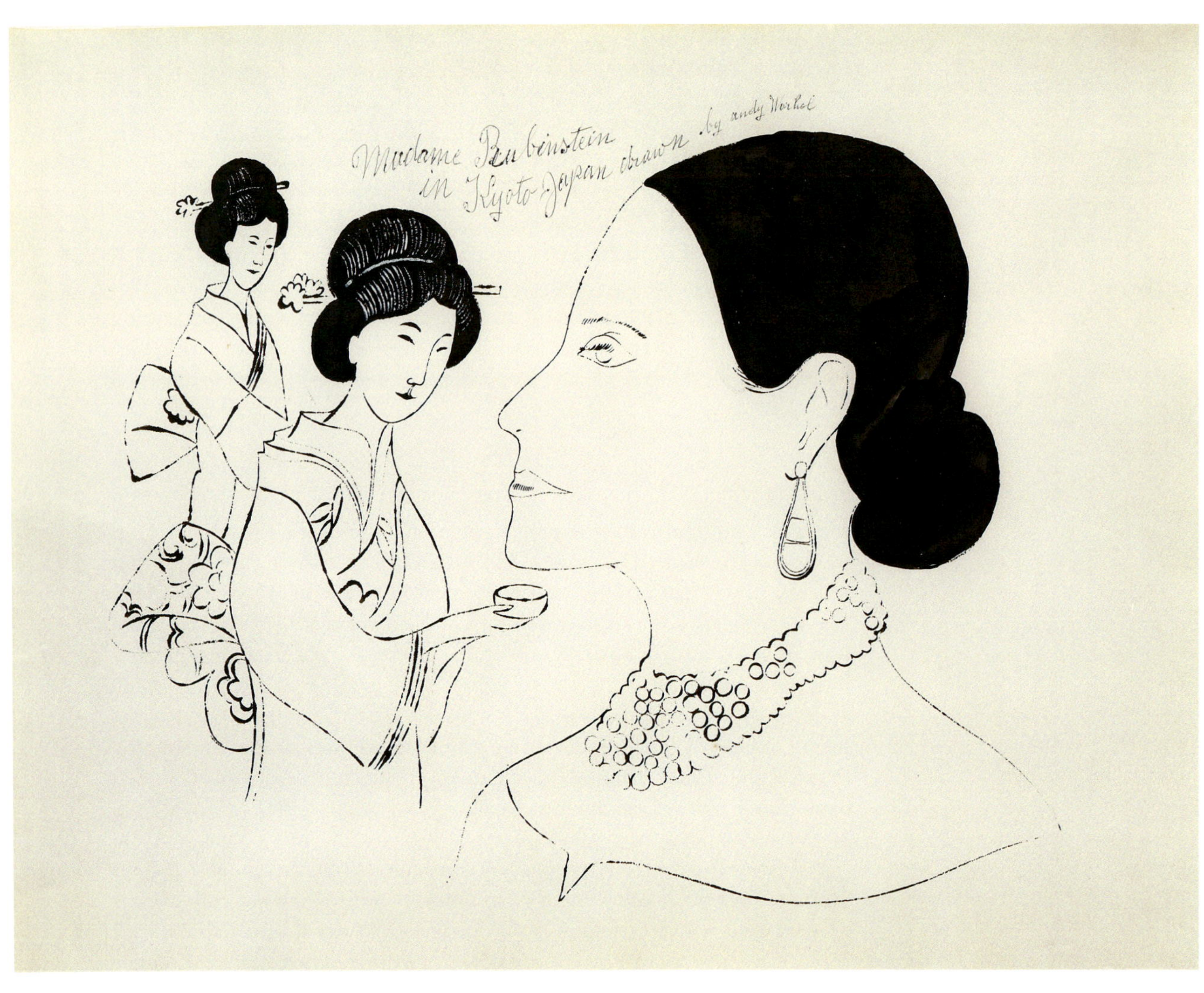

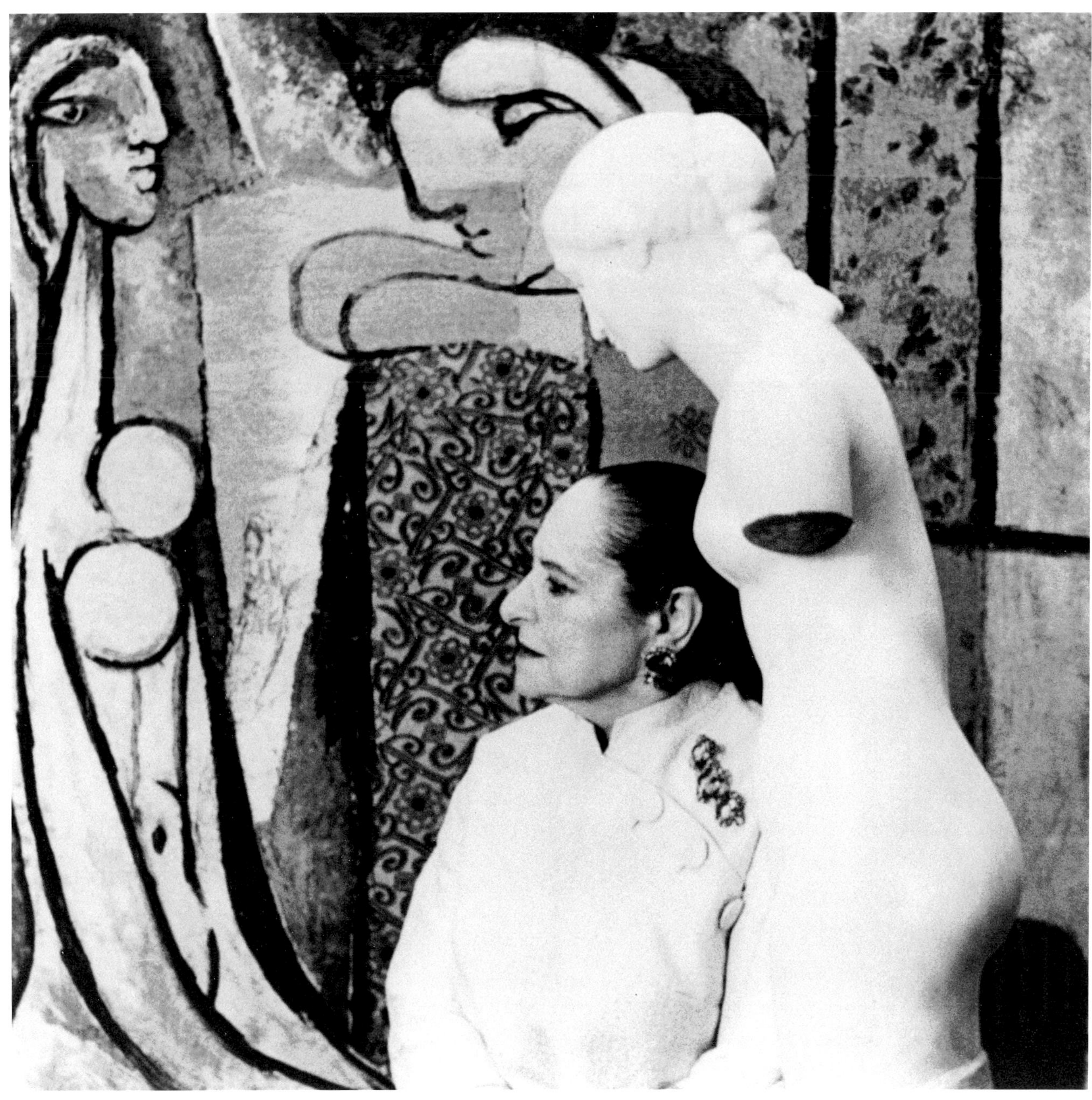

Rubinstein seated in front of Picasso's tapestry, *Confidence*, 1934, alongside Nadelman's *Classical Figure*, 1910.

Overleaf: Pablo Picasso
Twelve untitled portraits of Helena Rubinstein, from a series of more than thirty, 1955
Pencil and conté crayon on paper, each 17¼ × 12⅝ in. (43.8 × 32.1 cm)
Himeji City Museum of Art, Japan

The suite of drawings, seen together, constitutes an assemblage of faces, a parade of selves.

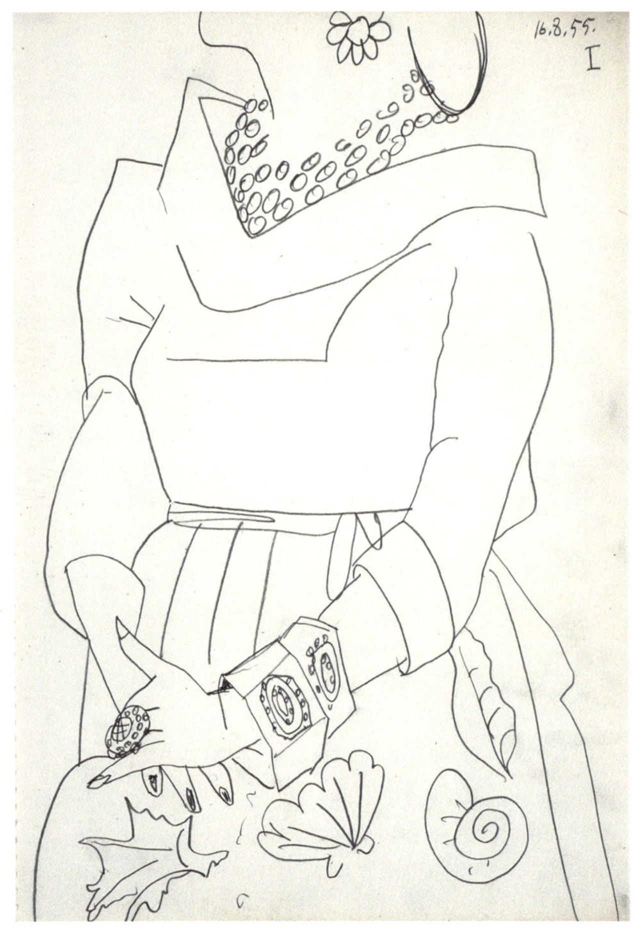
16.8.55.
I

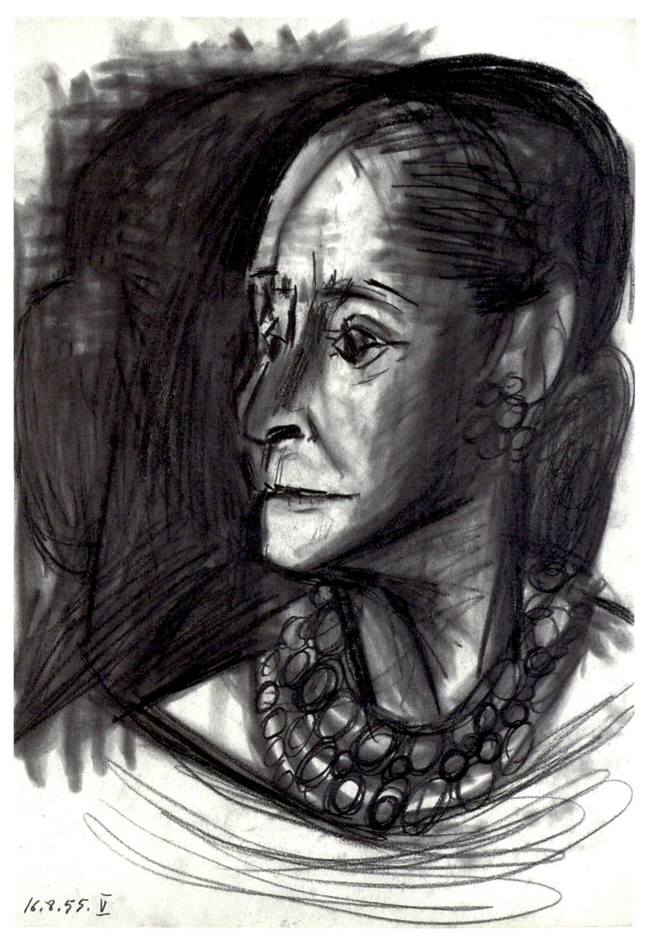
16.8.55. V

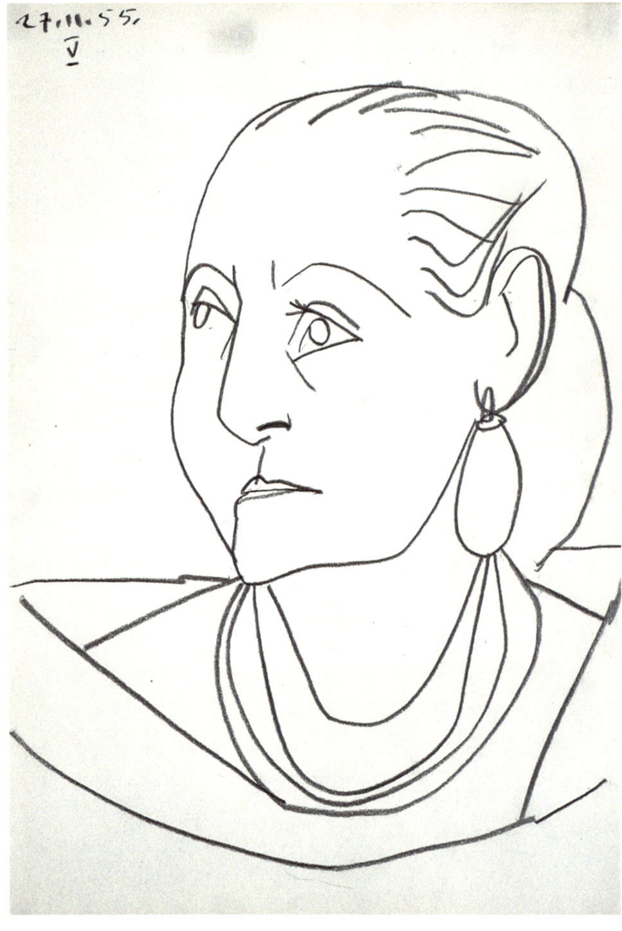
27.11.55.
V

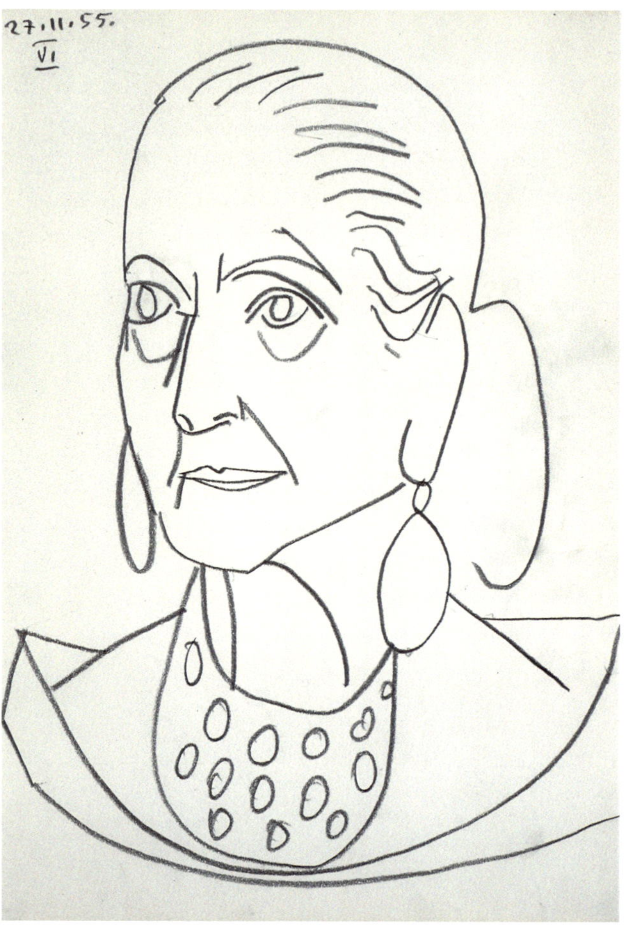
27.11.55.
VI

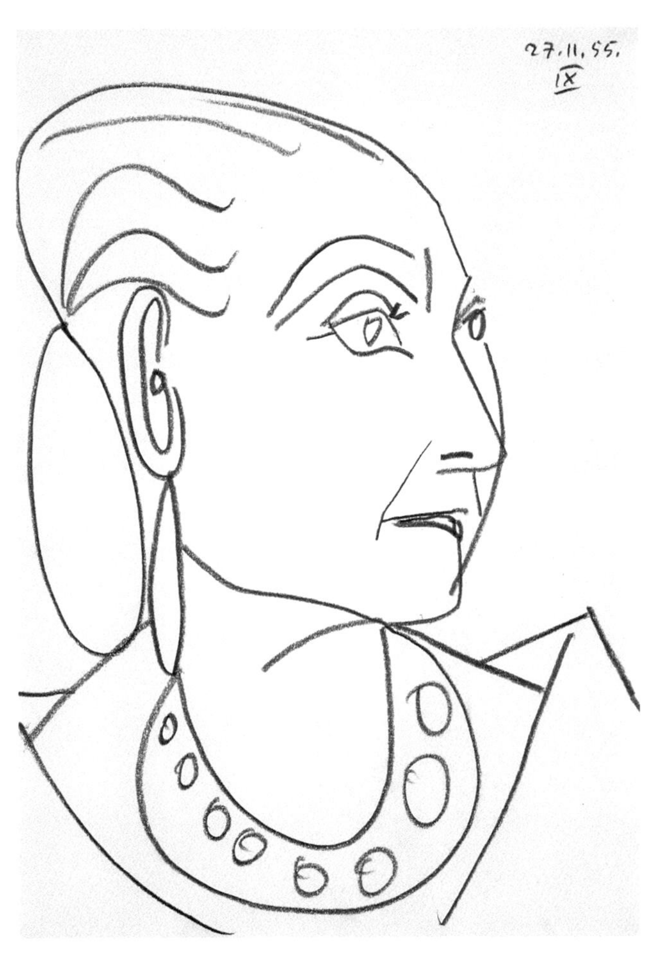
27.11.55.
IX

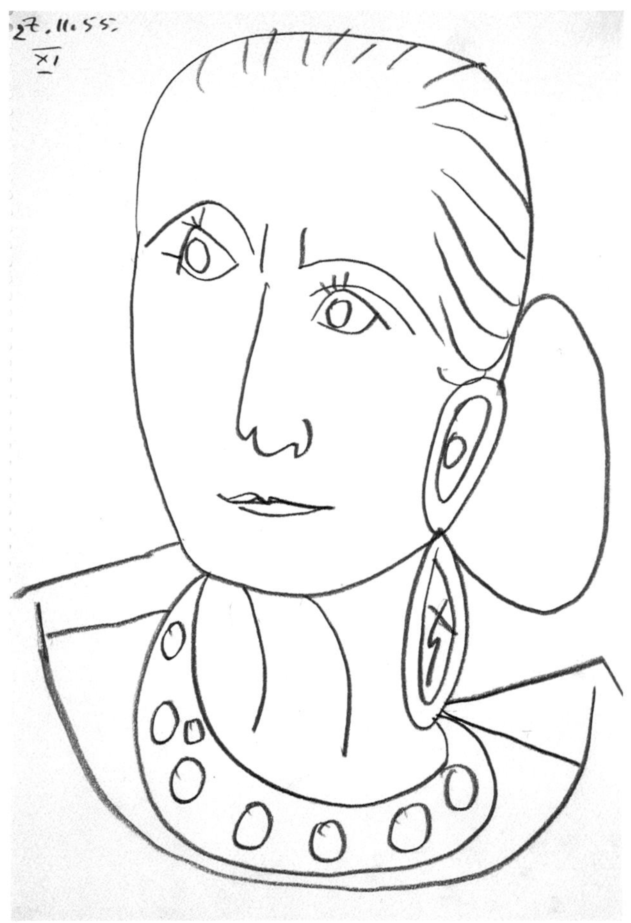
27.11.55.
XI

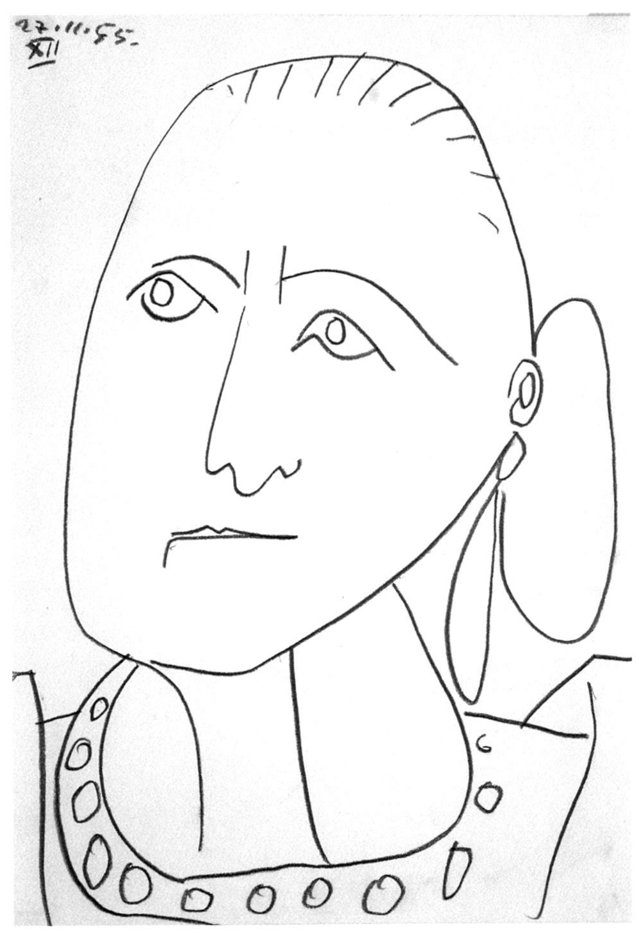
27.11.55.
XII

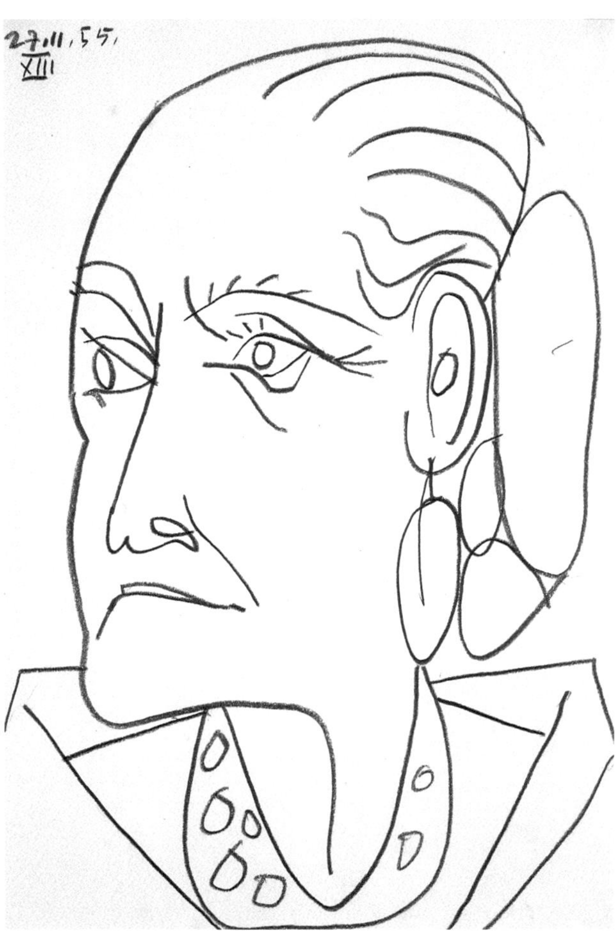
27.11.55.
XIII

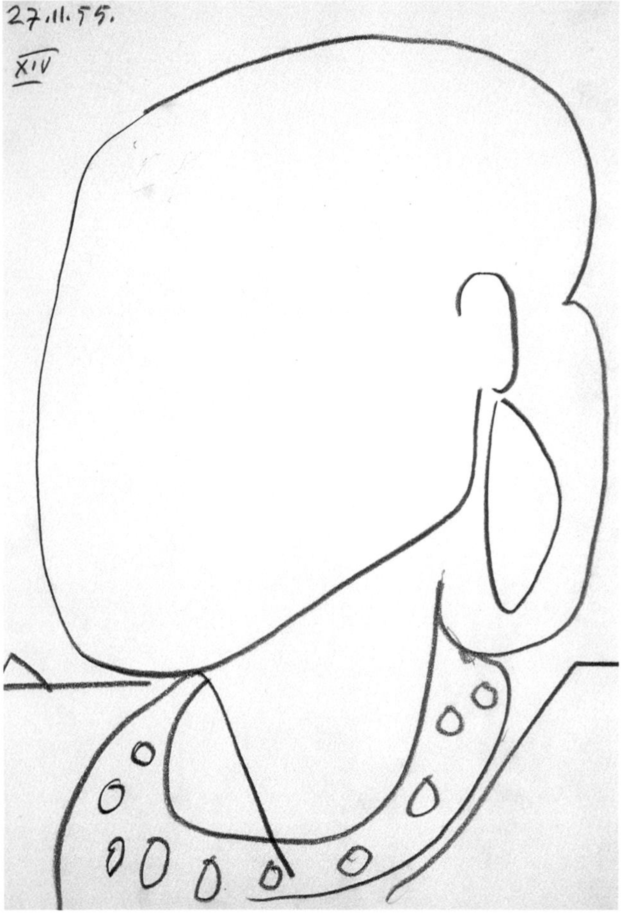

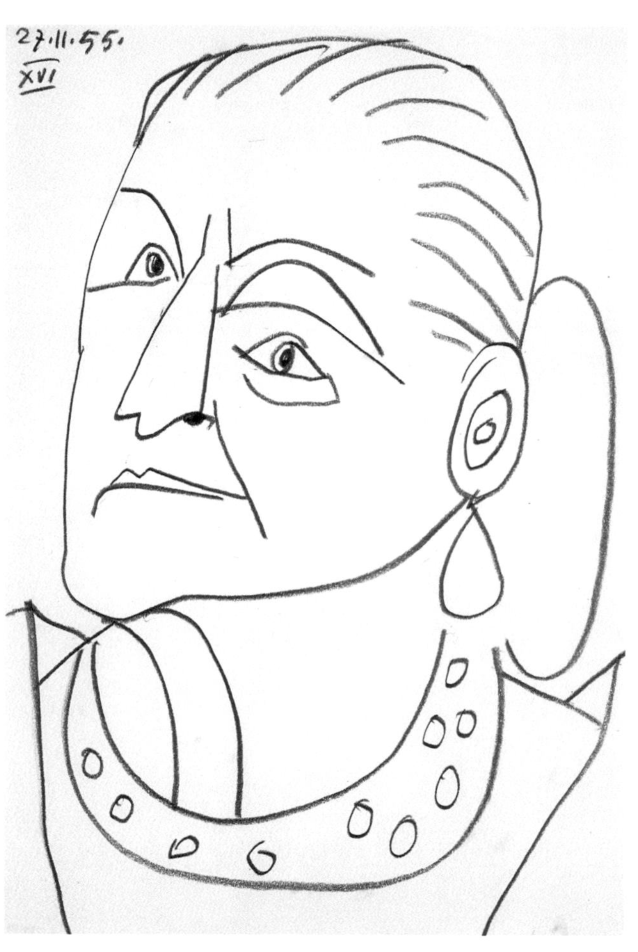
27.11.55.
XVI

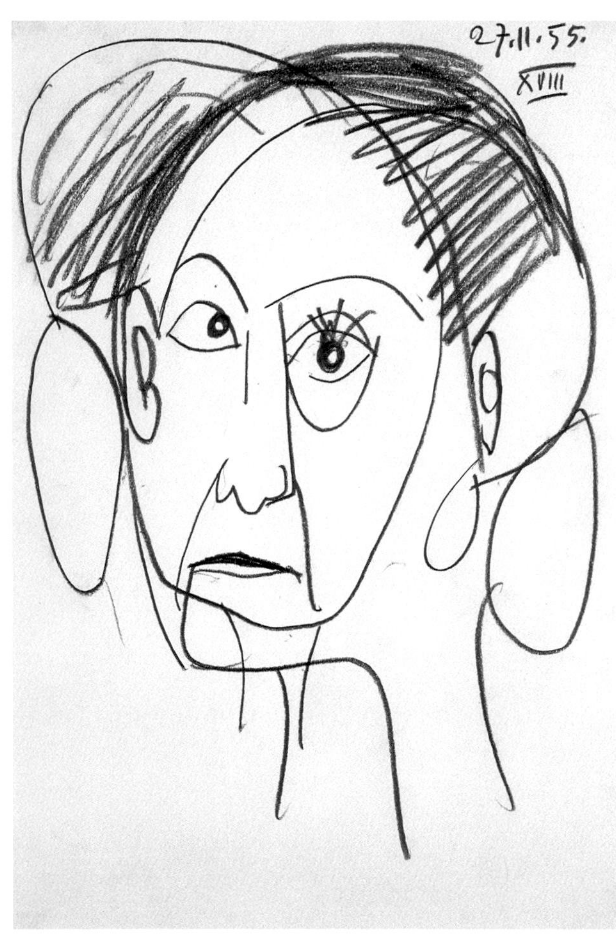
27.11.55.
XVIII

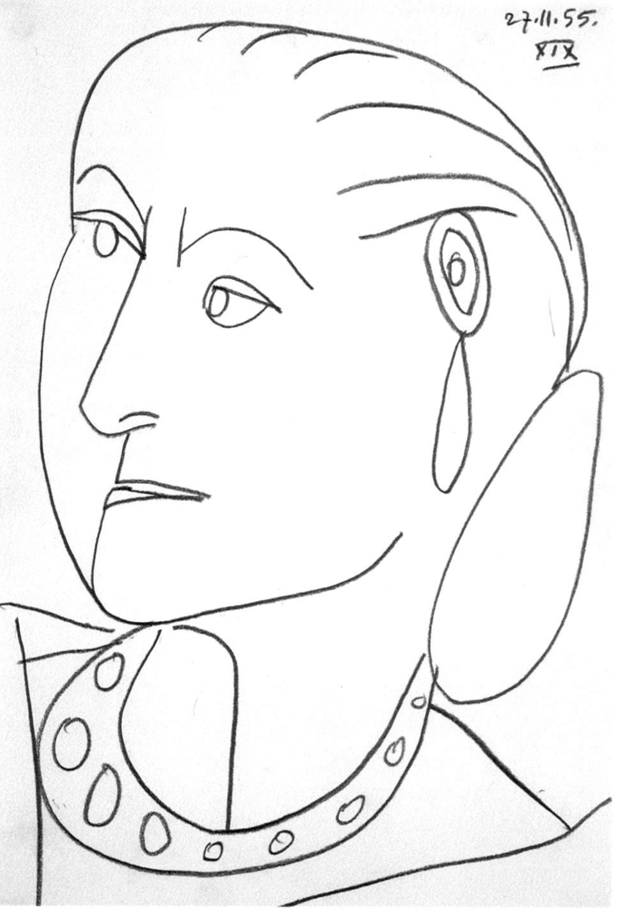
27.11.55.
XIX

a playful extrapolation of Hicks's clean, modernist look, allowed for a constant dialogue between decor and art. "I hope Mr. Hicks learned from me, as I did from him," Madame noted in her memoir.[112]

But it was the manner in which Madame influenced taste, while developing her own aesthetics of ethnicity, that distinguished her. What has often been glossed over as bad taste—certainly by the austere standards of mid-century modernism—was rather the fruition of a woman who cultivated eccentricity, who refused to obey the rules of the game or respect the usual boundaries, whether between distinct historical periods, between private and public space, between commerce and culture, or between Western and non-Western art.

That portraits dominated her several collections reflects her lifelong engagement with faces, her championing of individuality, and her belief in the potential for self-transformation. Her runaway eclecticism and sentimentality led to wildly uneven acquisitions, but among the works she chose there are some gems—her Picassos, Max Ernst's *Two Sisters*, Kees van Dongen's *Woman with Necklace*, Amedeo Modigliani's *Woman with a Blue Scarf*, Brancusi's *Mlle Pogany*, Miró's *Portrait*, Willem de Kooning's *Elegy*. These works speak, in their ways, to the intricacies of identity and the potential for change (see pages 154–59).

The Ideal Mirror

Objects, as the saying goes, can be either used or possessed. Yet, to the extent that Madame's collections became part of her persona, and were often made public, they evolved in a particularly personal way. The impulse to collect is driven by more than the affection for certain objects. Beauty is a value in itself, but for the collector it can also be quantified. The act of accruing can be read as having some ulterior psychological meaning. In Madame's case, collecting embodied her sense of self. Just as she regarded her jewelry as a form of protection, so it can be argued that her many possessions provided her with unconditional companionship.

It was a salient characteristic of Rubinstein to allow her private life to be coopted by her career. She deliberately made her domestic space public and lived most fully in the public eye. Despite her many siblings and cousins, her tens of thousands of employees, the throngs of her friends and acquaintances, Madame was more solitary than social. Perhaps because she could never depend on her family to take the reins of her business, she maintained sole control until her death.

Her independence, established early, had always defined her. As a girl she had had to shoulder domestic duties, helping her mother care for her seven younger siblings. Her favorite diversion from household drudgery had been to walk from Kazimierz to the Rynek, a renowned medieval square in Krakow, not far from the Rubinstein house. She would spend time at its Cloth Hall, designed in the fourteenth century as a center for the textile trade. The immense building, filled with merchants' stalls, had reigned for centuries as one of the great markets of Europe, where all kinds of treasures were bought and sold. And it was there that the young Helena, threading her way among the endless booths, examining myriad objects—amber, glass, dolls, linens—had become enthralled with things. There, in the Cloth Hall of her youth, her enduring delight in rummaging and collecting had been kindled.[113]

This lasting, formative experience—one associated with being unburdened by family—resonates in her devotion to collecting. Human relationships, as she was the first to admit, were rarely fulfilling. But she

112 Rubinstein, *My Life for Beauty*, 112.
113 See Woodhead, *War Paint*, 31.

Rubinstein's apartment at 216, boulevard Raspail, Paris, 1933, showing paintings by Miró, Ernst, and Picasso, several Bakota reliquary figures, a Fang head, and a Baule drum.

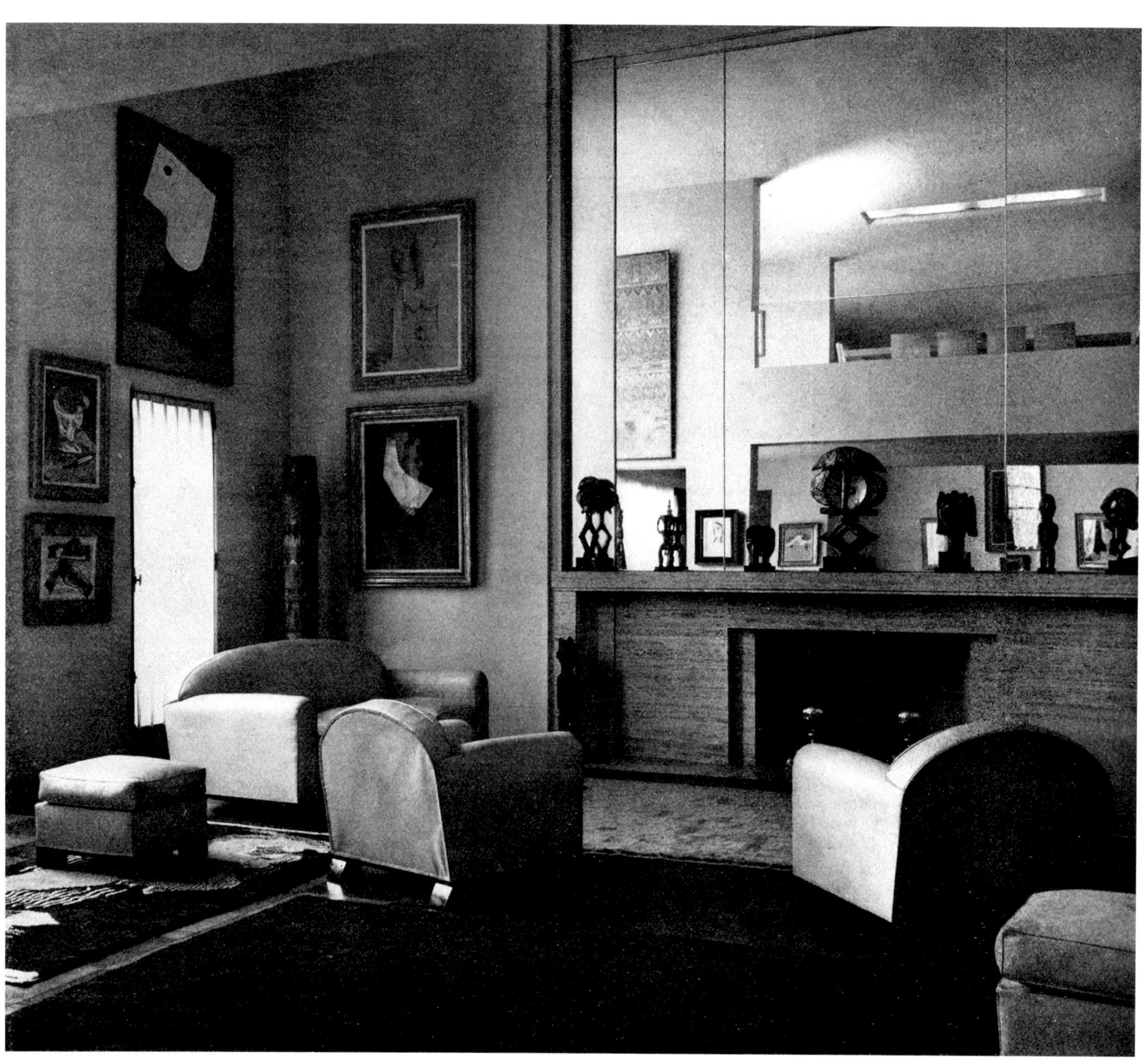

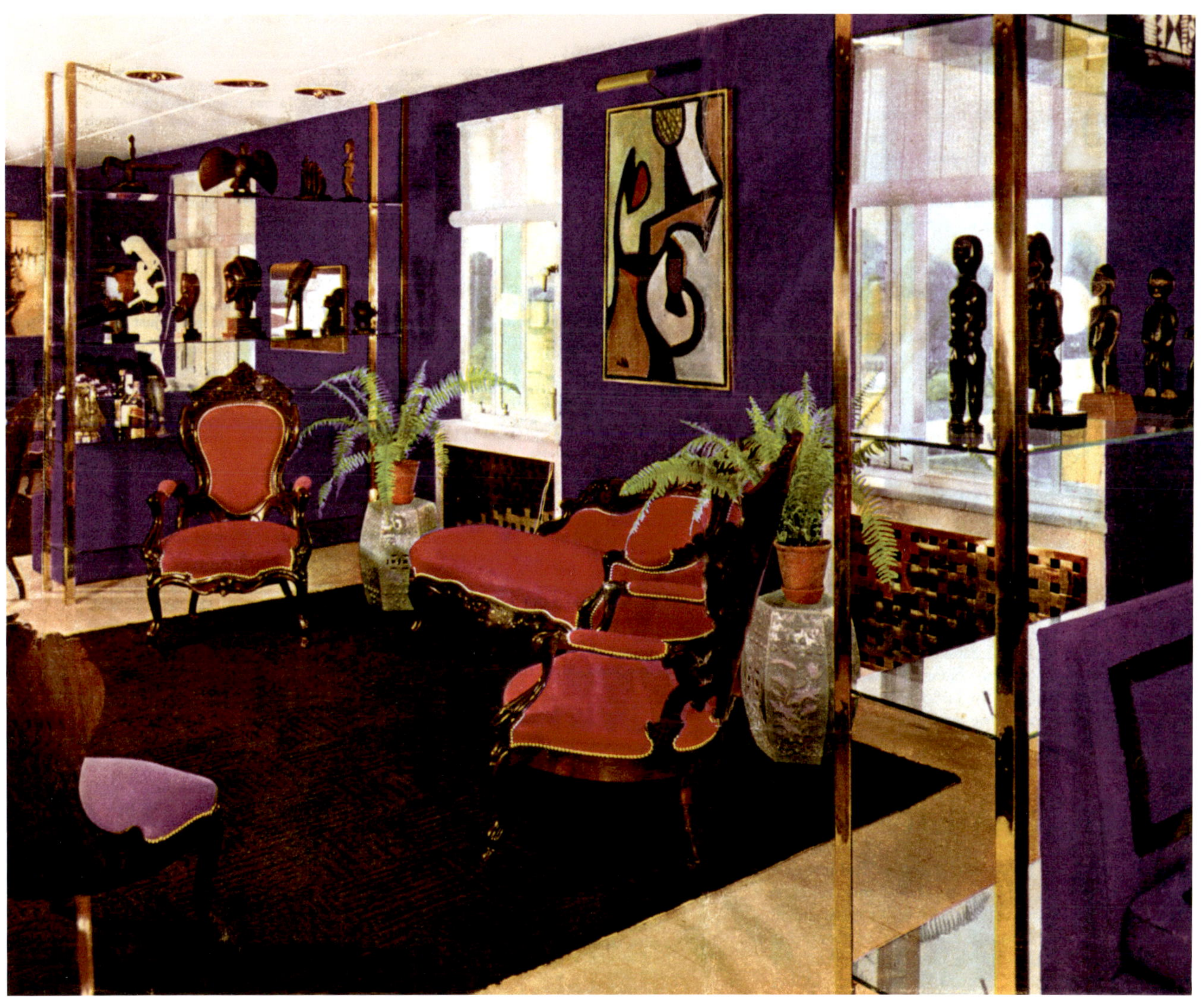

Rubinstein's London apartment, designed by David Hicks, c. 1961. In the center of the purple wall is a painting by Jean-Michel Atlan. African sculptures line the glass shelves, and cerise Belter chairs make up the ensemble.

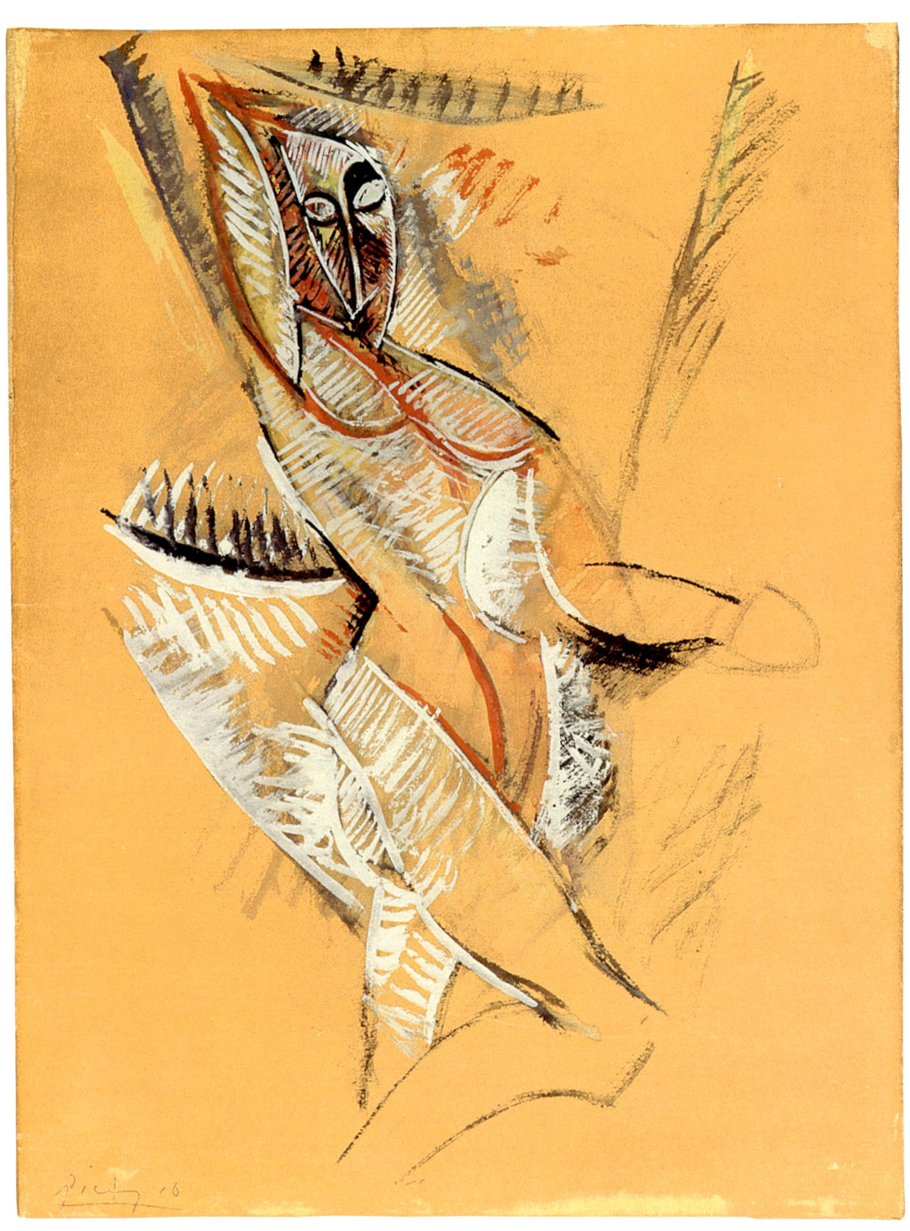

Pablo Picasso
Study for *Nude with Drapery*, 1907
Gouache on paper, mounted on canvas, 12 × 9¼ in.
(30.5 × 23.5 cm)
Private collection

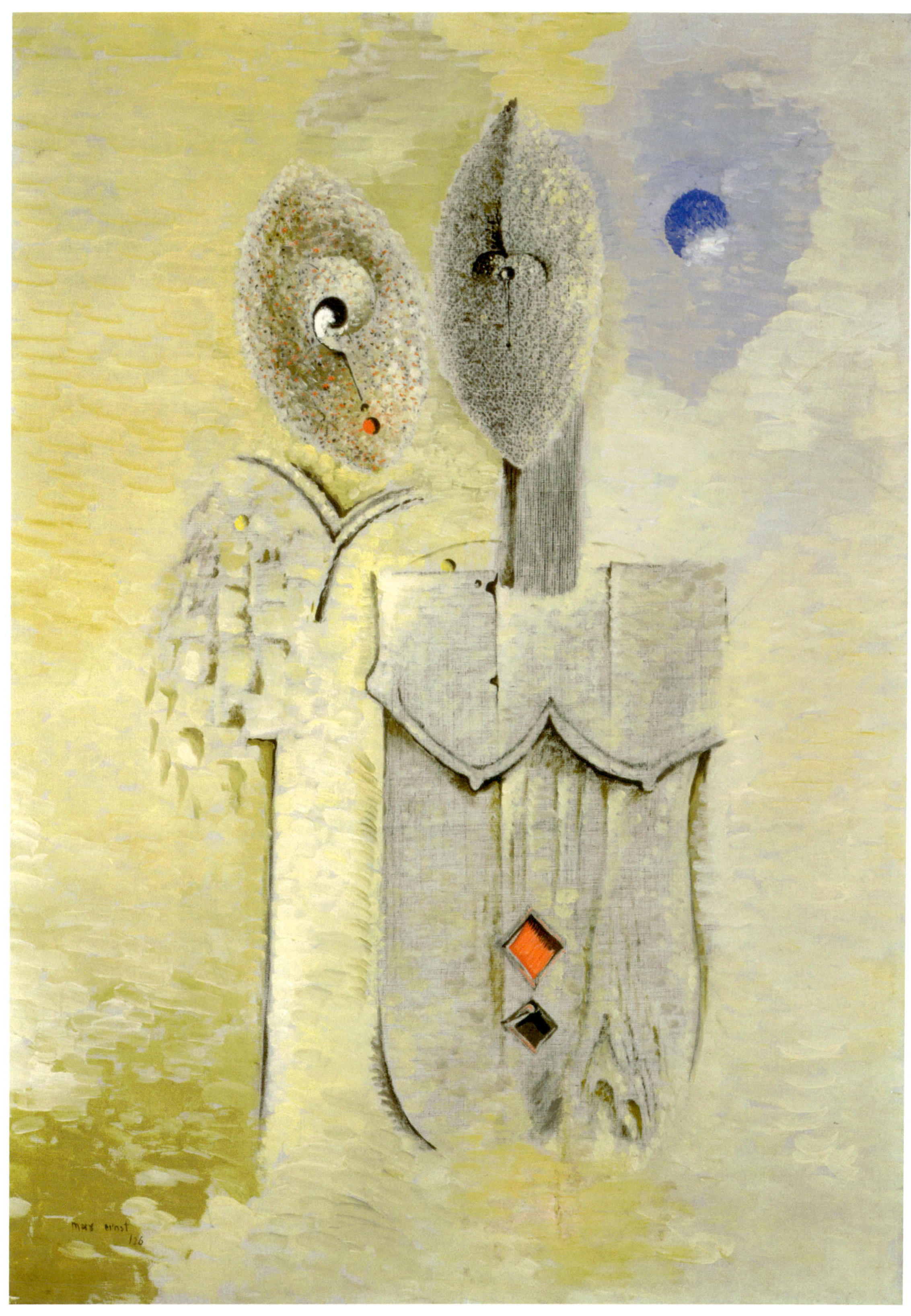

Max Ernst
Two Sisters, 1926
Oil on canvas, 39⅜ × 28¾ in. (100 × 73 cm)
The Menil Collection, Houston

Ernst's Surrealist image of two sisters must have appealed to Rubinstein, whose own sisters worked for her and caused her endless exasperation.

Kees van Dongen
Woman with Necklace–Red Ground, 1905
Oil on canvas, 39 × 31 in. (99.1 × 78.7 cm)
Location unknown

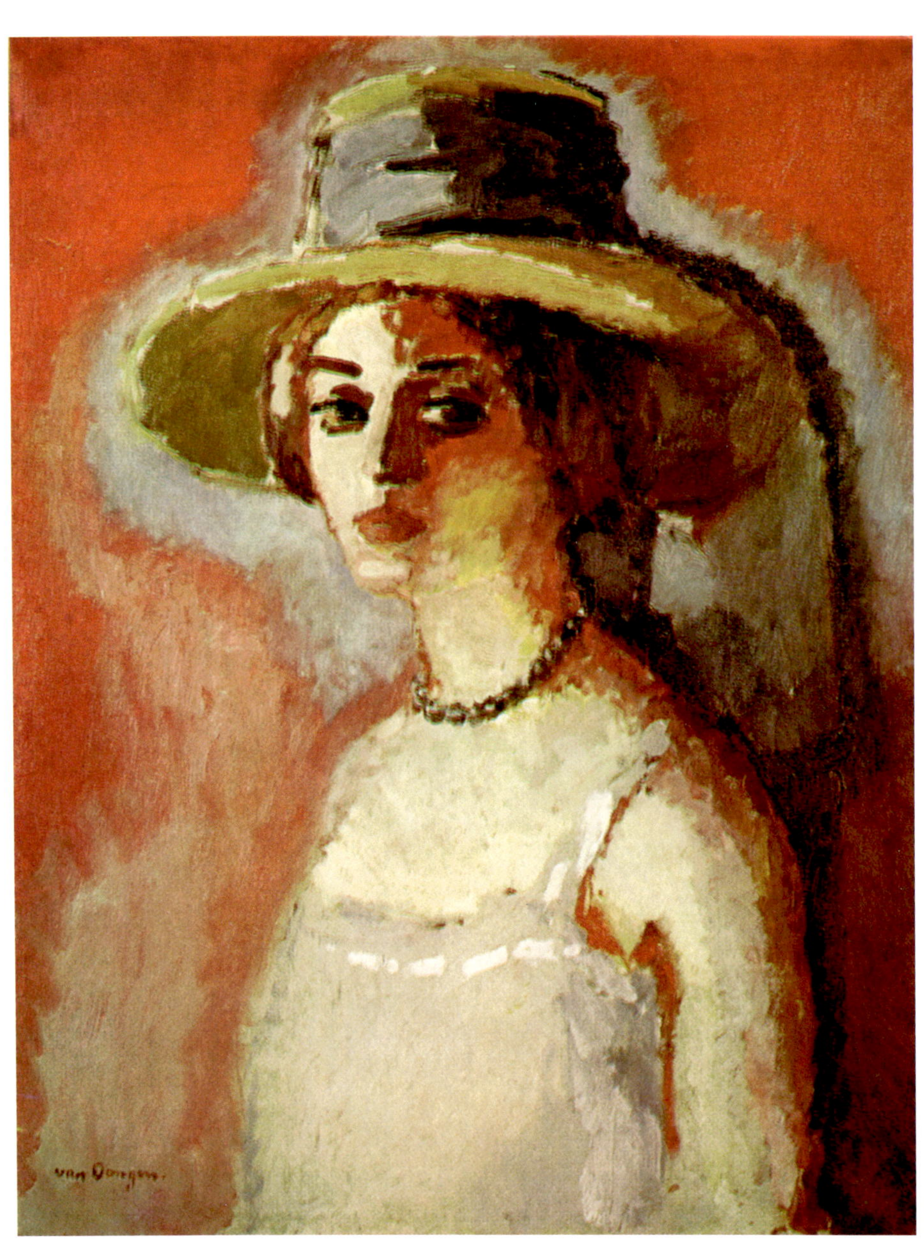

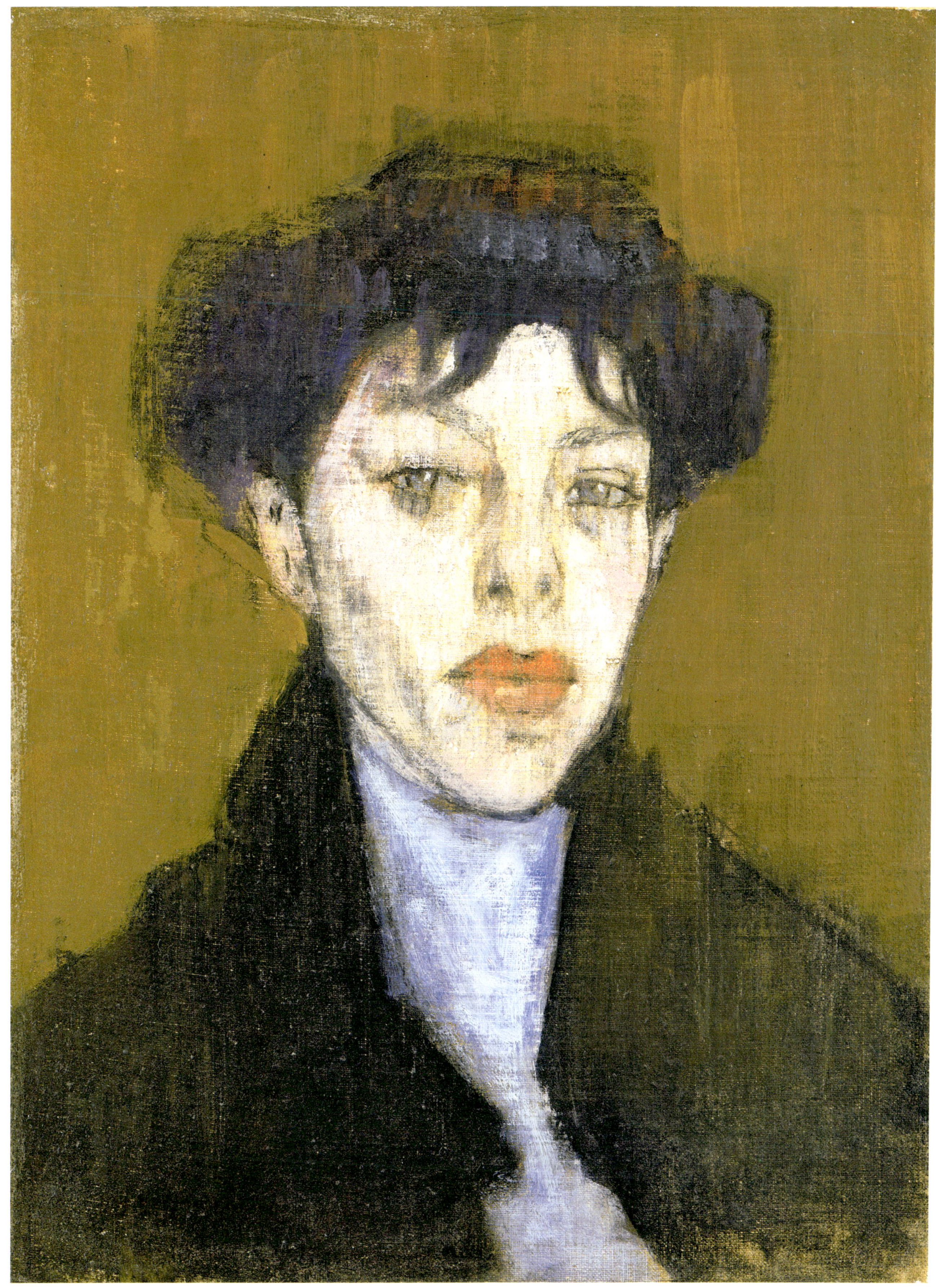

Amedeo Modigliani
Woman with a Blue Scarf, c. 1906
Oil on canvas, 12½ × 9½ in. (31.8 × 24.1 cm)
Location unknown

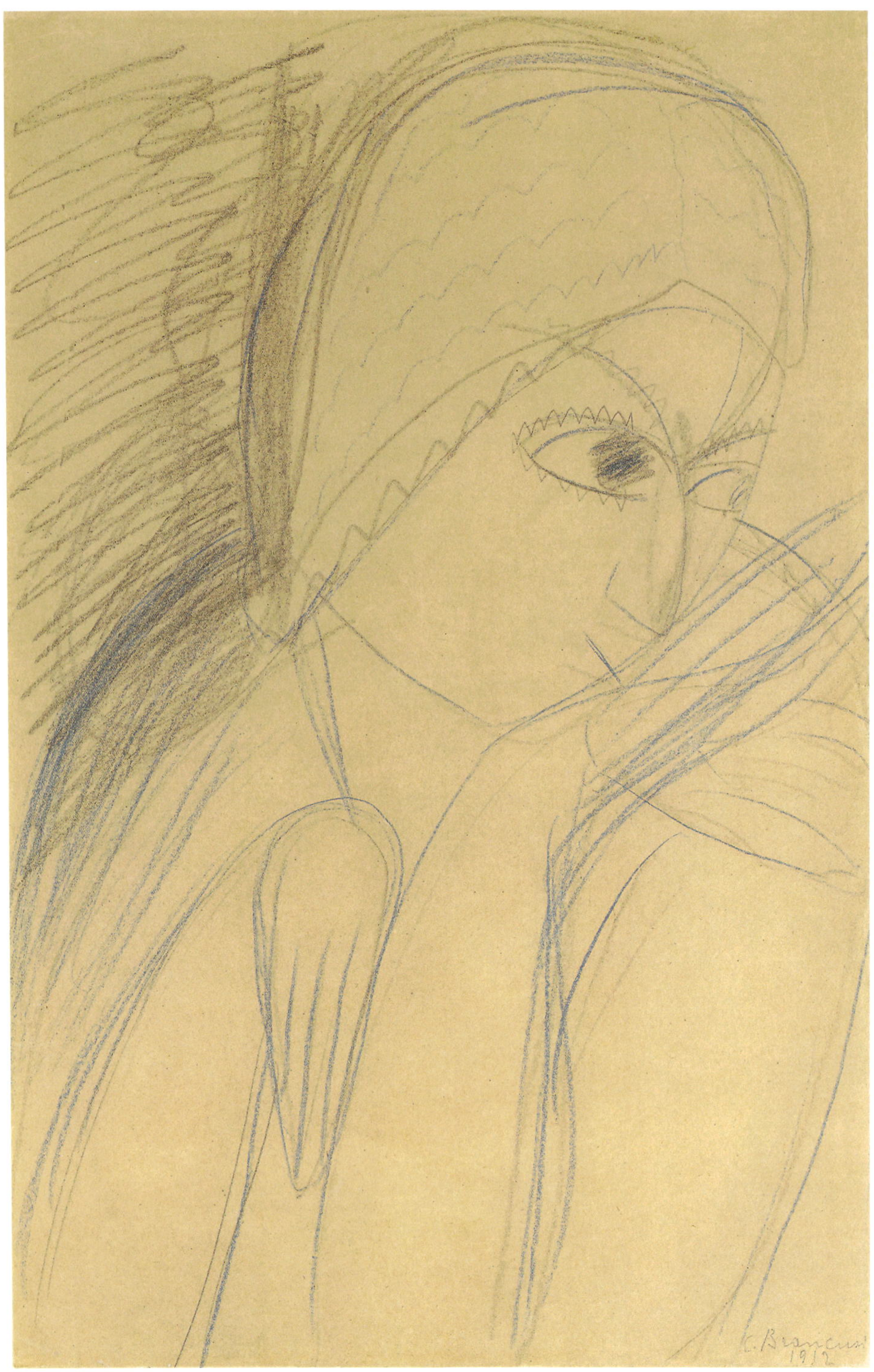

Constantin Brancusi
Mlle Pogany, 1912
Blue wax crayon and pencil on paper
18½ × 12⅝ in. (47 × 32.1 cm)
Private collection

Willem de Kooning
Elegy, 1939
Oil on Masonite, 40¼ × 47¾ in.
(102.2 × 121.3 cm)
Private collection

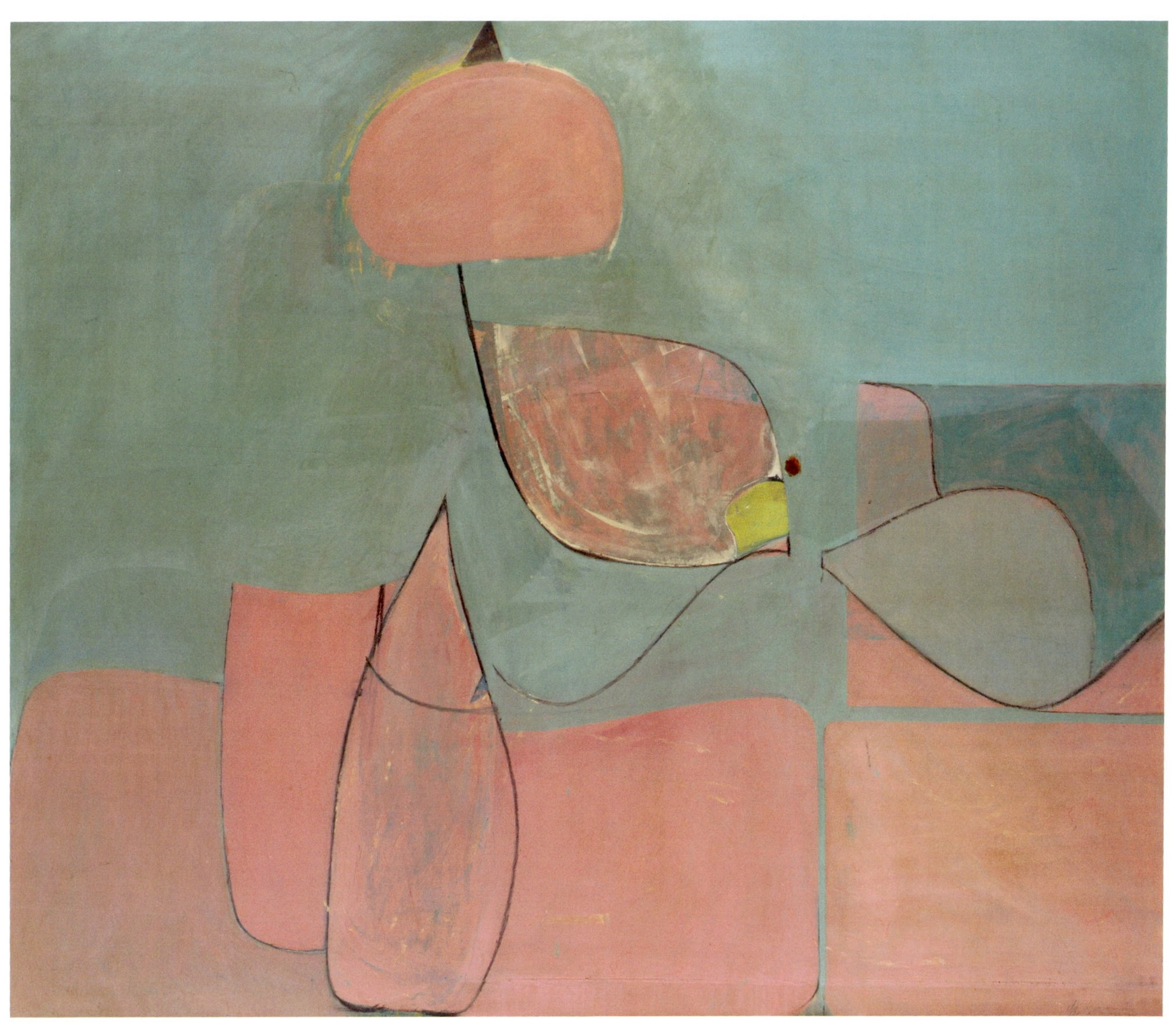

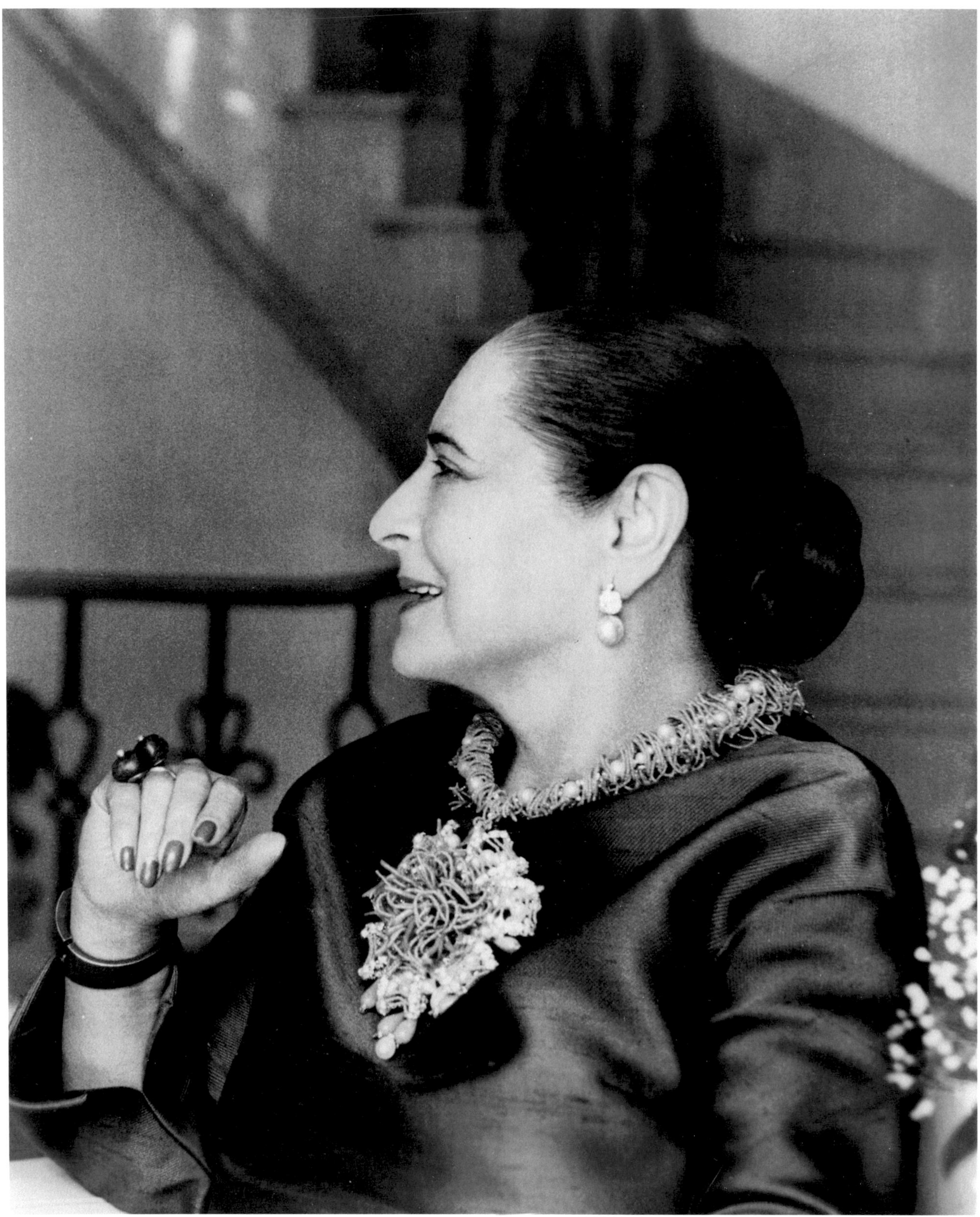

Rubinstein's passion for haute couture scarcely diminished even in her nineties, when she became an early champion of Yves Saint Laurent, first when he worked at the House of Dior, and then when he presented his first collection under his own name, in 1962, when she purchased this deep purple silk and wool ensemble with neckline and pendant embroidered in coral, pearls, and silver.

recognized that collecting had multiple purposes and motives, and the value of objects might be measured in many ways, from their intrinsic beauty to the status they conveyed to the commercial uses to which they might be put.

Helpful in further understanding the psychology of collecting is the philosopher Jean Baudrillard's exploration of the subject:

> *The objects that occupy our daily lives are in fact the objects of a passion, that of personal possession . . . the objects in our lives, as distinct from the way we make use of them at a given moment, represent something much more, something profoundly related to subjectivity . . . a mental realm over which I hold sway, a thing whose meaning is governed by myself alone. . . .*
>
> *Any thing can be possessed, invested in, or, in terms of collecting, arranged, sorted and classified. The object thus emerges as the ideal mirror: for the images it reflects succeed one another while never contradicting one another. Moreover, it is ideal in that it reflects images not of what is real, but only of what is desirable. . . . I am able to gaze on it without its gazing back at me. This is why one invests in objects all that one finds impossible to invest in human relationships.*[114]

For Baudrillard, the object as "ideal mirror" reflects the meanings its owner invests it with—ideas, symbols, emotions, whatever is personal. The notion of "not what is real, but only what is desirable" returns us to the world of self-invention, of beauty, and of art—in short, to the world of cosmetics.

Whatever ulterior symbolism her collecting may have served, the ideal mirror, for Madame, was also a tool of trade. She used it to change the reality of generations of women by enabling them to see themselves as they wished to be. Today we take that subjectivity for granted, but the sense of individuality she fostered was new and profound in the early twentieth century. She advocated a sense of exceptionality in a world that discouraged nonconformity. The ideal of freedom that she offered women allowed them to be modern and to understand the fundamental principle that one's identity is a matter of choice.

114 Jean Baudrillard, "The System of Collecting," *Cultures of Collecting*, ed. John Elsner and Roger Cardinal (London: Reaktion Books, 1994), 7, 11.

selected bibliography

Archives

Helena Rubinstein Foundation archive, Fashion Institute of Technology, State University of New York, Special Collections.

Helena Rubinstein archive, L'Oréal Luxe, Paris.

Publications

"A Beauty Salon in Art Moderne." *Good Furniture*, 30, no. 5 (May 1928): 242–44.

"And What's More." *Vogue* 101, no. 9 (May 1, 1943): 80.

"A Tiny, Tireless Tycoon of Beauty." *Life* 56, no. 20 (May 15, 1964): 115-16, 118.

Baldwin, Neil. *Man Ray: American Artist* (New York: Clarkson N. Potter, 1988).

Baudelaire, Charles. "On the Ideal and the Model." In *Art in Paris 1845–1862: Salons and Other Exhibitions*. Jonathan Mayne, trans. and ed. London: Phaidon Press, 1965.

——. *The Painter of Modern Life and Other Essays*. Jonathan Mayne, trans. and ed. London: Phaidon Press, 1964.

Baudrillard, Jean. "The System of Collecting." In John Elsner and Roger Cardinal, eds. *Cultures of Collecting*. London: Reaktion Books, 1994, 7–24.

"Beauty Specialist Displays Her Nadelmans." *Art Digest* 6 (April 15, 1932): 15.

Brandon, Ruth. *Ugly Beauty: Helena Rubinstein, L'Oréal, and the Blemished History of Looking Good*. New York: HarperCollins, 2011.

Breward, Christopher, Becky Conekin, and Caroline Cox, eds. *The Englishness of English Dress*. Oxford: Berg, 2002.

"The Business of Beauty Is the Business of Rubinstein." *Life* 2, no. 9 (March 1, 1937): 39.

Charles-Roux, Edmonde. *Chanel and her World: Friends, Fashion, Fame*. London: Hachette-Vendome, 1981.

Clifford, James. "Negrophilia," in Denis Hollier, *A New History of French Literature*. Cambridge, MA: Harvard University Press, 1989, 901–8.

——. *The Predicament of Culture: Twentieth-Century Ethnography, Literature, and Art*. Cambridge, MA: Harvard University Press, 1988.

Clifford, Marie J. "Helena Rubinstein's Beauty Salons, Fashion, and Modernist Display." *Winterthur Portfolio* 38, no. 2–3 (Summer-Autumn, 2003): 83-108.

"Collector's Fantasy." *Vogue* 92, no. 4 (August 15, 1938): 120–23.

Collins, Amy Fine. "The Reign of Helena Rubinstein," *House & Garden* 164, no. 11 (November 1992): 144–47, 198–99.

De Castelbajac, Kate. *The Face of the Century: 100 Years of Makeup and Style*. New York: Rizzoli, 1995.

de Grazia, Victoria, ed., with Ellen Furlough. *The Sex of Things: Gender and Consumption in Historical Perspective*. Berkeley: University of California Press, 1996.

De Peyster Kip, Carola. "Worn Out and Repaired." *Harper's Bazaar* 71 (February 1937): 102–3.

"Designed for Dining." *House & Garden* 93, no. 4 (April 1, 1948): 126–31.

de Wolfe, Elsie. *The House in Good Taste*. New York: Century, 1913. Repr. New York: Rizzoli, 2004.

Einstein, Carl. *Negerplastik, von Carl Einstein; mit 116 Abbildungen*. Munich: K. Wolff, 1920.

"Elie Nadelman: Sculptor of Modern Life." Press release, Whitney Museum of American Art, New York, 2003.

Ewen, Stuart. *All Consuming Images: The Politics of Style in Contemporary Culture*. Rev. ed. New York: Basic Books, 1988.

Fabe, Maxene. *Beauty Millionaire: The Life of Helena Rubinstein*. New York: T. Y. Crowell, 1972.

Fitoussi, Michèle. *Helena Rubinstein: The Woman Who Invented Beauty*. Sydney: HarperCollins, 2012.

Flanner, Janet. "Des diverses formes de beauté." *L'Oeil* 34 (October 1957): 24–31.

Gilroy, Paul. " 'To Be Real': The Dissident Forms of Black Expressive Culture." In Catherine Ugwu, ed. *Let's Get It On: The Politics of Black Performance*. Seattle: Bay Press, 1995, 12–33.

Gray, Allison, "People Who Want to Look Young and Beautiful." *The American Magazine* 94 (December 1922): 32–33, 161–64.

Grossman, Wendy A. *Man Ray, African Art, and the Modernist Lens*. Washington, DC: International Art and Artists, 2009.

Haskell, Barbara. *Elie Nadelman: Sculptor of Modern Life*. Exh. cat. New York: Whitney Museum of American Art, 2003.

Hegger, Grace. "Beauty Bought and Paid For." *Vogue* 46, no. 10 (November 15, 1915): 68, 116.

"Helena Rubinstein Dies Here at 94." *New York Times* (April 2, 1965): 1, 32.

"Helena Rubinstein in Her Paris Home." *House & Garden* 73, no. 1 (January 1938): 50–51.

Hollander, Anne. "The Modernization of Fashion." *Design Quarterly* 154 (Winter 1992): 27–33.

Hulten, Pontus, Natalia Dumitresco, and Alexandre Istrati. *Brancusi*. New York: Harry N. Abrams, 1987.

"It's a Beautiful Day." *Vogue* 89, no. 2 (January 15, 1937): 74–77, 116–17.

James, T. F. "Princess of the Beauty Business." *Cosmopolitan* 146 (June 1959): 38–44.

Jones, Geoffrey. *Beauty Imagined: A History of the Global Beauty Industry*. New York: Oxford University Press, 2010.

——. *Beauty Imagined: A History of the Global Beauty Industry*. Oxford: Oxford University Press, 2010.

Kachur, Lewis. *Displaying the Marvelous: Marcel Duchamp, Salvador Dalí, and Surrealist Exhibition Installations*. Cambridge, MA: MIT Press, 2001.

Kear, Jon. "Vénus Noire: Josephine Baker and the Parisian Music-Hall." In Michael Sheringham, ed. *Parisian Fields*. London: Reaktion Books, 1996, 46–70.

Kent, Jacqueline C. "Charles Frederick Worth: The Father of Haute Couture." In *Business Builders in Fashion*. Minneapolis: Oliver Press, 2003, 21–37.

Kieffer, Elaine Brown. "Madame Rubinstein: The Little Lady from Krakow Has Made a Fabulous Success of Selling Beauty." *Life* 11, no. 6 (July 21, 1941): 36–40, 43–45.

Kirstein, Lincoln. *The Sculpture of Elie Nadelman*. New York: The Museum of Modern Art, 1948.

Kuznetsov, Alexander. *Pavel Tchelitchew: Metamorphoses*. Stuttgart: Arnoldsche, 2013.

Long, Christopher. *Paul T. Frankl and Modern American Design*. New Haven, CT: Yale University Press, 2007.

Mannes, Marya. "African Art in the Rubinstein Collection." *International Studio* 92, no. 384 (May 1929): 55–56.

Man Ray. *Self Portrait*. London: Andre Deutsch, 1963.

Martin, Richard. *Fashion and Surrealism*. New York: Rizzoli, 1987.

"Mme. Rubinstein's Living Art Blocks Fifth Avenue Traffic." *Life* 2, no. 9 (March 1, 1937): 40.

Mumford, Lewis. "The Sky Line: The City of the Future." *New Yorker* 12, no. 47 (January 9, 1937): 48; 50–51.

Nadelman, Elie. "Notes for a Catalogue." *Camera Work* 32 (October 1910): 41. Repr. in Lincoln Kirstein, *Elie Nadelman*. New York: Eakins Press, 1973, 265.

"New Paris Apartment of Madame Helena Rubinstein." *Vogue* 82, no. 10 (November 15, 1933): 52–53.

O'Higgins, Patrick. *Madame: An Intimate Biography of Helena Rubinstein*. New York: Viking Press, 1971.

"On Her Dressing-Table." *Vogue* 45, no. 9 (May 1, 1915): 82, 84.

Peiss, Kathy. "Making Up, Making Over: Cosmetics, Consumer Culture, and Women's Identity." In Victoria de Grazia, ed., with Ellen Furlough. *The Sex of Things: Gender and Consumption in Historical Perspective*. Berkeley: University of California Press, 1996, 311–36.

——. *Hope in a Jar: The Making of America's Beauty Culture*. New York: Henry Holt, 1998.

Perry, Gill. *Women Artists and the Parisian Avant-Garde: Modernism and "Feminine" Art, 1900 to the Late 1920s*. Manchester, UK: Manchester University Press, 1996.

Portraits of Helena Rubinstein. New York: Metropolitan Museum of Art, 1976.

Portraits d'Helena Rubinstein. Paris: Musée des Arts Décoratifs, 1977.

Reed, Christopher, ed. *Not At Home: The Suppression of Domesticity in Modern Art and Architecture*. London: Thames and Hudson, 1996.

Rubin, William, ed. *"Primitivisim" in Twentieth Century Art: Affinity of the Tribal and the Modern*. New York: Museum of Modern Art, 1984.

Rubinstein, Helena. "Beauty—A Real Definition." In *Arts and Decoration* 19, no. 1 (May 1923): 86–87.

——. "Exterior Decoration." *Arts and Decoration* 18, no. 3 (January 1923): 52, 56.

——. *Food for Beauty*. New York: Ives Washburn, 1938.

——. *My Life for Beauty*. New York: Simon and Schuster, 1964, rev. ed., 1966.

——. *The Art of Feminine Beauty*. New York: Horace Liveright, 1930.

——. "Why I Love Jewels." Typescript, n.d. Helena Rubinstein archive, L'Oréal Luxe, Paris.

Schiaparelli, Elsa. *Shocking Life: The Autobiography of Elsa Schiaparelli*. London: V & A Publications, 2007.

Scranton, Philip. ed. *Beauty and Business: Commerce, Gender, and Culture in Modern America*. New York: Routledge, 2001.

Slesin, Suzanne. *Over the Top: Helena Rubinstein, Extraordinary Style, Beauty, Art, Fashion, Design*. New York: Pointed Leaf Press, 2006.

Smith, Terry. *Making the Modern*. Chicago: University of Chicago Press, 1993.

Sontag, Susan. *On Photography*. New York: Farrar, Straus and Giroux, 1977.

Sparke, Penny. "The 'Ideal' and the 'Real' Interior in Elsie de Wolfe's 'The House in Good Taste of 1913.'" In *Journal of Design History* 16, no. 1 (January 2003): 63–76.

Swerling, Jo. "Profiles: Beauty in Jars and Vials." *New Yorker* 4, no. 19, (June 30, 1928): 20–23.

Tashjian, Dickran. *A Boatload of Madmen: Surrealism and the American Avant-Garde, 1920–1950*. New York: Thames and Hudson, 1995.

Tobias, Andrew. *Fire and Ice: The Story of Charles Revson—The Man Who Built the Revlon Empire*. New York: William Morrow, 1976.

Trachtenberg, Alan. *Reading American Photographs*. New York: Hill & Wang, 1989.

True, James, "Policies that Built World-Wide Sales for Helena Rubinstein." *Sales Management* 24 (November 22, 1930): 298–99, 325–27.

"The Vanity Box." *Theatre Magazine* 28, no. 214 (December 1918): 376.

Vaughan, Hal. *Sleeping With the Enemy: Coco Chanel's Secret War*. New York: Knopf, 2011.

Wall, Florence E. *The Principles and Practice of Beauty Culture*, 4th ed. New York: Keystone Publications, 1961.

Warburton, Nigel. *Ernö Goldfinger: The Life of an Architect*. London: Routledge, 2004.

Woodhead, Lindy. *War Paint: Madame Helena Rubinstein and Miss Elizabeth Arden—Their Lives, Their Times, Their Rivalry*. Hoboken, NJ: John Wiley & Sons, 2003.

index

Page numbers in *italics* refer to illustrations.

advertising, 11, *45*, 46, 56, *58–59*, 66, *70*, *71*, *75*, *78–86*, 97, *106*
African art, 9, 20, *25*, *27*, 30, *31*, *34–36*, *44*, *47*, 89, 90, *91–96*, *110*, 111, *114–16*, *152*, *153*
anti-Semitism, 29
Arden, Elizabeth, 17, 20, *29*, 29–30, 46, *70*, 87, 117, 143, 145
Art Deco, 87, 99–100, *127*, 143
Art Moderne, *75*, 99–100
Atlan, Jean-Michel, 145, *153*
Australia, 19, 33, 52, 55–56, *57*
avant-garde, 62, 89, 121, 136

Baker, Josephine, *89*, 89–90
Bakst, Léon, 66
Balenciaga, *106*, 136
Ballets Russes, 61, 62, 66
Bara, Theda, 29, *30*
baroque, 46, *124*, 128
Barré, Martin, 145
Baudelaire, Charles, 90, 97
Baudrillard, Jean, 161
Bauhaus school, *75*, *81*, 100
Bayer, Herbert, *75*, *81*
Beaton, Cecil, *29*, *51*, 61, *63*, *100*, 121
beauty industry, 17, 29, 46, 143, 145
beauty salons and services, 19, 29, *33*, 46, *55–56*, *71*, *75*, *75–78*, 97, 111, 121, 143
Beauvais tapestry, 99
Beckman, Rosalie Silberfeld (aunt), 52
Beerbohm, Max, 56
Belle Epoque, 17, 61
Benjamin, Ashley, 87
Benois, Alexandre, 66
Bérard, Christian, *32*
Bernhardt, Sarah, *111*
Bonwit Teller, 100, 121
Brancusi, Constantin, 33, *37*, 89–90, 99, 143, 151, *158*
Braque, Georges, 99, *104*
Brauner, Victor, *110*
Breton, André, 139

celebrity photography, 46
Chagall, Marc, *27*, *112–13*
Chanel, Coco, 17, 29, 61, *63*, 111
Chareau, Pierre, 99, *99*
Chicago salon, *71*, 99, *99*
classical Greece, *71*, *74*, 111, 117, 139
Cocteau, Jean, 121
collecting, psychology of, 33, 151, 161
cosmetics packaging and design, 121, *126–27*, 143
cosmetics use by women, 29, 55, *80*, 89, 90, 143
Cubism, *40*, 90, *103*, 145
Cutting, Mrs. R. Fulton, II, *110*
Cuttoli, Marie, 99, *101*

Dalí, Salvador, *32*, *47*, *107*, 121, *138–42*, 139, 143
De Chirico, Giorgio, 117, *119*
Degas, Edgar, *111*
de Kooning, Willem, *75*, *110*, 151, *159*
de Predis, Ambrogio, *78*
d'Erlanger, Catherine, 61
designer fashion, *19*, 62, 100, *107*, 111, *111*, *113*, 121, 145, *160*. *See also specific designers*
Deskey, Donald, 100, *105*
De Stijl school, 100
de Wolfe, Elsie, 19, *19*
Diaghilev, Sergei, 61, 62
Dior gown, *111*
Dobell, William, *134*, 136
Doucet, Jacques, 62, *63*
Dufy, Raoul, *32*, 62

Eisenstaedt, Alfred, *112*
Epstein, Jacob, 90, *91*
Ernst, Max, 151, *152*, *155*

femininity, 19, 52, 55, *70*, 136
feminism, 17, 30, 52, 55
Fini, Leonor, *130*
Folies-Bergère night club, 89
Frank, Jean-Michel, *33*, 117
Frankl, Paul T., *75*, 87, 100, *105*
Freud, Sigmund, 52

glass collection, 33, *44*
Goldfinger, Ernö, 87, *88*, 89, 99
Gordon, Witold, 87
Gourielli-Tchkonia, Artchil (second husband), 19, 100, *112*

Hagborg, August, *57*
Harlem Renaissance, 89, 90
Helleu, Paul César, 56, *60*, 62, *70*, *71*
Hicks, David, 145, 151, *153*
high fashion. *See* designer fashion; interior design; *specific designers*
Hoffmann, Josef, *105*
House of Gourielli, 19
House of Worth, 62, *63*

inclusiveness. *See* multiculturalism
individualism, 12, 19–20, 161
interior design, 19–20, 62, 66, *70*, *75*, 87, 89, 100, 117, 121, 128, 145. *See also salons and residences under cities*

Jazz Age, *63*, 89
jewelry, *16*, 20, *32*, *48*, 97, 111, *111*, 136, 145, 151, *160*

Kahlo, Frida, 20, *22*
Kane, Martine, 117, *118*, 121
Kesslere, George Maillard, *49*, 111
Klimt, Gustav, 52
Krakow, 30, 52, 128, 151

Latin American art, 9, 20, 30, *34–35*, 128, *131*
Lauder, Estée, 46
Laurencin, Marie, *32*, *133*, 136
Léger, Fernand, 33, *33*, *40*, 99, *105*, 117
Loewy, Raymond, 100
London: Grafton Street salon, 46, 66, 87, *88*, 89; move to, 56, 61; residence, 145, *153*
Loos, Adolf, 87
Lovet-Lorski, Boris, 99, *102*
Lurçat, Jean, *105*
Lykuski, Jacob, 56

Maar, Dora, *67*
magazine and newspaper ads. *See* advertising
magazine features, 100, *106–10*, 121, 128
Maison de Beauté Valaze (Melbourne), 55
Maison Myrbor (Paris), *33*, 99
Malone, Annie Turnbo, 17
Manet, Edouard, 117
Man Ray, *31*, *50*, 89, 121, *126–27*
Marcoussis, Louis Casimir, 99, *103*, *106*
masks, 9, *34–35*, 52, *85*, *95*, 111, *114*, *116*
masks, cosmetic, *71*, *75*, *75*, *85*
Matisse, Henri, *27*, 33, *40*, *42*, 99, *110*
Maugham, Somerset, 56
Medgyes, Ladislas, *68*, 117, *118*
miniature rooms, 117, *123–24*
Miró, Joan, *23*, 33, *39*, *41*, *75*, *106*, *110*, 151, *152*
modernism, *71*, *75*, 87, 89–90, 97, 100, 121, 151
Modigliani, Amedeo, *27*, *33*, 117, 151, *157*
Montenegro, Roberto, *32*, *48*
Morand, Paul, 61
multiculturalism, 12, 20, 33, 89, 90
Mumford, Lewis, 117
Munkácsi, Martin, *120*
Muray, Nickolas, *64*
Musée d'Ethnographie (Paris), 90
Museum of Modern Art (MOMA), 111, 117, 121

Nadelman, Elie, 33, *33*, *38*, 70–71, *72–74*, 87, *105*, *110*, 111, 117, *131*, *147*
negrophilia, 89, 90
Neoclassicism, 143
New York City: 49th Street beauty salon, *73*; 57th Street beauty salon, 97, 100, *105*; Fifth Avenue beauty salon, *33*, 46, 66, *73*, 117, *118–19*, 121, *124–25*, *129*; 49th Street beauty salon, *73*; Park Avenue apartment, *23*, *26–27*, 30, *47*, *69*, *105*, *107*, *110*, 128, *131*, 139; Rubinstein's move to, 29, 66, 70
New Zealand, 56

Oberon, Merle, *106*
Oceanic art, 9, 20, *25*, *27*, 30, *31*, *34–35*, 89, 90
Ogilvy, David, 143
O'Higgins, Patrick, 61, *65*, 145
opaline glass, 33, *44*
Op art, *75*, *86*
Orientalism, 62
Orloff, Chana, 99

Pallavicini, Federico, *23*, *129*
Paris: beauty salon, 46, 56, 61, 87, 90, 143; residences, *25*, 30, *36*, *44*, *65*, *67*, 90, *106*, *108*, 121, 128, *152*
Paterson's Gallery (London), 71
Paul, Bruno, *105*
Peiss, Kathy, 33
perfume and fragrance products, 19, *75*, *84*, 121, 143
photography and portraiture, 33, *43*, 55, 62, 90. *See also* Rubinstein, Helena
Picasso, Pablo, *27*, 33, *39*, 99, *107*, *125*, 136, 145, *147–50*, 151, *152*, *154*
Piero del Pollaiuolo, *125*
Poiret, Paul, 62, *64*, 99, 111
Portinari, Cândido, 20, *21*, *32*
postwar America, 143, 145
publications by Rubinstein, 19, *43*, 46, *98*

Ratton, Charles, 30
Revlon brand, 46, 143
Revson, Charles, 46, 143
Rivera, Diego, 20, *22*
Rouault, Georges, *27*
Rubinstein, Helena: biography of, 9, 17, 46; compared to Arden, 20, 29–30, *70*, 117; eccentricity of, 11, 20, 30, 62, 111, 145, 151; family photograph with mother and sisters, *54*; first marriage of, 56, 61, 136; Jewishness and, 29, 30, 33, 143; persona, 33–46, 151; photographs and portraits of, *16*, *18*, *22*, *25*, *28*, *32*, 33, *36*, 46, *47–51*, 52, *54–55*, *59–60*, *63–64*, *68–69*, *80*, *91*, *100–101*, *112–13*, *124*, 128, *132–35*, 136, *137–38*, 139, *144*, *146–50*, 151, *160*; second marriage of, 19, 100, *112*
Rubinstein, Mala (niece), *73*, 145
Russo, Margherita, *32*

Saint-Cloud, France, laboratory, *28*
Saint Laurent, Yves, 145, *160*
Schiaparelli, Elsa, *100*, 111, *113*, 121
Sert, Misia, 61–62
Shaw, George Bernard, 56
Silberfeld, Helena (aunt), 52
Simpson, Wallis, 121
Snow, Carmel, 111
Sontag, Susan, 52
Spratling, William, *48*
Steichen, Edward, *106*
Sterner, Harold, 117
Studio Dorland, *81*
Süe, Louis, *67*, 136, 143
suffragists, 29, *29*
Surrealism, 30, *31*, 56, 62, *67*, *85*, 117, *120*, 121, *130*, 139, 143
Sutherland, Graham, *32*, 128, *135*, 136
Sweeney, James Johnson, 111
Szivessy, András (later André Sive), 87

Tchelitchew, Pavel, *32*, *33*, *69*, *110*, 136, *137*
Terry, Emilio, 143
Titus, Edward (first husband), 11, 56, 61, 66, *70*, 136
Titus, Horace (son), 61
Titus, Roy (son), 46, 61

Valaze skin cream, *45*, 55–56, *58*, *78*, *82*, *127*
van Dongen, Kees, 151, *156*
Velázquez, Diego, *129*
Vertès, Marcel, *32*
Vienna, 52

Walker, Madam C. J., 17
Warhol, Andy, 145, *146*
Weston, Edward, 55
women's empowerment. *See* feminism
World War II, 143
Worth, Charles, 62

image credits, copyrights, and museum accession numbers

Every reasonable effort has been made to supply complete and correct credits; if there are errors or omissions, please contact the Jewish Museum so that corrections can be made in any subsequent edition.

Cover: Photograph by George Maillard Kesslere; image provided by the Helena Rubinstein Foundation Archives, Fashion Institute of Technology, SUNY, Gladys Marcus Library, Special Collections. Frontispiece, page 2: Artwork © Estate of Pablo Picasso / Artists Rights Society (ARS), New York; photograph by Béatrice Hatala, provided by Gagosian Gallery, New York. Page 15: See page 85. Page 16: Sculpture © Estate of Elie Nadelman; photograph by Alfredo Valente, image © SZ Photo, provided by The Image Works. Page 18: Photograph by George Maillard Kesslere; image provided by the Helena Rubinstein Foundation Archives, Fashion Institute of Technology, SUNY, Gladys Marcus Library, Special Collections. Page 19: Photograph by Baron de Meyer; image provided by the New York Public Library / Art Resource, New York. Page 21: Artwork © Artists Rights Society (ARS), New York / AUTVIS, São Paulo; image provided by Christie's Images / Bridgeman Images. Page 22 top: Artwork © Banco de México Diego Rivera Frida Kahlo Museums Trust, Mexico, D.F. / Artists Rights Society (ARS), New York; image provided by Bridgeman Images. Page 22 bottom: Photograph by Emmy Lou Packard; image provided by the Helena Rubinstein Foundation Archives, Fashion Institute of Technology, SUNY, Gladys Marcus Library, Special Collections. Page 23 top: Sculptures © Estate of Elie Nadelman; image provided by Stiftung F.C. Gundlach. Page 23 bottom: Photograph © Bettmann / Corbis. Page 24: Photograph by Jean Vincent; image reproduced in *Over the Top: Helena Rubinstein, Extraordinary Style, Beauty, Art, Fashion, Design*, courtesy of Pointed Leaf Press. Page 25: Image provided by the Helena Rubinstein Foundation Archives, Fashion Institute of Technology, SUNY, Gladys Marcus Library, Special Collections. Page 26: Photograph by George Maillard Kesslere, image reproduced in *Over the Top: Helena Rubinstein, Extraordinary Style, Beauty, Art, Fashion, Design*, courtesy of Pointed Leaf Press. Page 27 top: Image reproduced in *Over the Top: Helena Rubinstein, Extraordinary Style, Beauty, Art, Fashion, Design*, courtesy of Pointed Leaf Press. Page 27 bottom: Photograph by Gottscho-Schleisner, Inc.; image provided by the Library of Congress, LC-G613-57629. Page 28: Photograph © Boris Lipnitzki; image provided by Roger-Viollet / The Image Works. Page 29 bottom: Photograph provided by Corbis. Page 30: Photograph by Underwood & Underwood; image provided by Profiles in History / Corbis. Page 31: Artwork © Man Ray Trust / Artists Rights Society (ARS), New York / ADAGP, Paris / Telimage. Page 32: Image provided by the Helena Rubinstein Foundation Archives, Fashion Institute of Technology, SUNY, Gladys Marcus Library, Special Collections. Page 33: Sculptures © Estate of Elie Nadelman; photograph by Samuel H. Gottscho; image provided by the Museum of the City of New York. Page 34 top left: Brooklyn Museum, Gift of Princess Gourielli (Mme Helena Rubinstein) 53.149.3; image provided by Bridgeman Images. Page 34 top right: Image provided by Bridgeman Images. Page 34 bottom left: Photograph by Alison Duke. Page 34 bottom right: Photograph by Bradford Robotham. Page 35 left: Photograph by Alison Duke. Page 35 right: Photograph by Alison Duke. Page 36: Sculpture © Estate of Elie Nadelman, image reproduced in *Over the Top: Helena Rubinstein, Extraordinary Style, Beauty, Art, Fashion, Design*, courtesy of Pointed Leaf Press. Page 37: National Gallery of Art, Washington, DC, Given in loving memory of her husband, Taft Schreiber, by Rita Schreiber, 1989.31.3; artwork © Artists Rights Society (ARS), New York / ADAGP, Paris. Page 38 top: Collection of the New-York Historical Society, 2001.223a-d; artwork © Estate of Elie Nadelman. Page 38 bottom: Artwork © Estate of Elie Nadelman. Page 39 top left: Carnegie Museum of Art, Pittsburgh; Purchase: gift of the Howard Heinz Endowment, 66.13; artwork © Estate of Pablo Picasso / Artists Rights Society (ARS), New York; photograph provided by the Carnegie Museum of Art. Page 39 top right: The Metropolitan Museum of Art, New York, Jacques and Natasha Gelman Collection, 1998, 1999.363.60; artwork © Estate of Pablo Picasso / Artists Rights Society (ARS), New York; photograph by Malcolm Varon; image provided by The Metropolitan Museum of Art. Page 39 bottom: Metropolitan Museum of Art, Jacques and Natasha Gelman Collection, 1998, 1999.363.47; artwork © Successió Miró / Artists Rights Society (ARS), New York / ADAGP, Paris; photograph by Malcolm Varon; image provided by The Metropolitan Museum of Art. Page 40 top: The Museum of Fine Arts, Houston, Gift of Madame Helena Rubinstein, 53.10; artwork © Artists Rights Society (ARS), New York / ADAGP, Paris. Page 40 bottom left: The Museum of Modern Art, New York, Stephen C. Clark Fund, 1951, 128.1951; artwork © Succession H. Matisse, Paris / Artists Rights Society (ARS), New York; digital image provided by The Museum of Modern Art / licensed by SCALA / Art Resource, New York. Page 40 bottom right: Artwork © Artists Rights Society (ARS), New York / ADAGP, Paris. Page 41 left: Artwork © Successió Miró / Artists Rights Society (ARS), New York / ADAGP, Paris; photograph by Bradford Robotham. Page 41 right: Artwork © Successió Miró / Artists Rights Society (ARS), New York / ADAGP, Paris. Page 42: Metropolitan Museum of Art, Jacques and Natasha Gelman Collection, 1998, 1999.363.42; artwork © Succession H. Matisse, Paris / Artists Rights Society (ARS), New York; photograph by Malcolm Varon; image provided by The Metropolitan Museum of Art. Page 43: Photograph by Bradford Robotham. Page 44: Image provided by the Helena Rubinstein Foundation Archives, Fashion Institute of Technology, SUNY, Gladys Marcus Library, Special Collections. Page 45: Sculptures © Estate of Elie Nadelman; image and text © Hearst Corporation. Page 47: Photograph by Herbert Gehr; image provided by Time Life Pictures / Getty Images. Page 48 top: Image provided by Art Resource, New York. Page 48 bottom: Los Angeles County Museum of Art, California, Gift of Goddard Family in Memory of Phyllis Goddard, M.2012.189.1; digital image provided by Museum Associates / LACMA, licensed by Art Resource, New York. Page 49: Image provided by Sotheby's New York. Page 50: Artwork © Man Ray Trust / Artists Rights Society (ARS), New York / ADAGP, Paris, image reproduced in *Over the Top: Helena Rubinstein, Extraordinary Style, Beauty, Art, Fashion, Design*, courtesy of Pointed Leaf Press. Page 51: Images provided by Condé Nast. Page 53: Image provided by the Helena Rubinstein Foundation Archives, Fashion Institute of Technology, SUNY, Gladys Marcus Library, Special Collections. Page 54: Image provided by the Helena Rubinstein Foundation Archives, Fashion Institute of Technology, SUNY, Gladys Marcus Library, Special Collections. Page 57: Image provided by the National Library of Australia. Page 58 top: Image provided by the National Library of Australia. Page 58 bottom: Image provided by the Mary Evans Picture Library / The Image Works. Page 59: Image provided by Condé Nast. Page 60: Image provided by the National Portrait Gallery, Smithsonian Institution / Art Resource, New York. Page 63 top left: Image provided by the Helena Rubinstein Foundation Archives, Fashion Institute of Technology, SUNY, Gladys Marcus Library, Special Collections. Page 63 top right: Image provided by the Helena Rubinstein Foundation Archives, Fashion Institute of Technology, SUNY, Gladys Marcus Library, Special Collections. Page 63 bottom left: Photograph by George Maillard Kesslere; image provided by the Helena Rubinstein Foundation Archives, Fashion Institute of Technology, SUNY, Gladys Marcus Library, Special Collections. Page 63 bottom right: Image provided by the Helena Rubinstein Foundation Archives, Fashion Institute of Technology, SUNY, Gladys Marcus Library, Special Collections. Page 64: Artwork © Nickolas Muray Photo Archives; image provided by George Eastman House, International Museum of Photography and Film. Page 65: Photograph by Jean Vincent, image reproduced in *Over the Top: Helena Rubinstein, Extraordinary Style, Beauty, Art, Fashion, Design*, courtesy of Pointed Leaf Press. Page 67: Artwork © Artists Rights Society (ARS), New York / ADAGP, Paris, image reproduced in *Over the Top: Helena Rubinstein, Extraordinary Style, Beauty, Art, Fashion, Design*, courtesy of Pointed Leaf Press. Page 68: Photograph by Herbert Gehr; image provided by Time Life Pictures / Getty Images. Page 69: Photograph by Samuel H. Gottscho; image provided by the Museum of the City of New York. Page 72: National Gallery of Art, Washington, DC, Gift of Robert P. and Arlene R. Kogod, 1975.79.1; artwork © Estate of Elie Nadelman. Page 73 top: Sculptures © Estate of Elie Nadelman; image provided by Condé Nast. Page 73 bottom: Image provided by the Helena Rubinstein Foundation Archives, Fashion Institute of Technology, SUNY, Gladys Marcus Library, Special Collections. Page 74 top left: Allen Memorial Art Museum, Oberlin College, Oberlin, Ohio, Mrs. F. F. Prentiss Fund, 1968.16; artwork © Estate of Elie Nadelman. Page 74 top right: Hirshhorn Museum and Sculpture Garden, Smithsonian Institution, Washington, DC, Gift of Joseph H. Hirshhorn, 1966, 66.3783; artwork © Estate of Elie Nadelman. Page 74 bottom left: Artwork © Estate of Elie Nadelman. Page 74 bottom right: Artwork © Estate of Elie Nadelman; photograph by Jerry L. Thompson / Art Resource, New York. Page 75: Image provided by Acme, © Corbis. Page 76 top: Photograph © Lusha Nelson / Corbis; image provided by Condé Nast Archive / Corbis. Page 76 bottom: Photograph by Anton Bruehl; image provided by Condé Nast. Page 77 top: Image provided by Acme, © Corbis. Page 77 bottom: Photograph © Lusha Nelson / Corbis; image provided by Condé Nast Archive. Page 78 top: Image provided by Acme, © Corbis. Page 78 bottom: Image reproduced in *Life* magazine, July 21, 1941. Page 79: Image provided by the National Library of Australia. Page 80 left: Image provided by the Helena Rubinstein archive, L'Oréal Luxe, Levallois-Perret, France. Page 80 right: Image provided by the Hearst Corporation. Page 81: Image provided by the Helena Rubinstein archive, L'Oréal Luxe, Levallois-Perret, France. Pages 82–83: Image provided by Condé Nast. Page 88 top: Photograph by Bryan & Norman Westwood; image provided by the Royal Institute of British Architects, 5150. Page 88 bottom: Image provided by the Royal Institute of British Architects, 13294. Page 89: Photograph by George Hoyningen-Huene, © Horst P. Horst, courtesy of Staley-Wise Gallery; image provided by Archives Charmet / Bridgeman Images. Page 91: Image provided by the Helena Rubinstein Foundation Archives, Fashion Institute of Technology, SUNY, Gladys Marcus Library, Special Collections. Page 92: Indiana University Art Museum, 77.87; photograph by Michael Cavanagh and Kevin Montague. Page 93 top left: Photograph provided by Christie's Images / Bridgeman Images. Page 93 top right: Photograph provided by Sotheby's New York. Page 93 bottom left: Photograph provided by Sotheby's New York. Page 93 bottom right: Photograph provided by the Hood Museum of Art, Dartmouth College, Hanover, New Hampshire. Page 94: Photograph provided by Sotheby's New York. Page 95 top left: Photograph © Atlantic Art Partners; Photograph by Peter Zeray, Metropolitan Museum of Art. Page 95 bottom right: The Metropolitan Museum of Art, New York,

The Michael C. Rockefeller Memorial Collection, Bequest of Nelson A. Rockefeller, 1979, 1979.206.296; image provided by The Metropolitan Museum of Art / Art Resource, New York. Page 96 top right: Photograph provided by Sotheby's New York. Page 96 bottom left: Photograph provided by Sotheby's New York. Page 96 bottom right: Photograph provided by Sotheby's New York. Page 98 top: Photograph by Bradford Robotham. Page 98 bottom left: Image provided by the Helena Rubinstein Foundation Archives, Fashion Institute of Technology, SUNY, Gladys Marcus Library, Special Collections. Page 99: Images reproduced in *Over the Top: Helena Rubinstein, Extraordinary Style, Beauty, Art, Fashion, Design*, courtesy of Pointed Leaf Press. Page 100: Image provided by the Helena Rubinstein Foundation Archives, Fashion Institute of Technology, SUNY, Gladys Marcus Library, Special Collections. Page 101: Photograph © Boris Lipnitzki, provided by Roger-Viollet / The Image Works. Page 102: Photograph by Bradford Robotham. Page 103: Yale University Art Gallery, New Haven, Connecticut, Charles B. Benenson, B.A. 1933, Collection, 2006.52.94. Page 104: Artwork © Artists Rights Society (ARS), New York / ADAGP, Paris. Page 105 top: Nadelman sculpture © Estate of Elie Nadelman; image provided by the Helena Rubinstein archive, L'Oréal Luxe, Levallois-Perret, France. Page 105 bottom: Nadelman sculpture © Estate of Elie Nadelman; image provided by the Helena Rubinstein Foundation Archives, Fashion Institute of Technology, SUNY, Gladys Marcus Library, Special Collections. Page 106 left: Photograph by George Hoyningen-Huene, © Horst P. Horst, courtesy Staley-Wise Gallery, image provided by Mary Evans / National Magazines / The Image Works. Page 106 right: Artwork © Estate of Edward Steichen / Corbis; image provided by the Conde Nast Archive. Page 107 left: Photograph by Horst P. Horst; image provided by Condé Nast. Page 107 right: Photograph by Horst P. Horst; image provided by Condé Nast. Pages 108–9: Photographs by Carlo Bavagnoli. Page 110 top: Photograph by Horst P. Horst; image provided by Condé Nast. Page 110 bottom: Sculptures © Estate of Elie Nadelman; photograph by John Rawlings; image provided by Condé Nast. Page 111: Image provided by the Helena Rubinstein Foundation Archives, Fashion Institute of Technology, SUNY, Gladys Marcus Library, Special Collections. Page 112 top: Artwork © Artists Rights Society (ARS), New York / ADAGP, Paris. Page 112 bottom: Photograph by Alfred Eisenstaedt; image provided by Time Life Pictures / Getty Images. Page 113 left: Artwork © Artists Rights Society (ARS), New York / ADAGP, Paris; image provided by Christie's Images / Bridgeman Images. Page 113 right: Photograph © Boris Lipnitzki; image provided by Roger-Viollet / The Image Works. Page 114 right: Image provided by Bridgeman Images. Page 115: Photograph by Drew Bolton. Page 116: Photograph by George Maillard Kesslere; image provided by the Helena Rubinstein Foundation Archives, Fashion Institute of Technology, SUNY, Gladys Marcus Library, Special Collections. Page 118: Image reproduced in *Life* magazine, July 21, 1941. Page 119 top: Photograph by Samuel H. Gottscho; image provided by the Museum of the City of New York. Page 119 bottom: Artwork © Artists Rights Society (ARS), New York / SIAE, Rome; photograph by Stefan Altenburger, Zurich. Page 120: Image provided by the Hearst Corporation. Page 124 bottom: Photograph by Anton Bruehl; image provided by Condé Nast. Page 125 top left: Image provided by SCALA / Art Resource, New York. Page 125 top right: Image reproduced in *Life* magazine, March 1, 1937. Page 125 bottom: Image reproduced in *Life* magazine, March 1, 1937. Page 126: Artwork © Man Ray Trust / Artists Rights Society (ARS), New York / ADAGP, Paris. Page 127 top left: Photograph by Bradford Robotham. Page 127 top right: Photograph by Bradford Robotham. Page 127 bottom left: Image provided by the Helena Rubinstein archive, L'Oréal Luxe, Levallois-Perret, France. Page 127 bottom right: Photograph by Bradford Robotham. Page 129: Photograph by Gottscho-Schleisner, Inc.; image provided by the Library of Congress, LC-G612- 52663. Page 130: Artwork © Artists Rights Society (ARS), New York / ADAGP, Paris; photograph by Jochen Littkemann, Berlin. Page 131: Image reproduced in *Over the Top: Helena Rubinstein, Extraordinary Style, Beauty, Art, Fashion, Design*, courtesy of Pointed Leaf Press. Page 132: Sculpture © Estate of Elie Nadelman; image provided by the Helena Rubinstein Foundation Archives, Fashion Institute of Technology, SUNY, Gladys Marcus Library, Special Collections. Page 133: Artwork © Artists Rights Society (ARS), New York / ADAGP, Paris; image provided by Sotheby's New York. Page 134: Artwork © Sir William Dobell Art Foundation, licensed by Copyright Agency Viscopy Ltd.; image provided by Bridgeman Images. Page 135: Artwork © Estate of Graham Sutherland; image provided by Sotheby's New York. Page 137: Image provided by Sotheby's New York. Page 138: Artwork © Salvador Dalí, Fundació Gala-Salvador Dalí, Artists Rights Society (ARS), New York. Page 139: Artworks © Salvador Dalí, Fundació Gala-Salvador Dalí, Artists Rights Society (ARS), New York. Pages 140–42: Artworks © Salvador Dalí, Fundació Gala-Salvador Dalí, Artists Rights Society (ARS), New York. Page 144: Photograph © Steve Shapiro / Black Star. Page 146: Williams College Museum of Art, Gift of Richard F. Holmes, Class of 1946, M.2005.17.37; artwork © The Andy Warhol Foundation for the Visual Arts, Inc. / Artists Rights Society (ARS), New York. Page 147: Sculpture © Estate of Elie Nadelman; image provided by the Helena Rubinstein Foundation Archives, Fashion Institute of Technology, SUNY, Gladys Marcus Library, Special Collections. Pages 148–50: Artworks © Estate of Pablo Picasso / Artists Rights Society (ARS), New York. Page 152: Photograph by Buffotot, Paris. Page 153: Image © Estate of David Hicks. Page 154: Artwork © Estate of Pablo Picasso / Artists Rights Society (ARS), New York. Page 155: Artwork © Artists Rights Society (ARS), New York / ADAGP, Paris. Page 156: Artwork © Artists Rights Society (ARS), New York / ADAGP, Paris. Page 157: Image provided by Bridgeman Images. Page 158: Artwork © Artists Rights Society (ARS), New York / ADAGP, Paris, image provided by Christie's Images / Bridgeman Images. Page 159: Artwork © The Willem de Kooning Foundation / Artists Rights Society (ARS), New York. Page 160: Image provided by the Helena Rubinstein Foundation Archives, Fashion Institute of Technology, SUNY, Gladys Marcus Library, Special Collections.